Dieter Hillert (Ed.)

Linguistics and Cognitive Neuroscience

Linguistische Berichte
Sonderheft 6/1994

Dieter Hillert (Ed.)

Linguistics and Cognitive Neuroscience

Theoretical and Empirical Studies on Language Disorders

Westdeutscher Verlag

Linguistische Berichte

Forschung Information Diskussion

Alle *redaktionellen* Zuschriften und Sendungen erbitten wir nur an die verantwortliche Redaktion der Linguistischen Berichte, z. Hd.: Professor Günther Grewendorf, Johann Wolfgang Goethe-Universität Frankfurt, Institut für Deutsche Sprache und Literatur II, Gräfstr. 76, D-60486 Frankfurt am Main.

Mitteilungen, die für das LB-Info bestimmt sind, schicken Sie bitte immer an die Teilredaktion LB-Info, zu Händen von Prof. Dr. Herwig Krenn, Romanisches Seminar der Ruhr-Universität Bochum bzw. Herrn Klaus Müllner, Postfach 21 51, D-65779 Kelkheim.

Die Linguistischen Berichte erscheinen sechsmal im Jahr. Jahrgangsumfang ca. 480 S.

Jährlich erscheint ein Sonderheft, das je nach Umfang berechnet und den Abonnenten bei Bezug im Jahr des Erscheinens mit einem Nachlaß gegen Rechnung geliefert wird.

Bezugsbedingungen

Jahresabonnement (1994)	DM 139,– / öS 1084,– / sFr 139,–
Zweijahresabonnement (1994/95)	DM 250,– / öS 1950,– / sFr 250,–
Jahresabonnement priv. (1994)	DM 79,– / öS 616,– / sFr 80,90x
Zweijahresabonnement priv. (1994/95)	DM 142,– / öS 1108,– / sFr 145,30x
Einzelheftpreis	DM 25,– / öS 195,– / sFr 26,–
	jeweils zuzüglich Versandkosten

Alle Bezugspreise und Versandkosten unterliegen der Preisbindung.

Satz: ITS Text und Satz GmbH, Herford

ISSN 0935-9249
ISBN 978-3-531-12600-5 ISBN 978-3-322-91649-5 (eBook)
DOI 10.1007/978-3-322-91649-5

Inhalt

Dieter Hillert
Introduction . . . 7

Angela D. Friederici, Herbert Schriefers
The Nature of Semantic and Morphosyntactic Context Effects on Word Recognition in Young Healthy and Aphasic Adults . . . 9

Jean Gagnon, Pierre Goulet, Yves Joanette
Activation of the Lexical-semantic System in Right-brain-damaged Right-handers . . . 33

Harold Goodglass
Category-Specific Lexical Dissociations . . . 49

Helgard Kremin
Selective Impairments of Action Naming: Arguments and a Case Study . . . 62

Helen Leuninger, Jörg Keller
Some Remarks on Representational Aspects of Language Production . . . 83

Pierre Marcie, Michel Roudier, François Boller
Spontaneous Language and Impairment of Communication in Alzheimer's Disease . . . 111

Penny A. Prather
The Time Course of Lexical Activation in Fluent and Nonfluent Aphasia . . . 128

Arturo Hernandez, Elizabeth Bates
Interactive/Activation in Normal and Brain-damaged Individuals: Can Context Penetrate the Lexical 'Module'? . . . 145

Lewis P. Shapiro, Cynthia K. Thompson
On Lexical Properties, Syntax, and Brain Damage . . . 168

Lorraine K. Tyler
Morphological Deficits in Aphasia: Problems of Representation, Access or Integration? 202

Kerry Kilborn
On-line Integration of Grammatical Information in Wernicke's and Broca's Aphasia 219

David Swinney, Edgar Zurif
The Neurological Organization of Lexical and Structural Operations in Sentence Comprehension: Findings and Methodological Considerations 234

Dieter Hillert, Douglas F.H. Burrington, Gautam A. Gupta
Automatic Semantic Activation for Lexical Perception: Normal and Disordered Processing 245

The Authors 269

Introduction*

The purpose of this special issue of *Linguistische Berichte* is to provide a collection of representative papers on issues currently discussed in Linguistics and Cognitive Neuroscience. The collection represents a mixture of state-of-the-art research as well as of new experimental findings investigating grammatical and semantic processing in normal and neurologically-impaired speakers/hearers. A range of different methodologies are presented: representational issues of linguistic information in terms of levels of linguistic descriptions (e.g., trace theory or thematic roles) or in terms of linguistic units (e.g., semantically transparent derived words vs. semantically opaque derived words) are considered as well as processing issues of linguistic information in terms of psychological notions (e.g., automatic vs. controlled processing), in terms of neuropsychological notions (e.g., lexical dissociations), or even in terms of neurological notions (e.g., anatomical features).

This special issue is mainly concerned with the question of how language is processed in fluent and non-fluent aphasics, that is, how structural descriptions of different linguistic representations (e.g., phonology, morphology, syntax, semantics, and discourse) are used to provide assumptions about how native language is processed in normal and neurologically-impaired speakers/hearers. The methodological approaches selected by the authors in this issue are qualitatively divergent and considering the broad research field of language, cognition and the brain, it is important to get evidence from different approaches to shed more light on the nature of language disorders after brain-damage. This general view, however, does not imply that it is possible to investigate specific hypotheses by using different research methodologies. For example, the question of whether sentential context affects initial lexical access for comprehension can only be examined by using real-time techniques which permit one to probe within a time span in which context-free automatic lexical access occurs. Off-line methods such as meta-linguistic judgment tasks do not provide a technique to tap into the real-time process of natural language processing. Instead, these provide error scores which may result from non-specified informational resources which are not necessarily part of the language domain. The task should require the speaker/hearer's response to be closely tied in time to the input of the relevant speech unit.

However, in the attempt to find in behavioral terms an explanation for impaired language processing or impaired cognitive processing in general it is important not to focus on a unitary research strategy but to include within an experimental design a number of control tasks. With respect to the example given above – real-time lexical access for comprehension – off-line tasks are irrelevant for the interpretation of the real-time data. In the case of neurologically-impaired patients it seems particularly important to consider control tasks which allow one to get an overall view of the processing deficits. Other illustrative examples are investigations looking at dissociations of cognitive pathways or routes in group and single-case studies. The question is whether it is possible to compare several studies with each other which seem to investigate identical hypotheses but use slightly different methods within a paradigm. For example, lexical priming tasks are in principle not comparable when such factors as stimulus onset asynchrony, interstimulus interval, number of subjects, patients' syndromes, stimulus material, modalities, etc. are varying. To avoid such methodological flaws it is necessary not to run ad hoc studies the criteria of which are not or hardly comparable with the criteria of other studies reported in the literature. Another methodological weakness might be that research mostly focuses on a certain subject pool. To compare just normal and aphasic language processing with respect to the factors "age", may be too limited, that is, in order to regard aphasic speech as a deviation from normal language processing it is important not to consider only other kinds of experimental groups or subjects (e.g., bilingual aphasics, 2nd language learners, child language) but also cross-linguistic findings. For example, when we address certain issues concerning the temporal course of automatic processing of linguistic units it is obvious that questions such as whether a 2nd language learner processes certain linguistic segments similar as certain neurologically-impaired patients may be particularly relevant. Of course, the scource of deviated language processing compared to "prototypical" language processing (adult native speaker) is qualitatively different but in behavioral terms both kinds of deviated processing might be similar or identical. Thus, for a psycholinguistic diagnosis it does not matter which neurological changes caused impaired or altered cognitive processing. Let us now turn to the selected topics of this special issue.

The wide range of methodologies and methods as well as of questions and answers allows us not to cluster the papers according to certain criteria: types of lexical dissociations in different modalities and in different diagnostic groups and subjects (Goodglass; Kremin), the diagnosis of Alzheimer's disease on the basis of spontaneous speech (Marcie, Roudier & Boller), form-based errors in normal speakers (Leuninger & Keller), derivational morphology in two agrammatic patients (Tyler); real-time processing of grammatical and sentential-semantic processing in Broca's and Wernicke's aphasics (Friederici & Schriefers; Kilborn; Shapiro & Thompson; Swinney & Zurif), and real-time processing of lexical-semantics in right-handed right-brain-damaged patients (Gagnon, Goulet & Joanette) and of lexical semantics and sentential semantics in Anomia (Hernandez & Bates) and in Broca's and Wernicke's aphasics (Prather; Hillert, Burrington & Gupta).

Dieter Hillert San Diego, May 1994
(Guest Editor)

Note

* The editorial work of this special issue was supported by a fellowship of the Alexander von Humboldt Foundation (Feodor Lynen program VB2-FLF) to the guest editor. He is grateful to Allen I. Selverston for his invitation to work at the University of California, San Diego, and to Elizabeth Bates, Jeffrey L. Elman and David Swinney for providing facilities in the Departments of Cognitive Science, Linguistics and Psychology.

The Nature of Semantic and Morphosyntactic Context Effects on Word Recognition in Young Healthy and Aphasic Adults*

Angela D. Friederici, Herbert Schriefers, Berlin

1 Introduction

The process of word recognition is central in the study of language comprehension. To model this process, researchers consult normal as well as pathological language behavior. One of the main questions addressed in the context of adequately modelling language comprehension is, whether and how semantic and syntactic context information influences lexical access.

Two distinct views have been formulated with respect to the process of word recognition in sentential context. These are mainly based on experimental findings from normal comprehension behavior. One position claims that lexical access is autonomous, i.e., independent from context information (e.g., Forster 1979; Tanenhaus, Carlson & Seidenberg 1985). The alternative view holds that sensory input and context information interact to such an extent that context information changes activation levels of lexical elements even before any sensory input is available (e.g., Morton 1969, 1979; McClelland & Rumelhart 1981; Rumelhart 1978). A position between these two extremes takes sentential context information to play a role, but only in a late stage of lexical processing. In the first stage, analysis of a word is assumed to activate a set of candidate words. This activation cannot be influenced by contextual information. In the next stage, this set is reduced and eventually a single candidate is selected. Contextual influences are assumed to be operative at this second stage, be it in spoken word recognition (see Marslen-Wilson 1984, 1987; Zwitserlood 1989), or in visual word recognition (Rueckle & Oden 1986; and Sanocki et al. 1985).

In addition to the general question of contextual influences on the recognition of words, the proposed models different with respect to whether and how semantic and syntactic processes can be differentiated. While most models holding the lexical-access-is-autonomous position claim these two processes to be distinct, interactive models do not. Data from subjects with circumscribed brain lesions and resulting specific language

* This research was supported by the Alfried Krupp von Bohlen- und Halbach-Stiftung and by the Max-Planck-Institut für Psycholinguistik. We thank Heinrich Mundt, Katja Kühn and Jochen Nieradt for running the experiments.

impairments are of particular relevance in discussing this issue. Earlier reports suggested that aspects of semantic and syntactic knowledge are selectively affected by circumscribed lesion in the left hemisphere (e.g., Zurif & Caramazza 1976). More recent studies rather seem to indicate that semantic and syntactic processing mechanisms are differentially affected by different left hemisphere lesions (e.g., Swinney, Zurif & Nicol 1989; Friederici 1985).

In the present study we will investigate the influence of sentential context on visual word recognition in young healthy adults and compare their performance to that of subjects suffering from brain lesions causing non-optimal central processing conditions. First, we will report two experiments with young adults, in which we investigate if and how semantic plausibility versus implausibility and morphosyntactic correctness versus incorrectness of the context affects lexical access, and to what extent these two factors interact during word recognition. Then, we will study, if and how a reduction in the central language processing capacity caused by central brain lesions affects semantic and morphosyntactic processes. This experiment involves adult subjects with focal brain lesions, resulting in a *specific* reduction of central processing capacities. In particular, we will investigate a group of agrammatic Broca's patients, who are characterized as suffering from a selective computational deficit in the syntactic domain, and compare them with a group of aphasic control subjects and a group of normal controls.

Before reporting these experiments, we shall discuss recent findings on sentential context effects on word recognition in young healthy subjects, as well as the relevant evidence on sentence context effects in aphasic subjects.

2 Sentence context effects in word recognition

2.1 Semantic and syntactic context effects in young healthy subjects

There are quite a number of empirical studies of sentence context effects on word recognition in healthy subjects (e.g., Goodman, McClelland & Gibbs 1981; Schuberth & Eimas 1977; Stanovich & West 1983; Swinney 1979; Tanenhaus, Leiman & Seidenberg 1979). However, we will restrict our discussion to some selected papers which are of particular interest for the present study, as they systematically evaluated the effect of syntactic context on word recognition also under investigation here.

Marslen-Wilson & Tyler (1980) studied the effect of sentential context on spoken word recognition in a word monitoring task. Monitoring latencies were shorter for words in normal sentences than for words in so-called syntactic prose (i.e., sentences which are syntactically, but not semantically intact). Words in sentences with so-called scrambled prose (i.e., sentences which are neither syntactically nor semantically intact) had the longest monitoring latencies. From these findings, the authors concluded that sentence context does affect word recognition and, furthermore, that the effects of syntactic and semantic context are additive.

Wright & Garrett (1984) investigated influences of syntactic sentence context on visual word recognition, using a lexical decision task. Their results in combination with results from a replication study, using an additional neutral baseline condition (West & Stanovich 1986), showed a facilitatory effect for syntactically (and semantically) correct sentences and an inhibitory effect for sentences whose syntax was incorrect. The combined results support the idea of syntactically based context effects.

Recently, O'Seaghdha (1989) investigating context effects on word recognition, using a lexical decision task, showed that facilitatory effects, due to associative-lexical relatedness between a word (e.g., author) in the context phrase and the target word (e.g., *BOOK*) in a word string (e.g., *the author of the BOOK*), can be obtained only for phrases which are syntactically coherent. Scrambled word lists with the same words (e.g., *the author the of BOOK*), in contrast, did not produce any facilitatory effect. These results suggest an interaction between associative-lexical and syntactic factors, as the relatedness effect is present only in phrases with a coherent syntactic structure. Simpson et al. (1989) obtained similar results with a naming task. A semantic relatedness effect was only found for syntactically coherent sentences, but not for scrambled sentences. However, in contrast to O'Seaghdha (1989), they found only facilitation in the related condition, but no inhibition in the unrelated condition, as compared to a neutral baseline context. When comparing context effects of normal sentences, semantically anomalous, but syntactically coherent sentences, and scrambled word lists on the processing of word targets, Simpson et al. (1989) found a significant related-unrelated difference only for normal sentences. From these findings the authors conclude that there are genuine sentence context effects which are not reducible to intralexical priming effects. The combined findings suggest that syntactic *and* semantic coherence are a prerequisite for sentence context effects on word recognition (see also Stanovich et al. 1985).

The nature of semantic and morphosyntactic effects, their possible interaction, as well as their potential additivity under normal processing conditions will be investigated in Experiment 1 and 2.

2.2 Context effects in subjects with central brain lesions

A critical test for the distinctiveness of semantic and syntactic processes will include subjects who suffer from central brain lesions associated with *specific* language breakdowns. A processing limitation for syntactic processes, in particular, appears to be the prime characteristic of agrammatic Broca's aphasia (Friederici & Kilborn 1989; Hagoort 1990; Prather et al. 1991; Swinney, Zurif & Nicol 1989). Their language behavior has been described as the result of a central syntactic deficit (e.g., Berndt & Caramazza 1980), or as the result of a specific deficit concerning the temporal structure of language processes (e.g., Baum 1988; Blumstein, Milberg & Shier 1982; Friederici 1985; Friederici & Kilborn 1989; Hagoort 1990; Milberg, Blumstein & Dworetzky 1987; Prather et al. 1991; Shankweiler et al. 1989; Tyler & Cobb 1987) with syntactic processes being affected in particular (Blumstein et al. 1991; Haarmann & Kolk 1991a; Friederici 1988; Swinney, Zurif & Nicol 1989).

This latter position is compatible with the idea that the comprehension behavior seen in agrammatic Broca's aphasics is a reflection of an impairment in the retrieval of syntactic information which, in normal subjects, is fast and automatic (Friederici 1988). Activation of syntactic information, though possible in principle, is not automatic in Broca patients and, therefore, delayed with respect to the activation of lexical-semantic information. This delay, in turn, is the cause for the observed difficulties in the structural assignment of lexical elements (see also Haarmann & Kolk 1991b). Empirical evidence in support of this claim includes the demonstration that monitoring times for closed class elements carrying syntactic information are dramatically delayed compared to open class elements (Friederici 1985), and the finding that agrammatic Broca's aphasics, though sensitive to syntactic violations in sentences, are seriously slowed down in detecting such violations (Friederici & Kilborn 1989; Huber et al. 1990). Additional support for the view that syntactic information is not activated automatically in these patients is provided by experiments demonstrating that Broca's aphasics, but not normal controls, are able to ignore sentential context information in a cross-modal lexical decision task upon instruction (Kilborn & Friederici 1994). A study by Blumstein and coworkers (Blumstein et al. 1991) of syntactic priming effects, provides additional evidence for the view that Broca's aphasics display impairments primarily in the automatic language processing routines.

The combined data indicate that there is a slower-than-normal availability of linguistic information in patients with lesions in the Broca's area and that syntactic information, in particular, is not activated in a fast, automatic and obligatory fashion. These patients may, therefore, provide a possibility to investigate the nature of morphosyntactic processes and their interaction with semantic processes under the condition of a limited capacity specific to the syntactic processing domain. This will be done in Experiment 3.

3 The present experiments

In the present experiments we investigate the effect of sentential context varying semantic and syntactic dimensions on the recognition of visually presented words in healthy young adults and aphasic adults.

3.1 Sentence contexts used in the present experiments

The stimulus material used in the experiments were sentences containing semantic and syntactic violations. The sentences in the syntactic violation condition, however, only carry a minimal morphosyntactic error. This is in contrast to early studies on syntactic context effects discussed above. O'Seaghdha (1989) and Simpson et al. (1989) used contexts of scrambled lists of words and compared those with semantically and syntactically coherent contexts. In the present experiments, the structure of the sentence context remains intact, and only a minimal morphosyntactic error is introduced. The syntactically correct sentences and the morphosyntactically incorrect sentences differ only in one aspect, namely, the definite article. (1) gives an example of a correct sentence (the target word is indicated by uppercase letters, i.e., *BRIEF/LETTER*), (2) gives the corresponding morphosyntactically incorrect sentence. (2) is only incorrect by virtue of the definite article *"das"* which marks accusative neuter. Given that *"Brief"* is a masculine noun, a correct sentence requires the article *"den"* which marks accusative masculine, as in (1).

(1) *Er schreibt den BRIEF*
(He writes the (accusative masc.) letter)

(2) **Er schreibt das BRIEF*
(He writes the (accusative neuter) letter)

In addition, we introduced a so-called neutral baseline similar to the one used, for example, by Stanovich & West (1979), McClelland & O'Regan (1981), Simpson et al. (1989). We are aware of the problem to determine a neutral baseline, but chose the present one in analogy to the studies cited (for a general discussion of this issue see also Jonides & Mack (1984) and Neely (1990)). An example of the neutral baseline used in the present experiments is given in (3).

(3) **Jetzt sehen Sie BRIEF*
(Now you see LETTER)

There is a clear associative-lexical relation between the verb and the target noun in (1) and (2). Note that no additional associative-lexical relation is present in the sentences, as all sentences contain a pronoun in subject position. The important questions with respect to the three sentence types presented so far are (a) whether there is a difference between (1) and (2) with faster reaction time for (1), suggesting a morphosyntactic effect, and (b) whether we obtain a facilitation in (1) relative to the baseline (3), but not in (2). This latter result would suggest that a minimal disruption in morphosyntactic coherence can lead to an elimination of a facilitatory effect in the sentence context.
In addition to the syntactic manipulation, we introduced a manipulation of the semantic appropriateness of the context (Experiment 1, conditions (4) and (5)). This was done by replacing the verb in (1) and (2) by a different transitive verb. This verb was chosen such that the noun target (e.g., *BRIEF/LETTER*) following the verb represents a violation of the verb's selectional restriction. For instance, instead of the verb *schreiben/write*, the verb *fahren/drive* is inserted into sentences (1) and (2), thus yielding:

(4) *Er fährt den BRIEF*
(He drives the (accusative masc.) letter)

(5) **Er fährt das BRIEF*
(He drives the (accusative neuter) letter)

Note two things about this situation. First, the verb and the noun in (4) and (5) are not only unrelated; rather, the sentences are semantically anomalous. We would expect this semantic anomaly to be reflected in inhibition for the lexical decision on the target noun. Second, this semantic anomaly is completely crossed with morphosyntactic in-/coherence. This situation opens the possibility to investigate the relative influences of

the syntactic and the semantic aspects of the sentence context on word recognition. The main points of interest are (a) whether the two influences are additive, or whether an inappropriate semantic sentence context has the same influence on target processing, irrespective of the morphosyntactic correctness of the sentence, and (b) whether the corresponding patterns differ across the different groups.
Experiment 2 attempts to clarify the specific question whether potential syntactic effects observed under the different semantic relations between verb and noun (positive relations/negative relations) are dependent upon the presence of the conditions with semantically incoherent sentences. Therefore, we replaced these sentences ((4) and (5)) by sentences with semantically neutral verb-noun relations as in (6) and (7). Sentence (6) is semantically neutral and syntactically correct. Sentence (7) is also semantically neutral but syntactically incorrect.

(6) *Er sucht den Brief*
(He searches the (accusative masc.) letter)

(7) **Er sucht das Brief*
(He searches the (accusative neuter) letter)

This will allow us to investigate if and to what degree semantic inappropriateness introduced in the remaining Experiments influences potential semantic and syntactic effects.
As the design and materials are the same across all Experiments (with only slightly modified materials in Experiment 2), we will first describe the design and the materials in general (for the modification introduced in Experiment 2, see Experiment 2).

3.2 Design and Materials

In each of the experiments there were 10 target nouns, 5 of masculine gender and 5 of neuter gender. Each of the 5 nouns occurred in each of the 5 context conditions mentioned above. In the neutral baseline condition the target noun followed the sentence *Jetzt sehen Sie* (*now you see*). Despite the problems associated with defining a given context as "neutral", we will, however, call this condition "neutral" for the presentation of the results. We will come back to the problem of an appropriate neutral baseline in the discussion section.
In the semantically *and* syntactically correct condition (see (1) above) the noun followed a sentence of the form pronoun+verb+article. The target noun always fulfilled the selectional restriction of the verb, and was thus a close associate of the verb (e.g., *Er schreibt den Brief / He writes the letter*). This condition will hereafter be referred to as +SYN+SEM. In the syntactically incorrect condition (see (2) above) the same context sentence was used, but the article preceding the target noun was not correct. When the target noun was masculine, the article was the article for accusative neuter (*das*). When the target noun was neuter, the article was accusative masculine (*den*). This condition will be referred to as –SYN+SEM. In the (see (4) above) semantically incorrect condition the verb of the +SYN+SEM condition was substituted by a different verb.

This verb was selected such that the target noun violated the verb's selectional restrictions (e.g., *Er fährt den Brief / He drives the letter*). This condition will be referred to as +SYN–SEM. In the semantically and syntactically incorrect condition (see (5) above) the same verb as in the preceding context condition was used, but moreover the article was changed such that it did not agree with the target noun in gender (e.g., *Er fährt das Brief / He drives the letter*). This condition will be referred to as –SYN–SEM.
In the conditions (1), (2), (4), and (5) each verb served in the +SYN+SEM and –SYN+SEM condition for one target noun and, in the +SYN–SEM and the –SYN–SEM conditions for a different target noun. Therefore, altogether ten different transitive verbs were used (see Appendix 1 for a listing of the materials).
In addition to these ten (target nouns) times five (context conditions) trials with word targets, fifty additional trials with nonword targets were constructed. These nonword trials were constructed as follows. First, from each of the ten target nouns a nonword was derived by changing one letter. All nonwords were legal nonwords according to the rules of German phonology and spelling. Each resulting nonword was randomly assigned to one of the fifty context sentences of the word trials. In addition, ten practice trials were constructed. None of the words, nonwords or verbs of the practice trials occurred in the word or nonword trials.
The resulting onehundred word and nonword trials were randomized under the restriction that the repetition of the same target word in the five different context conditions was counterbalanced across the ten targets. Furthermore, the randomizations were constructed under the restriction that (i) the same target word was not allowed to occur in direct succession, (ii) a target word and its derived nonword were not allowed to occur in direct succession, and (iii) the same response (word vs. nonword) would not occur more than three times in direct succession.

4 Experiments

4.1 Experiment 1: Semantic and syntactic context effects in young adults

In Experiment 1 we will investigate the influence of semantic and morphosyntactic violations upon word recognition.

Subjects: Twenty-two students, all native speakers of German, participated in the experiment. They had a mean age of 23 with a range from 19 to 26.

Materials and Procedure: Materials have already been described above. Subjects were tested individually. They were seated in front of a MULTISYNCH computer screen with a panel with two pushbuttons in front of them. The primes and the targets were presented as black letters on a white background. Context sentences were presented in lower case (except for the first letter of the sentence) and targets in capital letters. The time course of a trial was as follows. First, a fixation cross appeared in the middle of the screen for 220 msec. This was followed by a period of 100 msec during which the screen stayed blank. Then the context sentence including the article was presented for 750 msec, followed by a 'blank period' of 220 msec, the target followed this period and remained on the screen for 1550 msec. By pressing either the left or the right pushbutton, the subject indicated his word-/nonword decision. The reaction time from the onset of the target to the button press was automatically registered by a computer. 2000 msec after the target had vanished from the screen the next trial started with the presentation of the fixation cross. Fixation cross, context sentence, and target always appeared centered in the middle of the screen.

Results

All trials with an incorrect lexical decision were excluded from further analysis. All reaction times more than two standard deviations away from the corresponding subject's and item's mean were replaced by estimates following the procedure recommended by Winer (1971). This was the case for 1.45 % data points. Table 1 gives the mean lexical decision times (in msec) for the word targets in the five different context conditions, and the corresponding percentage of incorrect lexical decisions.

For the data of the present and the following experiments two sets of analyses were computed, one including and one excluding the neutral baseline condition. The latter analysis treats the remaining four conditions as the full crossing of the two factors Semantics (+SEM vs. –SEM) and Syntax (+SYN vs. –SYN) and therefore allows for a direct test of the potential additivity of the two factors. The former analysis treats the five experimental conditions as five levels of one single factor. Hereinafter, we will refer to these two analyses as the two-factor and the one-factor ANOVA, respectively. Given the ongoing discussion in the literature about what constitutes a "neutral" baseline, we perform both analyses for each experiment.

The one-factor ANOVA with the five context conditions revealed a significant main effect of Context Condition ($F(4,84) = 17.42$, $p < .0005$, $MSe = 7587$). Comparisons between the five context conditions were performed by means of a Newman-Keuls test. This test revealed the following pattern. The +SYN+SEM condition is significantly faster than all four remaining context conditions. The +SYN–SEM and the –SYN–SEM conditions are both significantly slower than the baseline and the –SYN+SEM conditions. No other differences were significant.

The corresponding two-factor ANOVA revealed significant main effects of the Semantic and the Syntax factor ($F(1,21) = 39.5$, $p < .0005$, $MSe = 512.3$, and $F(1,21) = 18.3$,

Table 1 Mean lexical decision times and error percentage (in parentheses) for Experiment 1

neutral	+SYN+SEM	–SYN+SEM	+SYN–SEM	–SYN–SEM
611 (0.0)	576 (0.9)	611 (0.0)	633 (0.5)	639 (0.5)

$p < .0005$, $MSe = 977.6$, respectively), and a significant interaction of these two factors ($F(1,21) = 4.94$, $p < .05$, $MSe = 924.8$).
Due to the small number of items in each condition, item analyses were carried out by the non-parametric Wilcoxon-Tests, with items as the replication dimension. For the present experiment, these non-parametric item analyses revealed that +SYN+SEM is significantly different from +SYN–SEM ($p < .05$) and from –SYN–SEM ($p < .05$).

Discussion

What can be seen in the present experiment is the following. There is a clear facilitation effect for the +SYN+SEM condition compared to the baseline. The same positive semantic relation between verb and target noun, however, fails to show a comparable effect, when the target noun is preceded by a gender incongruous definite article (–SYN+SEM vs. baseline). When considering the present baseline to represent a neutral one, we would have to take these results to suggest a facilitory effect in the case of syntactically and semantically coherent context, and no effect when the syntactic context is incoherent due to a local morphosyntactic violation, i.e., gender violation.
One interpretation of these results would view these findings to indicate that a minimal morphosyntactic violation, in this case incorrect gender (–SYN+SEM vs. baseline) is able to wipe out a semantic facilition effect seen in the coherent sentences (+SYN+SEM vs. baseline). This would mean that semantic coherence alone is not enough to produce a facilitation effect between two lexical elements when these are presented in a sentential context which is morphosyntactically incoherent, be it due to a mismatch between definite article and target noun, as in the present experiment, or be it due to a syntactically unstructured context as reported by O'Seaghdha (1989). Moreover, these results raise the question to what extent the facilitation effect observed between +SYN+SEM and the baseline could be syntactic in nature.
However, the data can also be interpreted in a different fashion. The pattern observed for the +SYN+SEM and the –SYN+SEM conditions could be taken to reflect a pure morphosyntactic effect, i.e., a gender marking effect similar to the one reported by Grosjean, Dommergues and Cornu (submitted) for French. The finding of an inhibitory effect for the semantically incorrect sentences (+SYN–SEM) compared to the baseline, without an additional inhibition for the –SYN–SEM vs. the +SYN–SEM condition suggests that semantic, but not syntactic aspects have an inhibitory influence on the lexical decision. Thus, when considering the neutral baseline, the data seem to be in accordance with the view that syntactic processes are highly automatic, as automatic processes have been defined as being connected with facilitation effects, but not inhibitory effects (Posner & Snyder 1975; Schneider & Shiffrin 1977; Shiffrin & Schneider 1977). By contrast, semantic processes are facilitatory *and* inhibitory in nature. This view is put to test in Experiment 2.
The interpretation whether the observed effects are indeed inhibitory or facilitatory, certainly depends on the baseline chosen. At least with respect to the present baseline, the results from this experiment suggest that facilitation effects can only be observed when the context is semantically *and* morphosyntactically correct. Inhibitory effects

are observed in the presence of selectional restriction violations, irrespective of morphosyntactic variations. A morphosyntactic mismatch alone does not inhibit target processing relative to the baseline, suggesting that morphosyntactic aspects of processing are rather located in the facilitatory domain. In summary, the results of Experiment 1 lend themselves to two different possible interpretations. The first interpretation assumes a semantic facilitation effect (+SEM+SYN vs. baseline) which is eliminated in the case of morphosyntactic incorrectness (–SYN+SEM vs. baseline). The second interpretation attributes the facilitation effect in the +SYN+SEM condition to morphosyntactic facilitation, thus assuring that the semantic relatedness between the verb and the noun in this condition does not genuinely contribute to this facilitation effect.

4.2 Experiment 2: Syntactic violation effects in semantically normal sentences in young adults

In Experiment 2 we will study which of the interpretations for the facilitation effect observed in Experiment 1 holds. Here, we will use semantically correct sentences which contain either a strong or a relatively neutral semantic relation between the context verb and the noun target. This will also provide a possibility to test the influence of semantic relatedness upon syntactic processes.

Subjects: Eighteen students, all native speaker of German, participated in the experiment. Their mean age was 24.9 years with a range from 19 to 35.

Material and Procedure: The materials used in this experiment differed from that of Experiment 1 in one important respect. The sentence types (4) and (5) which contained a semantic anomaly in the relation between the verb and target noun were replaced by sentences with a neutral verb-noun relation (see (6) and (7) above. This means that in these sentences the verbs used have no strong selectional restrictions (e.g., *suchen/search, nehmen/take, kaufen/buy etc.*). Sentence type (6) contains no morphosyntactic violation, whereas sentence type (7) contains an article preceding the target which is not compatible with the gender of the target word. Thus, the materials used in Experiment 2 consist of five conditions, three conditions already used in Experiment 1, (+SYN+SEM, -SYN+SEM and the so-called neutral baseline condition), and in addition a semantically neutral, syntactically coherent condition (+SYNøSEM), and a condition with semantically neutral verb-noun relatedness and a morphosyntactic violation (–SYNøSEM).
Apart from the replacement of the critical verbs all other aspects of the material construction were identical to those described in 3.2. The procedure was the same as in Experiment 1.

Results

All trials with an incorrect lexical decision were excluded from further analysis. All reaction times more than two standard deviations away from the corresponding

Table 2 Mean lexical decision times and error percentage (in parentheses) for Experiment 2

neutral	+SYN+SEM	-SYN+SEM	+SYNøSEM	-SYNøSEM
552 (3.0)	537 (4.5)	569 (3.0)	533 (2.5)	559 (4.5)

subject's and item's mean were replaced by estimates following the procedure recommended by Winer (1971). This was the case for 1.5 % of the data points. Table 2 gives the mean lexical decision times (in msec) for the word targets in the five different context conditions, and the corresponding percentage of incorrect lexical decisions.
In the one-factor ANOVA the main effect of context conditions was significant ($F(4,76) = 4.12$, $p < .005$, $MSe = 1070$). Newman-Keuls tests ($p < .05$) revealed that the lexical decision times for the +SYN+SEM and for +SYN–SEM condition were faster than the –SYN+SEM and the –SYN–SEM condition. The difference between +SYN+SEM and –SYN+SEM replicates the data from Experiment 1. The difference between neutral and +SYN+SEM is similar to Experiment 1 at a descriptive level, but the facilitation for the semantically and morphosyntactically coherent over the neutral condition is not statistically reliable. The two-factor ANOVA showed a significant main effect of the Syntactic factor ($F(1,19) = 17.3$, $p < .0005$, $MSe = 947.9$), but neither a main effect of the Semantic factor nor an interaction of these two factors (both F's smaller 1).
As in Experiment 1, item analyses were carried out using the Wilcoxon-Test. The analyses also show that the two conditions with intact syntax (+SYN+SEM and +SYNøSEM) differ significantly from those with incorrect syntax (–SYN+SEM and –SYNøSEM, $p < .05$).

Discussion

The pattern of lexical decision times for those sentences with a strong semantic relation between context verb and noun target (+SYN+SEM vs. –SYN+SEM) is very similar to those sentences in which a strong semantic relation is absent (+SYNøSEM vs. –SYNøSEM). This similarity strongly suggests that the faster lexical decision times for the +SYN+SEM compared to the –SYN+SEM condition seen in Experiment 1 and in Experiment 2 are not a semantic relatedness effect, but primarily a morphosyntactic coherence effect similar to the one reported by Grosjean and coworkers (Grosjean, Dommergues & Cornu, submitted) for isolated article-noun combinations.
The combined findings from Experiment 1 and 2 indicate that the fastness of processing for the targets in semantically and morphosyntactically correct sentences (+SYN+SEM) is mainly due to the syntactic coherence, and is not carried by the semantic relatedness between verb and target noun. This contrasts with the results of O'Seaghdha (1989) who found a genuine effect of semantic relatedness in syntactically correct sentences. This difference to the present results might be due to the type of words establishing

the semantic relation (noun to noun in O'Seaghdha, and verb to noun in the present study) and/or the degree of semantic relatedness introduced.

Given the baseline used in the present experiments, our results suggest that morphosyntactic coherence leads to a facilitatory effect and that morphosyntactic incoherence, in turn, does not lead to an inhibitory effect. Moreover, they indicate that semantic violations produce inhibitory effects which are independent of the morphosyntactic correctness vs. incorrectness of the sentence.

The nature of the morphosyntactic and semantic context effects will further be investigated using subjects with central limitations of language processing due to specific brain lesions. Given the different properties of semantic and syntactic processes discussed above, these processes may be differentially affected by central brain lesions. Agrammatic Broca's aphasics whose deficit has been characterized as a loss of automaticity in the syntactic processing domain (e.g., Friederici 1988) or the language processing domain in general (e.g., Blumstein et al. 1991) will be of particular interest when investigating the nature of sentential context effects.

4.3 Experiment 3: Sentence context effects in Broca aphasics

Experiment 3 investigated whether differential syntactic and semantic context effects can be observed in subject groups suffering from computational deficits as a result of central brain lesions. A group of Broca's aphasics, who are assumed to suffer from a computational deficit in the syntactic domain, was tested in Experiment 3. A group of Wernicke patients who are assumed to demonstrate deficient lexical and/or integration processes served as aphasic controls and a group of age-matched healthy subjects as normal controls.

Subjects: Eight agrammatic Broca's aphasics (mean age 47.8: range 37-57) and five Wernicke's aphasics (mean age 63.4: range 48-76) were tested. The patients were classified according to the Aachen Aphasia Test (Huber et al. 1983). All Broca patients suffered from a lesion in the anterior part of the left hemisphere, all Wernicke patients from a lesion in the posterior part of the left hemisphere. Two patients from each group were excluded from the analysis as their error rates were too high. The criterium for exclusion was more than 50 % errors in one of the five conditions. Individual histories of all patients are displayed in Appendix 2.

A group of normal older subjects served as age-matched controls for the aphasic subjects. Seventeen adults between 45 and 74 years of age (mean age 57 years) participated in the experiment.

Procedure: The procedure for the group of normal controls was the same as in Experiment 1. The procedure for the aphasic subjects was similar to Experiment 1 with the following changes. Each trial was initiated by the experimenter. The prime stayed on the screen until the subject pressed the right button of a two-button panel to indicate that he or she had read the sentence prime. The prime was substituted by a fixation cross which stayed on the screen for 500 msec. The fixation cross was then replaced by the target which stayed on the screen until the subject had taken the lexical decision.

The next trial was initiated by the experimenter when he felt that the subject was ready for it. The change in the procedure also required a different procedure for data replacement in this experiment. Since we figured that reaction times above 3000 msec could not be taken as an on-line measure, reaction times over 3000 msec were treated as missing values.

Results

All trials to which subjects had given an incorrect lexical decision were excluded from analysis. Furthermore, for the normal control subjects all reaction times more than two standard deviations from the corresponding subject's and item's mean were substituted by estimates using the procedure recommended by Winer (1971). This was the case for 2.1 % of the data for the normal subjects.

For the aphasic subjects all reaction times above 3000 msec, all reaction times that exceeded two standard deviations from the corresponding patient's mean, and all errors were replaced by the mean of all valid reaction times of this patient in the given condition. Table 3 gives the mean reaction times (in msec) for the two patient groups and the control group as a function of context condition. In addition, Table 3 gives the percentage of data points excluded from analysis according to the above mentioned criteria, and the percentage of wrong lexical decisions (the erroneous lexical decisions being a subset of the excluded data points). Individual patient data are listed in Appendix 3.

Separate one- and two-factor ANOVAs were carried out for each patient group and the normal control group. In the one-factor ANOVA for the age-matched normal controls the main effect for context conditions was significant ($F(4,64) = 28.94$, $p < .0005$, $MSe = 7844$). Newman-Keuls test revealed that +SYN+SEM had faster lexical decision times than all remaining context conditions. This pattern was also found in the non-parametric item analysis (all p's < .05). Furthermore, the two context conditions with

Table 3 Mean lexical decision times and error percentage (in parentheses ( )) and total number of data replaced (in brackets [ ]) for Experiment 3

	neutral	+SYN+SEM	-SYN+SEM	+SYN-SEM	-SYN-SEM
BROCA	1497 (10.0) [18.3]	1367 (0.0) [8.3]	1431 (5.0) [13.3]	1636 (0.0) [8.3]	1479 (3.3) [8.3]
WERNICKE	1378 (4.0) [12.0]	1299 (8.0) [10.0]	1455 (0.0) [6.0]	1452 (6.0) [0.0]	1399 (3.3) [14.0]
NORMAL CONTROLS	629 (4.7)	578 (1.2)	619 (0.6)	669 (3.5)	663 (2.4)

selectional restriction violations (+SYN–SEM; –SYN–SEM) had significant longer reaction times than the neutral condition and the –SYN+SEM condition as revealed by Newman-Keuls statistics. These latter two differences did, however, not reach significance in the non-parametric item analysis. The two-factor ANOVA revealed significant main effects of Semantics and Syntax ($F(1,16) = 79.9$, $p < .0005$, MSe = 956.5, and $F(1,16) = 5.2$, $p < .05$, MSe = 961.8, respectively), and a significant interaction of these two factors ($F(1,16) = 13.8$, $p < .005$, MSe = 665.7).
The one-factor ANOVA for Broca's aphasic showed a significant main effect for context condition ($F(4,16) = 3.24$, $p < .05$). Newman-Keuls tests revealed significant differences between the +SYN–SEM and the +SYN+SEM conditions on the one hand, and between the +SYN–SEM and –SYN+SEM conditions on the other hand. No other difference was significant. The non-parametric item analysis gave the same pattern of significant differences (all p's < .05). The two-factor ANOVA for the Broca's aphasics showed a significant main effect for the Semantics ($F(1,5) = 24.6$, $p < .005$, MSe = 6079.4), and a significant interaction of Syntax and Semantics ($F(1,5) = 7.9$, $p < .05$, MSe = 9267.8), but no main effect of Syntax ($F(1,5) < 1$).
The one-factor ANOVA for Wernicke's aphasics, by contrast, showed no significant effect of context conditions ($F(4,12) = 1.71$, $p > 0.1$). The two-factor ANOVA showed no main effects of the semantic or the syntactic factor (both $F(1,4) < 1$), nor an interaction of these factors ($F(1,4) = 2.5$, $p = .20$, MSe = 22119).

Discussion and further comparisons

The performance of both aphasic groups clearly differs from that of the normal age-matched controls. This difference holds for the facilitation and inhibition effect in the one-factor ANOVA as well as for the interaction of the Semantic and the Syntactic factor in the two-factor ANOVA. For the one-factor analysis, the normal age-matched controls showed a facilitation effect for the grammatical sentences (+SYN+SEM) and an inhibition effect for the two conditions violating selectional restrictions (+SYN–SEM and –SYN–SEM). Moreover, their performance in the –SYN+SEM condition did not differ significantly from the neutral baseline. The two-factor ANOVA revealed that a semantic violation leads to a prolongation of lexical decision time irrespective of morphosyntactic correctness vs. incorrectness, whereas morphosyntactic correctness plays a role for semantically correct sentences.

Wernicke's aphasics

For Wernicke's aphasics no specific sentential context effect was obtained. This was also confirmed in the one-factor and the two-factor analysis. A direct comparison of the two-factor analyses for Wernicke's and normal control subjects in an ANOVA with the factors Group (Wernicke vs. normal controls), Semantics and Syntax revealed significant main effects of Group ($F(1,20) = 38.9$, $p < .005$, MSe = 234414), Semantics ($F(1,20) = 11.6$, $p < .005$, MSe = 4452.8), and an interaction of Semantics and Syntax

(F(1,20) = 12.8, p < 005, MSe = 4955.5). The Semantics by Syntax interaction, however, is dependent on the factor Group, as revealed by the Group by Semantics by Syntax interaction (F(1,20) = 5.2, p < .05, MSe = 4955.5). This interaction is due to the presence of a syntax by semantics interaction for normal controls and the absence of such an interaction for Wernicke's aphasics.
This result for the Wernicke patients is compatible with the findings of Hagoort (1990) who reported no sentential-semantic context effects in a group of Dutch speaking Wernicke's aphasics in an on-line ambiguity resolution experiment. In a similar paradigm, Swinney, Zurif and Nicol (1989) found a pattern of Wernicke's aphasics' behavior resembling that of normal control subjects. Blumstein et al. (1991), in contrast, found a normal facilitory syntactic priming effect for within-phrase syntactic dependencies, but no effects for across-phrase syntactic dependencies for Wernicke's patients. Whether and how patients from this group deviate from the normal pattern may well be a function of the severity of their language disturbance. The patients who participated in the present study showed severe problems with integrating the word target into the preceding sentential context.

Broca's aphasics

Broca's aphasics did show particular sentential context effects. Although they displayed a large interindividual variance with respect to the neutral baseline, their behavioral pattern with respect to the relation between the baseline and the critical conditions was very clear. Lexical decision times were dramatically slowed down when the context sentence contained a selectional restriction violation in an otherwise correct sentence prime (+SYN–SEM). Unlike for normal age-matched controls, however, a similar effect of a violation of selectional restriction was not observed for Broca's aphasics, when the selectional restriction violation appeared in a morphosyntactically incorrect (–SYN–SEM). Lexical decision times for this condition did not differ from the neutral baseline and the –SYN+SEM conditions. This observation is confirmed in a Group (Broca vs. normal controls) by Semantic by Syntax ANOVA. This ANOVA showed significant main effects of Group (F(1,21) = 124.8, p < .0001, MSe = 101854.5), and Semantics (F(1,21) = 103.4, p < 0.001, MSe = 2175.6), and a significant Semantics by Syntax interaction (F(1,21) = 29.4, p < .005, MSe = 2713.5). The Group by Semantics and the Group by Semantics by Syntax interactions are also significant (F(1,21) = 16.9, p < .005, MSe = 2175.6, and F(1,21) = 12.5, p < .005, MSe = 2713.5).
This latter interaction is of particular importance. It is a reflection of the fact that, for the normal age-matched controls, morphosyntactic in-/correctness plays a role for semantically correct sentences, but not for semantically incorrect sentences, whereas for Broca's aphasics precisely the reverse is true. Broca's aphasics only show an inhibition effect due to a violation of selectional restriction when the sentence is syntactically correct. The presence of a morphosyntactic violation (–SYN+SEM) wipes out the strong semantic inhibition effect observed for the syntactically correct sentences (+SYN–SEM). The pattern observed for the group of Broca's aphasics as a whole also holds for the individual patients (see Appendix 3) in so far as, leaving the neutral baseline

out of consideration, for five of the six subjects the +SYN–SEM condition yields the longest reaction times.

These data suggest that the Broca's aphasics tested in the present study suffering from circumscribed lesions in the anterior part of the left hemisphere are able to cancel the integration processes once they encounter a morphosyntactic violation.[1] This result strongly argues for a primacy of syntax in Broca's aphasics for the present task. The underlying process reflected in the observed patients' behavior may involve the following steps. When presented with a short sentential context and a subsequent word target, the integration of the target depends upon a checking mechanism which first checks the local morphosyntactic coherence. If the target matches the morphosyntactic constraints, semantic integration processes take place. These semantic integration processes can be successfully carried out in the +SYN+SEM condition, but do not lead to a positive result in the +SYN–SEM condition, thus yielding longer lexical decision times in the latter than the former condition. If the target does not match the morphosyntactic constraints, these patients' checking mechanism seems to be alerted, searching for further confirmatory or disconfirmatory information. If semantic aspects do suggest a possible integration, as in the –SYN+SEM condition, morphosyntactic inconsistencies are overruled and the target is successfully integrated into the sentence prime. If semantic aspects in addition to the syntactic aspects are disconfirmatory, any further integration seems to be cancelled, as the finding of faster reaction times for –SYN–SEM compared to +SYN–SEM indicates. This is in contrast to normal age-matched controls, who try to integrate the sentence final noun under all circumstances leading to prolonged lexical decision times in the +SYN–SEM and –SYN–SEM conditions.

The present demonstration of Broca's aphasics' 'hypersensitivity' to morphosyntactic aspects, such as gender, is compatible with a recent study investigating Broca's aphasics' ability to process gender information in French (Jarema & Friederici 1994). In this study agrammatic patients were tested for their sensitivity of grammatical gender (*le post / the post vs. la poste / the post office*) showing a surprisingly good performance. This result together with related findings provides strong evidence against the hypothesis of a central syntactic deficit in Broca patients. These results are compatible with the view that these patients are sensitive to syntactic violations, in principle, (e.g., Linebarger et al. 1983; Shankweiler et al. 1989), but unlike normals, they seem to deal with syntactic information in a non-automatic, controlled way. This could even lead to cancellation of semantic integrated processes in the presence of a morphosyntactic violation as in the present experiment.

General Discussion

The combined results suggest that semantic and morphosyntactic aspects of language processing are to be differentiated as they produce different effects on word recognition in young healthy adults and are differently affected by lesions in the anterior part of the left hemisphere.

Experiment 1 showed that semantic and morphosyntactic violations in the relation between a sentence context and a sentence final word target affect lexical decision times on the target differently. With respect to a so-called neutral baseline context (*now you see*) a facilitation effect was only present for those targets which were semantically related and morphosyntactically coherent with the context. Sentences whose context verb and target noun constituted a selectional restriction violation caused a clear inhibition compared to the neutral baseline. Interestingly, morphosyntactic violations alone had no effect compared to the baseline, nor did we observe an additive effect for sentences which carried both, a semantic and a morphosyntactic violation.

The nature of the facilitation effect seen in Experiment 1 was further specified in Experiment 2 which did not include sentences carrying semantic violations, but only two types of semantically correct sentences with either a strong or neutral semantic relation between context verb and target noun. As no effect of semantic relatedness was found in this experiment, we reasoned that the particularly fast lexical decision times observed for those sentences which were semantically and morphosyntactically correct are mainly due to the syntactic coherence and possibly to the semantic correctness, but definitely not due to the semantic relatedness alone. The presence of facilitatory syntactic effects and the absence of inhibitory syntactic effects was taken to indicate that the morphosyntactic processes under investigation are fairly automatic. Neither their initiation nor their execution directly depend upon semantic variables.

Experiment 3 studied semantic and syntactic processes under the condition of central language processing limitations induced by a circumscribed cortical lesion. Broca's aphasics who are characterized by a special deficit of processing syntactic information on-line, unlike normals, only showed a semantic inhibition effect for sentences which were morphosyntactically correct, but not for those which were morphosyntactically incorrect. This latter finding indicates first, that these patients are sensitive to morphosyntactic violations and second, that incorrectness of the morphosyntactic structure can lead to a cancellation of lexical integration processes. It appears that syntactic processes can change their normal status by the alteration of central processing conditions and become subject to and/or initiate controlled processes in patients with lesions in the anterior part of the left hemisphere.

In conclusion, the combined results show that semantic and syntactic factors normally interact in a very subtle way when lexical elements are integrated in sentential context. Syntactic effects seem to be independent of the strength of the semantic relation between a critical word in the prime and a given target, though not necessarily independent of the relation's correctness as defined by selectional restrictions. Thus, the observed effects are compatible with a view assuming lexical integration processes to be dependent upon both syntactic and semantic context without necessarily requiring their interaction. The determination of the relation between sentential context and the word to be integrated may be supported by a checking mechanism which checks the incoming word with respect to syntactic *and* semantic aspects independently (Norris 1986).

When language processing is limited by a particular type of cortical lesion, the nature of syntactic processing may be altered. Broca's aphasics suffering from brain lesions in the anterior part of the left hemisphere, in contrast to their aphasic controls, show sensitivity to morphosyntactic aspects, but in a very special way. The syntactic processes which appear to be fast, automatic and obligatory and also quite independent of controlled post-lexical semantic integration processes in normals, seem to have lost their normal status in Broca's aphasia and, therefore, can interfere with post-lexical integration processes. These latter data may suggest that the syntactic processes which are normally fast, automatic and obligatory are subserved by a distinct brain system located in the anterior part of the left hemisphere.

Appendix 1

Material used in Experiment 1 and 3

Er schreibt den Brief.
Er fährt den Brief.
Er schreibt das Brief.
Er fährt das Brief.
Jetzt sehen Sie Brief.

Er fährt das Auto.
Er näht das Auto.
Er fährt den Auto.
Er näht den Auto.
Jetzt sehen Sie Auto.

Sie näht den Rock.
Sie trinkt den Rock.
Sie näht das Rock.
Sie trinkt das Rock.
Jetzt sehen Sie Rock.

Er trinkt den Wein.
Er putzt den Wein.
Er trinkt das Wein.
Er putzt das Wein.
Jetzt sehen Sie Wein.

Sie putzt das Zimmer.
Sie kocht das Zimmer.
Sie putzt den Zimmer.
Sie kocht den Zimmer.
Jetzt sehen Sie Zimmer.

Sie kocht den Brei.
Sie bügelt den Brei.
Sie kocht das Brei.
Sie bügelt das Brei.
Jetzt sehen Sie Brei.

Sie bügelt das Hemd.
Sie liest das Hemd.
Sie bügelt den Hemd.
Sie liest den Hemd.
Jetzt sehen Sie Hemd.

Er liest den Roman.
Er wäscht den Roman.
Er liest das Roman.
Er wäscht das Roman.
Jetzt sehen Sie Roman.

Sie wäscht das Kleid.
Sie ißt das Kleid.
Sie wäscht den Kleid.
Sie ißt den Kleid.
Jetzt sehen Sie Kleid.

Er ißt das Brot.
Er schreibt das Brot.
Er ißt den Brot.
Er schreibt den Brot.
Jetzt sehen Sie Brot.

Material used in Experiment 2

Er sucht den Brief.
Er schreibt den Brief.
Er sucht das Brief.
Er schreibt das Brief.
Jetzt sehen Sie Brief.

Er malt das Auto.
Er fährt das Auto.
Er malt den Auto.
Er fährt den Auto.
Jetzt sehen Sie Auto.

Sie kauft den Rock.
Sie näht den Rock.
Sie kauft das Rock.
Sie näht das Rock.
Jetzt sehen Sie Rock.

Er lobt den Wein.
Er trinkt den Wein.
Er lobt das Wein.
Er trinkt das Wein.
Jetzt sehen Sie Wein.

Sie zeigt das Zimmer.
Sie putzt das Zimmer.
Sie zeigt den Zimmer.
Sie putzt den Zimmer.
Jetzt sehen Sie Zimmer.

Sie mag den Brei.
Sie kocht den Brei.
Sie mag das Brei.
Sie kocht das Brei.
Jetzt sehen Sie Brei.

Sie schenkt das Hemd.
Sie bügelt das Hemd.
Sie schenkt den Hemd.
Sie bügelt den Hemd.
Jetzt sehen Sie Hemd.

Er kennt den Roman.
Er liest den Roman.
Er kennt das Roman.
Er liest das Roman.
Jetzt sehen Sie Roman.

Sie holt das Kleid.
Sie wäscht das Kleid.
Sie holt den Kleid.
Sie wäscht den Kleid.
Jetzt sehen Sie Kleid.

Er liebt das Brot.
Er ißt das Brot.
Er liebt den Brot.
Er ißt den Brot.
Jetzt sehen Sie Brot.

Appendix 2: Individual Patient History

	Age	Etiology	Onset	Classification according to AAT		Token Test	Comprehension Score (AAT)
B1	37	Trauma	'77	Broca	100 %	19	104/120
B2	44	CV	'89	Broca	89 %	19	103/120
B3	49	CV	'83	Broca	100 %	25	80/120
B4	53	CV	'79	Broca	100 %	20	101/120
B5	50	CV	'88	Broca	96 %	4	120/120
B6	54	CV	'86	Broca	100 %	7	86/120
B7*	49	CV	'79	Broca	100 %	14	88/120
B8*	57	CV	'81	Broca	100 %	10	110/120
W1	70	CV	'79	Wernicke	99.6 %	27	109/120
W2	56	CV	'77	Wernicke	94.1 %	25	97/120
W3	76	CV	'78	Wernicke	93.1 %	9	90/120
W4	62	CV	'88	Wernicke	75.3 %	20	93/120
W5	53	CV	'88	Wernicke	99.5 %	29	70/120
W6*	48	CV	'86	Wernicke	100 %	22	81/120
W7*	50	CV	'90	Wernicke	99.0 %	20	91/120

* Patients were excluded from the analyses as error scores were too high.

Appendix 3: Individual subject data for aphasics: Lexical decision times in msec and percentage erroneous lexical decision

	neutral	+SYN+SEM	-SYN+SEM	+SYN-SEM	-SYN-SEM
BROCA					
B1	1836 (50.0)	1616 (0.0)	2015 (10.0)	1802 (0.0)	1958 (10.0)
B2	1341 (10.0)	1339 (0.0)	1405 (0.0)	1736 (0.0)	1447 (0.0)
B3	1868 (0.0)	1551 (0.0)	1670 (0.0)	1695 (0.0)	1620 (10.0)
B4	1478 (0.0)	1350 (0.0)	1412 (0.0)	1536 (0.0)	1448 (0.0)
B5	1103 (0.0)	985 (0.0)	966 (0.0)	1139 (0.0)	1095 (0.0)
B6	1182 (20.0)	1283 (0.0)	949 (20.0)	1317 (0.0)	1050 (0.0)
WERNICKE					
W1	872 (0.0)	776 (10.0)	924 (0.0)	857 (10.0)	795 (0.0)
W2	1015 (0.0)	980 (0.0)	986 (0.0)	1035 (0.0)	972 (0.0)
W3	1310 (10.0)	1103 (20.0)	1140 (0.0)	1209 (10.0)	1302 (0.0)
W4	1786 (0.0)	1779 (10.0)	2069 (0.0)	2047 (0.0)	2268 (0.0)
W5	1829 (10.0)	1726 (0.0)	1902 (0.0)	2042 (10.0)	1663 (10.0)

Note

1 We are aware of the discussion on the issue of single-case versus group studies and the problem of general statements concerning patient groups (e.g., Caramazza 1986; Zurif, Gardner & Brownell 1989), but we feel that the inclusion of lesion data and other neurological data will eventually reduce the apparent variance of patients classified only on behavioral grounds (see also Bates, Appelbaum & Allard 1991).

References

Bates, E., M. Appelbaum & L. Allard (1991): "Statistical constraints on the use of single cases in neuropsychological research". Brain and Language 40, 295 – 329.

Baum, S.R. (1988): "Syntactic processing in agrammatism: Evidence from lexical decision and grammaticality judgment tasks". Aphasiology 2, 177 – 135.

Berndt, R.S. & A. Caramazza (1980): "A redefinition of the syndrome of Broca's aphasia: Implications for a neuropsychological model of language". Applied Psycholinguistics 1, 225 – 278.

Blumstein, S.E., W. Milberg & R. Shier (1982): "Semantic processing in aphasia: Evidence from an auditory lexical decision task". Brain and Language 17, 301 – 315.

Blumstein, S.E., W.P. Milberg, B. Dworetzky, A. Rosen & F. Gershberg (1991): "Syntactic priming effects in aphasia: An investigation of local syntactic dependencies". Brain and Language 40, 393 – 421.

Caramazza, A. (1986): "On drawing inferences about the structure of normal cognitive systems from the analysis of patterns of impaired performance: The case for single-patient studies". Brain and Cognition 5, 41 – 66.

Forster, K.I. (1979): "Levels of processing and the structure of the language processor". In: W.E. Cooper & E. Walker, eds., Sentence Processing: Psycholinguistic studies presented to Merrill Garrett. Hillsdale, N.J.: Erlbaum.

Friederici, A.D. (1985): "Levels of processing and vocabulary types: Evidence from on-line comprehension in normals and agrammatics". Cognition 19, 133 – 167.

Friederici, A.D. (1988): "Agrammatic comprehension: Picture of a computational mismatch". Aphasiology 2, 279 – 284.

Friederici, A.D. & K. Kilborn (1989): "Temporal constraints on language processing: Syntactic priming in Broca's aphasia". Journal of Cognitive Neuroscience 1, 262 – 272.

Goodman, G.O., J.L. McClelland & R.W. Gibbs Jr. (1981): "The role of syntactic context in word recognition". Memory and Cognition 9, 580 – 586.

Grosjean, F., J. Dommergues & E. Cornu (submitted): "The gender marking effect in French spoken word recognition". Perception and Psychophysics.

Haarmann, H.J. & H.H.J. Kolk (1991a): "Syntactic priming in Broca's aphasics: Evidence for slow activation". Aphasiology 5, 247 – 263.

Haarmann, H.J. & H.H.J. Kolk (1991b): "A computer model of the temporal course of agrammatic sentence understanding: The effects of variation in severity and sentence complexity". Cognitive Science 15, 49 – 87.

Hagoort, P. (1990): Tracking the time course of language understanding in aphasia. Published Doctoral Diss., Catholic University of Nijmegen.

Huber, W., J. Cholewa, A. Wilbertz & A. Friederici (1990, October): What the eyes reveal about grammaticality judgments in aphasia. Paper presented at the 28th Annual Meeting of the Academy of Aphasia, Baltimore, Maryland, USA.

Huber, W., K. Poeck, D. Weniger & K. Wilmes (1983): Aachener Aphasie Test. Göttingen: Hogrefe.
Jarema, G. & A.D. Friederici (1994): "'Le' and 'la': Processing pronouns and articles in agrammatic aphasia". Brain and Language.
Jonides, J. & R. Mack (1984): "On the cost and benefit of cost and benefit". Psychological Bulletin 96, 29 - 44.
Kilborn, K. & A.D. Friederici (1994): "Cognitive penetrability of syntactic processing in Broca's aphasia". Neuropsychology 8, 1 - 8.
Linebarger, M.C., M.F. Schwartz & E.M. Saffran (1983): "Sensitivity to grammatical structure in so-called agrammatic aphasics". Cognition 13, 361 - 392.
Marslen-Wilson, W.D. (1984): "Function and process on spoken word recognition". In: H. Bouma & D.G. Bouwhuis, eds., Attention and Performance X: Control of Language Processes. Hillsdale, N.J.: Erlbaum.
Marslen-Wilson, W.D. (1987): "Functional parallelism in spoken word recognition". Cognition 25, 71 - 102.
Marslen-Wilson, W.D. & L. Tyler (1980): "The temporal structure of spoken language understanding". Cognition 8, 1 - 72.
McClelland, J.L. & J.K. O'Regan (1981): "Expectations increase the benefit derived from parafoveal visual information in reading words aloud". Journal of Experimental Psychology: Human Perception and Performance 7, 634 - 644.
McClelland, J.L. & D. Rumelhart (1981): "An interactive activation model of context effects in letter perception: Part 1. An account of basic findings". Psychological Review 88, 375 - 407.
Milberg, W., S.E. Blumstein & B. Dworetzky (1987): "Processing lexical ambiguities in aphasia". Brain and Language 31, 138 - 150.
Morton, J. (1969): "Interaction of information in word recognition". Psychological Review 76, 165 - 178.
Morton, J. (1979): "Word recognition". In: J. Morton & J.C. Marshall, eds., Structures and Processes. Psycholinguistic Series II. London: Paul Elek.
Neely, J.H. (1990): "Semantic priming effects in visual word recognition: A selective review of current findings and theories". In: D. Besner & G. Humphreys, eds., Basic Processes in Reading: Visual Word Recognition. Hillsdale, N.J.: Erlbaum.
Norris, D. (1986): "Word recognition: Context effects without priming". Cognition 22, 93 - 136.
O'Seaghdha, P.G. (1989): "The dependence of lexical relatedness effects on syntactic connectedness". Journal of Experimental Psychology: Learning, Memory and Cognition 15, 73 - 87.
Posner, M.I. & C.R.R. Snyder (1975): "Attention and cognitive control". In: R.L. Solso, ed., Information processing and cognition: The Loyola Symposium. Hillsdale, N.J.: Erlbaum.
Prather, P., L. Shapiro, E. Zurif & D. Swinney (1991): "Real-time examinations of lexical processing in aphasics". Journal of Psycholinguistic Research 20, 271 - 281.
Rueckle, J.G. & G.C. Oden (1986): "The integration of contextual and featural information during word identification". Journal of Memory and Language 25, 445 - 460.
Rumelhart, D.E. (1978): "Toward an interactive model of reading". In: S. Dornic, ed., Attention and Performance VI. Hillsdale, N.J.: Erlbaum.
Sanocki, T., K. Goldman, J. Waitz, C. Cook, W. Epstein & G.C. Oden (1985): "Interaction of stimulus and contextual information during reading: identifying words within sentences". Memory & Cognition 13, 145 - 157.
Schneider, W. & R.M. Shiffrin (1977): "Controlled and automatic human information processing: Detection, search, and attention". Psychological Review 84, 1 - 66.
Schuberth, R.E. & R.D. Eimas (1977): "Effects of context and the classification of words and nonwords". Journal of Experimental Psychology: Human Perception Performance 3, 27 - 36.
Shankweiler, D., S. Crain, P. Correll & B. Tuller (1989): "Reception of language in Broca's aphasia". Language and Cognitive Processes 4, 1 - 33.

Shiffrin, R.M. & W. Schneider (1977): "Controlled and automatic human information processing II. Perceptual learning, automatic attending and a general theory". Psychological Review 84, 127 - 190.
Simpson, G.B., R.R. Peterson, M.A. Casteel & C. Burgess (1989): "Lexical and sentence context effects in word recognition". Journal of Experimental Psychology: Learning, Memory and Cognition 15, 88 - 97.
Stanovich, K.E., R.G. Nathan, R.F. West & M. Vala-Rossi (1985): "Children's word recognition in context: Spreading activation, expectancy, and modularity". Child Development 65, 1418 - 1428.
Stanovich, K.E. & R.F. West (1979): "Mechanisms of sentence context effects in reading: Automatic activation and conscious attention". Memory and Cognition 7, 77 - 85.
Stanovich, K.E. & R.F. West (1983): "On priming by sentence context". Journal of Experimental Psychology: General 112, 1 - 36.
Swinney, D.A. (1979): "Lexical access during sentence comprehension: (Re)consideration of context effects". Journal of Verbal Learning and Verbal Behavior 18, 645 - 659.
Swinney, D., E. Zurif & J. Nicol (1989): "Effects of focal brain damage on sentence processing: An examination of the neurological organization of a mental module". Journal of Cognitive Neuroscience 1, 25 - 37.
Tanenhaus, M.K., G.N. Carlson & M.S. Seidenberg (1985): "Do listeners compute linguistic representations?" In: R. Dowty, L. Karttunen & R.A.M. Zwickey, eds., Natural language parsing: Psychological computational, and theoretical perspectives. Cambridge: Cambridge University Press.
Tanenhaus, M., J. Leiman & M. Seidenberg (1979): "Evidence for multiple stages in the processing of ambiguous words in syntactic contexts". Journal of Verbal Memory and Verbal Behavior 18, 427 - 440.
Tyler, L.K. & H. Cobb (1987): "Processing bound grammatical morphemes in context: The case of an aphasic patient". Language and Cognitive Processes 2, 245 - 262.
West, R.F. & K.E. Stanovich (1986): "Robust effects of syntactic structure on visual word processing". Memory and Cognition 14, 104 - 112.
Winer, B.J. (1971): Statistical Principles in Experimental Design. New York: McGraw-Hill.
Wright, B. & M. Garrett (1984): "Lexical decision in sentences: Effects of syntactic structure". Memory and Cognition 12, 31 - 45.
Zurif, E.B. & A. Caramazza (1976): "Psycholinguistic structures in aphasia: Studies in syntax and semantics". In: H. Whitaker & H.A. Whitaker, eds., Studies in Neurolinguistics. Volume I. New York: Academic Press.
Zurif, E., H. Gardner & H. Brownell (1989): "The case against the case against group studies". Brain and Cognition 10, 237 - 255.
Zwitserlood, P. (1989): "The locus of the effects of sentential-semantic context in spoken word processing". Cognition 32, 25 - 64.

Activation of the Lexical-semantic System in Right-brain-damaged Right-handers*

Jean Gagnon, Pierre Goulet, Yves Joanette, Montréal

A right hemisphere lesion can be the source of difficulties in the processing of words in right-handed individuals (Joanette, Goulet & Hannequin 1990). The research that have attempted to shed light on the nature of these difficulties have taken two orientations. One such orientation is the stream of research that has investigated the semantic nature of the lexical deficits among right-brain-damaged (RBD) subjects (Chiarello & Church 1986; Gainotti, Caltagirone & Miceli 1979, 1983; Gainotti, Caltagirone, Miceli & Masullo 1981; Joanette & Goulet 1986; Lesser 1974). These studies have tried to specify the semantic components that were affected following a right hemisphere lesion, such as the nonliteral meanings of words (Brownell, Potter, Michelow & Gardner 1984; Gardner & Denes 1973). Most of the time they have used tasks that required controlled or conscious processing of the lexical-semantic knowledge (e.g. written or oral comprehension tasks for single words, semantic judgment tasks, word fluency tasks, etc). Therefore, a second stream of research became more interested in the root cause of the semantic deficiencies found among RBD subjects than in the kind of semantic word components that were affected (Brownell & Molloy 1990; Joanette, Goulet & LeDorze 1988; Tompkins 1990). More precisely, these studies have attempted to determine whether the deficit in RBD subjects is attributable to difficulties in the use of the semantic knowledge or to a disruption of its organization.

These last studies were inspired by cognitive models, and particularly by the Two-processes theory, that contrasts "automatic" processes (Hasher & Zacks 1979; Posner & Snyder 1975a; Schneider & Shiffrin 1977) with "controlled" (Shiffrin & Schneider 1977), "conscious" (Posner & Snyder 1975a), or "effortful" (Hasher & Zacks 1979) processes. These two types of processes, automatic and controlled, are independent but may co-occur during the processing of information.

* The authors wish to thank Dominique Panet-Raymond and Elisabeth Ohashi for the translation of this paper, and Dieter Hillert who invited them to contribute to this special issue of Linguistische Berichte. They thank also the neuropsychologists and speech therapists of the Côte-des-Neiges, Jacques-Viger, Marie-Clarac and Villa-Médica hospitals, the "Association Québécoise des personnes aphasiques", and the subjects who collaborated to this study. This study was supported by grants from the Medical Research Council of Canada (PG-28) and the Fonds pour la Recherche en Santé du Québec.

A process is considered automatic when it occurs without intention, when the processing of stimuli is unconscious, and when no interference with any ongoing mental activity exists (Posner & Snyder 1975a). With respect to the semantic processing of words, such a process depends on the automatic spreading of activation within the lexical-semantic organization (Anderson 1976; Collins & Loftus 1975; Quillian 1962). This organization is generally thought of as a network of nodes corresponding to the conceptual representation of words in memory. The distance between nodes reflects the strength of the association between words. When a node is activated, the activation spreads rapidly and automatically to other semantically related nodes. Consequently, the processing of semantically related words occurring simultaneously or immediately following this initial activation becomes faster and easier than the processing of words that are not semantically related to the word that is at the origin of the initial activation. As this activation is automatic and depends only on the existence of semantic relatedness, it does not interfere with the processing of words unrelated to the initially activated nodes. Thus, the processing of related concepts is facilitated in the absence of any inhibition of unrelated concepts.

As for controlled, conscious or effortful processes, these are characterized primarily by strategies and conscious control, and by their high demand of attentional capacity (Hasher & Zacks 1979; Posner & Snyder 1975a; Schneider & Shiffrin 1977). Because these processes are capacity-limited, they can access only one memory location at a time without interference. To access a new concept, attention has to be displaced from one memory location to another. In a task requiring the semantic processing of a word, this displacement may be done strategically. Consequently, the processing of a word semantically-related to a stimulus initially reaching conscious awareness will be facilitated, thus benefiting from the use of a conscious strategy of semantic relatedness. In contrast, the processing of an unrelated stimulus will undergo negative interference as the strategy for relocalizing attention will need attentional resources, thus generating costs.

For more than 15 years, semantic priming techniques have represented a privileged means of studying the two types of activations (Neely 1977, 1991). Priming consists of the presentation of a stimulus, known as a *prime*, prior to or simultaneously to the presentation of a stimulus known as a *target*, which is the object of some processing. The use of *semantic* priming in the context of a lexical decision task revealed that a subject can decide more accurately and/or quickly that a series of letters constitutes a word when it is presented simultaneously or preceded by a semantically related word-prime (e.g. doctor-nurse) compared to a semantically unrelated word-prime (e.g. butter-nurse) (Meyer & Schvaneveldt 1971). This difference in the processing efficiency of semantically related and unrelated word-targets is known as the *priming effect*.

By modifying some aspects of the experimental conditions, it is possible to influence how subjects process the prime. Semantic automatic priming can be induced when conditions do not favor the active use of primes as valuable cues in predicting the nature of the target. On the contrary, priming is considered controlled when the conditions allow the subject to orient his attention to the prime and be aware of the relatedness between it and the target. Among the experimental factors that can be manipulated to induce either automatic or controlled priming there are: (a) the instructions given to the subject (Neely 1977); (b) the time interval between the prime and the target (Fischler & Goodman 1978; Neely 1977); (c) the probability that primes and targets are related (Fischler 1977; Tweedy et al. 1977). Under the automatic conditions, the lexical decision task is facilitated when targets and primes are related, without any detrimental effect on the processing of unrelated targets (Neely 1977). Thus, benefits are obtained without costs, which conforms to the predictions of the model proposed by Posner and Snyder (1975b). Under the controlled conditions, the processing of the target preceded by a related prime will be facilitated whereas the processing of a target preceded by an unrelated prime will be inhibited (benefits with costs). Facilitation and inhibition are usually assessed by the use of a neutral priming condition. Neutral primes typically consisted of either a string of Xs, the word "ready", the word "blank" or the word "neutral". Several authors have questioned the value of the neutral priming condition as a proper baseline for assessing facilitation or inhibition (see Neely 1991 for a critical review on semantic priming). But, this condition still remains the best way to obtain on-line indications about the automatic or effortful status of the priming effect induced.

Milberg and Blumstein (1981) were the first to refer to the Two-processes theory proposed by modern cognitivists to better understand the nature of lexical-semantic impairments in brain-damaged subjects.[1] Using a lexical decision task with priming deemed automatic, and a semantic judgment task requiring a more controlled processing, these authors demonstrated that the aphasics' semantic impairment reflected a difficulty in the controlled activation of lexical-semantic knowledge, in consciously accessing this knowledge, rather than its disintegration proper. In this study, aphasics were impaired in the semantic judgment task but their semantic knowledge was preserved and accessible in an automatic fashion as shown by an intact priming effect (Milberg & Blumstein 1981).

Neuropsychological domains, other than aphasiology, have also referred to the Two-processes theory in order to dissociate impairments at the representation level from those affecting access processes. For instance, this was the case when examining the semantic impairments found in patients suffering of dementia of Alzheimer's type (e.g., Chertkow, Bub & Seidenberg 1989). For their part, Joanette, Goulet & LeDorze (1988) were the first to describe lexical-semantic deficits among RBD subjects in light of the automatic-non automatic distinction. These authors undertook a temporal analysis of the performances of these subjects during a word fluency task. The results demonstrated that the exploration deficit of the lexicon starting from a semantic criteria (e.g. "animal" category) would depend primarily on the part of the task considered to be dependent on active research in the lexicon (the last 30 seconds) so that the initial stage, reflecting its automatic activation, would be preserved. The semantic character of the deficit was supported by the absence of a similar deficit when orthographic criteria were used (Joanette & Goulet 1986).

In line with the study of Joanette, Goulet & LeDorze (1988), other authors (Brownell & Molloy 1990; Tompkins 1990) had recourse to the priming techniques in order to understand the influence of the level of processing (automatic versus controlled) on the performances reported in the literature as being deficient among RBD subjects. For instance, the goal of the Brownell and Molloy's (1990) study was to investigate whether the trouble comprehending metaphorical and connotative meaning of words observed among RBD subjects (Brownell, Potter, Michelow & Gardner 1984) would always be present if the cognitive effort required by the task was reduced to a minimum. In order to answer this question, the authors submitted RBD subjects to a lexical decision task including an automatic priming context. The results demonstrated that the RBD subjects benefit just as much as normal subjects from the priming effect when prime-target pairs have a metaphorical relationship (e.g. cheap-stingy). The authors concluded that RBD subjects remain sensitive to this type of semantic relationship when the task does not require any conscious strategies or judgments.

Tompkins (1990) was also interested by the actual status of the disabilities of the RBD patients when they have to process metaphorical word meanings in semantic judgment tasks. She submitted RBD subjects to two conditions of semantic priming, one of automatic nature and the other of controlled nature. These two priming conditions were presented in the framework of a lexical decision task in which the targets, presented in the auditory modality, were ambiguous adjectives which had metaphorical and/or literal meanings. Tompkins (1990) also undertook a careful analysis of the controlled priming condition in order to investigate the capacity of the subjects to spontaneously develop strategic behaviors. In accordance with the conditions favoring a controlled priming, the experimenter insisted, in the presence of the subjects, on the nature and the validity of the semantic relation that existed between the prime and the target words presented during the task. The expectancies thus created within each subject were qualified as extrinsic since they would rest on strategies proposed by the examiner. These expectancies were evaluated by the intermediary of the three first prime-target semantically unrelated pairs presented during the experiment. They differed with intrinsic expectancies that would be generated by the subject himself. The intrinsic expectancies would develop, according to Tompkins (1990), as the subject runs into pairs in which the prime and the target are not semantically linked during the task. These same expectancies would therefore be founded on the capacity of the subject to recognize that the initial extrinsic expectations are not met and that he must change his initial strategy. Tompkins (1990) postulated that the elaboration of intrinsic expectations requires more effort and attentional resources than extrinsic strategies.

Tompkins (1990) reported that the priming effects obtained by the RBD subjects when processing metaphorical and literal meanings did not differ from those obtained by normal subjects in both conditions of priming. However, only normal subjects showed evidence of intrinsic expectancy during controlled priming. According to Tompkins (1990), these results show that RBD subjects do not demonstrate difficulty accessing the metaphorical or literal aspects of the meaning of words when such access is done relatively automatically or when these patients receive specific strategies. However, RBD patients do not have sufficient attentional resources to formulate their own strategies.

In her discussion of the results, Tompkins (1990) referred to a continuum that has also been proposed by Gagnon, Goulet, Joanette and Cardu (1988). She noted that a normal priming effect in RBD subjects on the controlled priming task contradicted the difficulties showed by these patients in the semantic judgment task used by Brownell et al. (1984). To explain this contrast, she suggested that RBD subjects' impairment was related to the amount of attentional resources required by each task considering a reduction in the available resource after a brain lesion. Thus, the controlled priming condition was situated somewhere between the automatic priming task and the semantic judgment task which were located at the poles of this continuum.

Tompkins also suggested that the dissociation found between the use of extrinsic and intrinsic strategies might be explained by reference to the same continuum of resource requirements. Her suggestion is based on her initial assumption according to which intrinsic strategic expectancies adopted during the controlled priming task require more attentional resources than the extrinsic expectancy initially imposed. However, some reservations can be put forward regarding the validity of this proposition. The measures reflecting the two levels of cognitive demands were both derived from the same controlled priming task. The actual strategies used by the subjects did not result from an experimental manipulation. The subjects were free to develop more or less effortful strategies and the experimenter had no control on the kind of strategies used. Recourse to intrinsic strategies rested on the relinquishment of the extrinsic strategy that did not guarantee the controlled status of the intrinsic attitude adopted by the subjects. A defective use of the extrinsic strategy with a more automatic intrinsic strategy adopted by the normal subjects might be coherent with the results reported by Tompkins (1990) for the controlled condition, particularly with respect to the absence of costs. Moreover, Tompkins' (1990) discussion of her findings on unrelated word-pairs is more relevant for the general abilities to use strategies than for the appreciation of the lexical-semantic disabilities in RBD subjects. From this perspective, it would have been interesting if Tompkins had undertook the same analysis and discussion with regard to the automatic condition.

In spite of the debatable nature of Tompkins' study, the hypothesis of a continuum governing lexical-semantic problems of RBD subjects still remains a promising vein of research. This hypothesis merits that future research attempt to better define the nature of the tasks which could constitute this continuum. This issue will be discussed later in this paper.

The main concern of the studies of Brownell and Molloy, and Tompkins was the processing of the metaphorical or connotative components of words. As for these components, Tompkins failed to find that RBD patients were impaired when they had to process the literal meaning of words. In fact, both studies failed to show that their RBD subjects suffered from a lexical-semantic disorder. However, none of these studies included a more conventional semantic task, such as a semantic judgment task, on which RBD subjects are usually deficient. Accordingly, none of these studies provided unquestionable information about the level of processing implicated in RBD subjects suffering from lexical-semantic impairments, particularly with regard to the processing of the literal processing of words. In contrast with these studies and in line with the suggestion made by Joanette, Goulet and LeDorze (1988), the present study[2] referred to the priming techniques and to a semantic judgment task to confirm that the difficulties of RBD subjects to process the literal meaning of words are due to a disturbance in the controlled use of lexical-semantic knowledge rather than to a disruption of the organization of this knowledge. A lexical decision task with automatic semantic priming allowed the evaluation of automatic activation of lexical-semantic knowledge. Similarly, a lexical decision task with controlled semantic priming, and a semantic judgment task allowed the evaluation of controlled activation of this knowledge.

Method

Subjects: The RBD group included ten right-handed French-speaking adults (≥ 79 on the Edinburgh Inventory; Oldfield 1971) aged between 44 and 83 years. All but one of the RBD subjects had suffered from a single vascular lesion limited to the right hemisphere and confirmed by the results of paraclinical (CT scan) and/or clinical neurological exams. The exception was a subject who had suffered a second stroke within the same hemisphere soon after the first. The time elapsed since the lesion varied from 40 to 96 days, with the exception of one subject (35 months). None of the RBD subjects exhibited signs of aphasia or intellectual deterioration according to their medical report. However, two patients suffered from unilateral left spatial neglect, two others from left homonymous hemianopia, whereas a fifth suffered from both these impairments.

An equivalent number of subjects free from neurological problems were paired, one to one, with the RBD subjects with respect to age, sex, and level of education. These subjects formed the normal control group. The two groups of subjects, RBD and normal, were also comparable with respect to the absence of a family history of left-handedness or ambidexterity. Table 1 reports the characteristics of each group of subjects.

Table 1 Characteristics of right-brain-damaged (RBD) and control subjects

Variables	Groups	
	RBD (n = 10)	Control (n = 10)
Age (years)	66.9 [11.5]	67.8 [9.8]
Sex (m/f)	2/8	2/8
Scolarity	7.9 [2.3]	8.6 [2.7]
Familial left-handedness or ambidexterity (yes/no)	9/1	7/3
Days post-onset	63.22 [14.87]	
Hospitalization (yes/no)	9/1	5/5

[ ]: standard deviation

Stimuli: The lexical decision (LD) tasks with semantic priming were elaborated from 120 "prime-target" pairs of 3 to 7 letters stimuli. Half of the targets (60/120) were concrete and imageable words (e.g., car) (Corbeil 1986). The other half were phonologically, morphologically and orthographically acceptable nonwords derived from the real words by letter substitutions (see Béland 1987). The target words and their paired nonwords were similar with respect to the number of letters, syllables, vowels and consonants that they included. The primes were either words or a series of four Xs in the neutral conditions.

To avoid any material specific effect, two versions of each type of priming task, automatic and controlled, were developed. Each version of a given priming condition, automatic or controlled, included different stimuli but, one version of the automatic priming task presented to a subject shared its stimuli with one of the versions of the controlled priming task presented to another subject and vice versa. Hence, the experiment was based on two protocols, A and B, each one incorporating one version of the automatic and the controlled priming tasks. These measures also assured the equivalency of the automatic and controlled priming protocols. Moreover, except for the series of Xs, each stimuli (word or nonword) was projected only once to each subject.

In summary, there were four priming tasks used. Each priming task (automatic and controlled) included 60 "prime-target" pairs. Half of these pairs had target words whereas the other half had nonwords as targets. The former were either of the semantically *related* type (R) (e.g. chaise-table), semantically *unrelated* type (UR) (e.g. chien-table), or of the *neutral* type (N) (e.g. XXXX-table). The R pairs included co-hyponymic words. These words were selected on the basis of the semantic category norms developed by Favreau and Segalowitz (1980). In order to put more emphasis on semantic relatedness than on strictly associative relationships, the R pairs were formed by matching a high category dominance item with a low category dominance item. All words in the R pairs were either moderately or weakly associated; none were highly associated. The UR pairs were made of unrelated words and they were similar to the R pairs in the number of letters (avg. for the primes: 5.5; avg. for the targets: 5.6), and word frequency (avg. for the primes: 56; avg. for the targets: 33) (Baudot 1970) of the words they incorporated. The N pairs were included to determine a baseline for the calculation of costs and benefits. In each priming task, the targets in the N pairs were comparable to those of other pairs with regard to the average number of letters (avg.: 5.7) and word frequency (avg.: 33) (Baudot 1970). For both automatic and controlled conditions, the thirty non-word target pairs were divided into 24 pairs in which the prime was a real word (e.g., coffret-chalime), and 6 pairs in which the prime was neutral (e.g. XXXX-turpon).

For automatic priming, the thirty pairs whose target was a real word were divided into 6 related pairs (25 % of the trials where the primes and targets were words), 18 unrelated pairs (75 %), and 6 neutral pairs. In the controlled priming condition, the thirty pairs whose target was a word were this time distributed inversely: 18 related pairs (75 %), 6 nonrelated pairs (25 %), and 6 neutral pairs.

With respect to the semantic judgment task, 12 pairs of co-hyponymic words (e.g., aigle-corbeau) were adapted from Chiarello and Church (1986) who reported that RBD subjects showed a semantic impairment on this material. Twelve other pairs of semantically unrelated words were constructed by interchanging the words from the twelve pairs of semantically related words. None of the words in this task (n = 24) were common to the semantic priming protocols. The words included in the semantic judgment task did not differ from those used in the LD tasks with semantic priming in terms of the average number of letters (avg.: 5) and mean word frequency (avg.: 33).

Apparatus and Procedure: The subjects were tested individually in the following order: 1) the semantic judgment task, 2) the automatic priming task, and 3) the controlled priming task. Half of the subjects of each group were tested with protocol A for the automatic and controlled priming conditions, whereas the other half were tested with protocol B.

For the semantic judgment task, the word pairs were presented orally and visually to the subjects. The words of each pair were presented above each other, in the centre of a white sheet of paper. The subjects had to indicate, by yes or no, "if the words of each pair go together". Each subject was warned that two words went together if they belonged to the same category. The task was illustrated by two examples.

Each priming task was preceded by explanations provided to the subjects: each subject was warned that the stimuli would be constituted of pairs and that the first stimulus might be a word or a series of Xs whereas the second item might be a word or a non-word. Then, subjects were instructed that they would have to decide as quickly and correctly as possible whether the second series of letters of each pair constituted a word or not. The instructions also advised the subject that they had to answer with the right hand by pressing one of two answer keys (yes-no). A time limit of 5000 ms was allotted for answering. The instructions provided before each of the priming conditions differed only with respect to the processing of the first stimulus of each pair (see below). Both of the priming conditions were illustrated with the help of 15 practice trials. During these trials, the subjects were informed of their performance. This practice session was repeated until the subject mastered the task.

For both priming tasks, the stimuli were presented visually using a "Macintosh SE" with the Psylab program version 0.85 (1988). The stimuli of each prime-target pair were presented one at a time, sequentially, at the centre of the screen. The prime was presented for 150 ms whereas the target for 2000 ms. Given that five brain-damaged subjects suffered from visual impairments, the prime presentation threshold permitting complete recognition was first determined individually (from 200 to 500 ms). An interval of 2000 ms separated each prime-target trial.

In the automatic priming condition, the time interval between prime and target was 300 ms. A relatively long prime-target interval was used because of the particular nature of the brain-damaged population. In addition, the instructions minimized the role of the prime by omitting to mention the possible presence of a semantic relation between the prime and the target. Inversely, in the controlled priming condition, the prime-target interval was raised to 1000 ms and the instructions insisted on the very probable semantic relation between the prime and target, and on the importance of using the prime to predict the nature of the target.

Results

The subjects produced so few errors on the priming tasks that parametric statistical analyses were impossible. Furthermore, only the number of errors for the UR pairs in the controlled priming condition was sufficient to allow a non parametric statistical comparison (Chi-square test) of performance between the two groups of subjects.

The average reaction time for the correct answers produced by each subject was calculated for each type of prime-target pair, for both priming conditions (automatic and controlled). These results were then submitted to an ANOVA with "Group" (brain-damaged and control) as a between-group factor and "Prime" (R, UR, and N) as a within-group factor. The priming effects, costs and benefits were evaluated by comparing the results obtained for the three types of pairs with the Newman-Keuls Mean Comparison Test ($\alpha = .05$).

The number of errors was also very small on the semantic judgment task. Accordingly, the performance of RBD and control subjects were analysed using non-parametrical statistics (Chi-square Test).

Automatic Priming: The mean reaction times for the RBD and control subjects for the three pair types during the automatic condition are reported in figure 1.

The control subjects answered more rapidly than the RBD subjects ($F_{(1;18)} = 24.83$, $p < 0.0001$). There was also a main effect of the "Prime" factor ($F_{(1;18)} = 6.79$, $p < 0.01$).

Figure 1 Mean reaction times for right-brain-damaged (RBD) and control subjects for the three pair types in the automatic priming condition

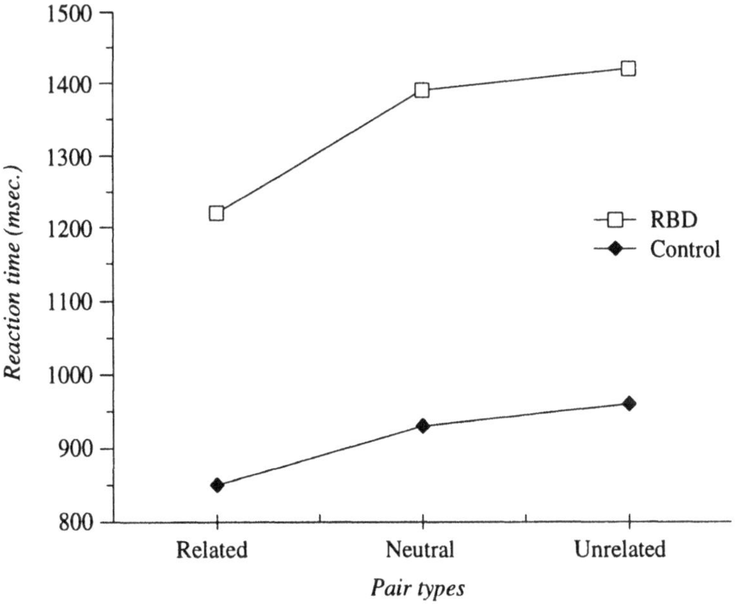

The reaction times for R pairs (1036 ms) were significantly shorter than for UR (1185 ms) or N (1154 ms) pairs. The reaction times for UR and N pairs did not differ significantly. The priming effect (149 ms) and the benefits (118 ms) were thus significant whereas the costs (-31 ms) were not. The interaction "Group X Prime" was not significant ($F_{(2;36)} = 0.62$, p = n.s.).
The only errors made concerned the UR pairs, thus suggesting the existence of costs. However, only six (3 RBD subjects and 3 controls) of the twenty subjects made one or more errors. The two groups of subjects distributed themselves identically in terms of the number of errors made for UR pairs in the automatic priming condition.

Controlled priming: The mean reaction times for the RBD and control subjects for the three pair types during the controlled condition are reported in figure 2.
There was a main effect of the Group factor, as the control subjects answered more rapidly than the RBD subjects ($F_{(1;18)} = 17.69$, $p < 0.001$). A significant effect of the nature of the prime ($F_{(1;18)} = 5.61$, $p < 0.01$) was also present. The reaction times were shorter for the R pairs (1057 ms) than for the UR (1303 ms) and the N (1220 ms) pairs. The reaction times for the UR and N pairs did not differ significantly. Thus, the priming effect (246 ms) and the benefits (163 ms) were significant whereas the costs (-83 ms) were not. The interaction "Group X Prime" was not significant ($F_{(2;36)} = 1.47$, p = n.s.).

Figure 2 Mean reaction times for right-brain-damaged (RBD) and control subjects for the three pair types in the controlled priming condition

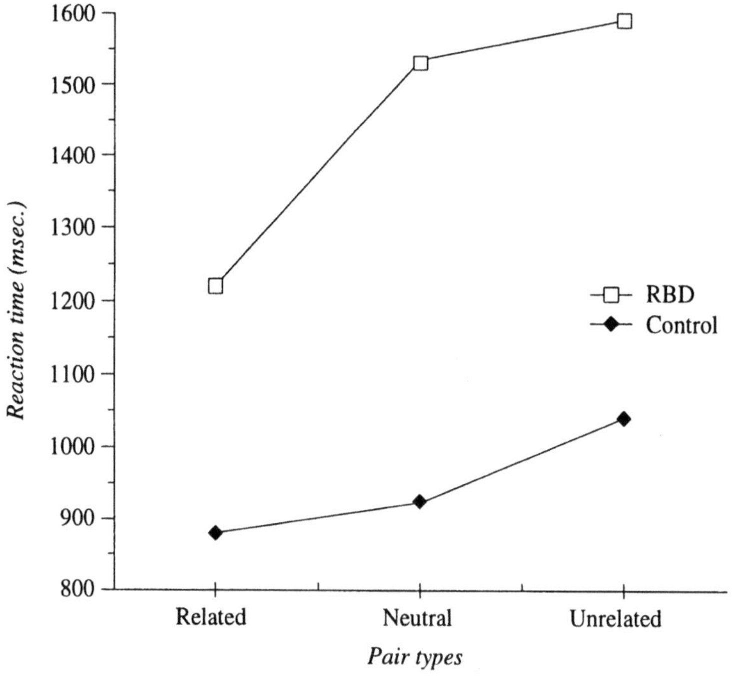

Table 2 Number of right-brain-damaged (RBD) and control subjects according to the number of errors produced on the unrelated pairs in the controlled priming condition

Groups	No of errors	
	0	1 or more
RBD	5	5
Control	8	2

Only two subjects produced an erroneous answer on the R and N pairs. One RBD subject made one error in the R pairs, whereas another RBD subject made two errors in the N pairs. The situation was slightly different for the UR pairs. Table 2 presents the distribution of RBD and control subjects according to the number of errors produced for this type of pair in the controlled priming condition. These distributions did not differ significantly ($\chi 2_{(0.05;1)} = 1.4$, p = n.s.).

Semantic judgment task: As shown in Table 3, a larger number of RBD subjects than controls produced a minimum of one error in the semantic judgment task ($\chi 2_{(0.01;1)} = 8.52$, $p < 0.01$). The RBD group produced fourteen errors whereas only four errors were produced by the control subjects. Most errors made by RBD subjects (11/14) as well as by controls (3/4) were false negatives. Among the errors of the RBD subjects, five were produced on the related pair "évier-poêle" (sink-stove) and four on the related pair "pêche-prune" (peach-plum). No word pair was particularly difficult for the control subjects.

Table 3 Number of right-brain-damaged (RBD) and control subjects according to the number of errors produced in the semantic judgment task

Groups	No of errors	
	0	1 or more
RBD	2	8
Control	7	3

Discussion

The right-handed subjects with a right-hemisphere lesion who participated in this study were just as sensitive as normal subjects to semantic priming as reflected by the priming effect and the analysis of costs and benefits. Aside from a nonspecific slowing of responses, the RBD subjects obtained significantly lower performances than those of the control subjects only on the semantic judgment task. Before concluding,

two points need to be addressed: 1) the automatic or controlled nature of the priming conditions obtained, and 2) the actual validity of the semantic judgment task.
The results on the automatic priming condition were expected and support the findings of other studies which had recourse to this technique with RBD subjects (Brownell & Molloy 1990; Tompkins 1990). However, in order to be able to draw a conclusion about the integrity of the semantic relationships within lexical-semantic knowledge, the automatic nature of semantic priming must be assured. Theoretically, this type of priming is only attributed to the automatic spreading of activation throughout the associative connections within lexical-semantic knowledge (Quillian 1962; Collins & Loftus 1975). This type of priming should thus produce benefits without costs (Posner & Snyder 1975b). The reaction times are congruent with this criterion. Regarding the number of errors, the results for N and R pairs showed that benefits were absent. A possible ceiling effect can account for this finding: as the N pairs do not incur any errors, the subjects could not improve their performance with R pairs. In contrast, the results for the N and UR pairs are congruent with the presence of costs. However, the errors produced on the UR pairs can be neglected because of infrequency and the small number of subjects responsable for these. To conclude, the automatic priming condition has indicated an automatic priming effect.
Contrary to what was expected, the RBD subjects were as sensitive as normals to the controlled priming effect. This finding matches the results reported by Tompkins (1990). However, the voluntary, effortful or strategic nature of the priming effect induced in the controlled priming condition is questionable. Theoretically, the strategic use of lexical-semantic knowledge should be reflected through the presence of both benefits (for R pairs) and costs (for UR pairs). The existence of costs is characteristic of the controlled nature of a priming condition. In the present study, the performance obtained with controlled priming resembled those obtained in the automatic condition. Controlled priming produced benefits without significant costs when reaction times were considered. With respect to the analysis of errors, the absence of benefits could be explained by the ceiling effect produced by the near perfect performance in the N trials. The costs were negligeable because only few errors were committed by few subjects for the semantically unrelated word pairs. To summarize, the absence of costs suggest that the experimental conditions (instructions, prime-target interval, proportion of R pairs) retained in order to produce controlled semantic priming probably may not have reached their goal. To discuss this issue more extensively, it would have been necessary to better document the subjects' behavior during controlled priming conditions. For instance, it would have been interesting to determine by other methods, such as a questionnaire, exactly how the subjects attempted to apply the anticipatory strategy suggested by the instructions for the task, towards the targets. For the moment, the status of the controlled priming conditions remains ambiguous.
The semantic judgment task was aimed at the evaluation of the subjects' capacity to recognize co-hyponymic relationships. As expected, the RBD's performance was significantly lower than that of the control subjects on this task. This difference confirms the findings already reported by Chiarello and Church (1986) following the application of a semantic judgment task comparable to that used here. This difference also supports other studies showing that RBD subjects demonstrate lexical-semantic difficulties in

semantic connotative/denotative judgment tasks (Brownell et al. 1984), in verbal fluency tasks (Joanette & Goulet 1986, 1988; Joanette, Goulet & LeDorze 1988; Laine & Niemi 1988), as well as for the comprehension of isolated words (Gainotti et al. 1979, 1981, 1983; Lesser 1974).

A detailed analysis of the results on the semantic judgment task was conducted in order to obtain more information about the exact nature of the difficulties manifested by the RBD subjects. This analysis showed that most errors concerned two word pairs: "évier-poêle" (sink-stove), "pêche-prune" (peach-plum). Despite the lack of any empirical evidence for such suggestion, the semantic relationship within the pair "évier-poêle" may differ from that involved by the other pairs. For instance, it may be more difficult to acknowledge that a sink is a piece of furniture at the same level as a stove, whereas the relationships within the other pairs are more obvious (e.g. "porc-veau" (pork-veal), "aigle-corneille" (eagle-crow)). This comment illustrates the importance that must be given to parameters such as the nature of the semantic relationship, the prototypicality of the items, and the semantic distance between two items of the same category when constructing semantic judgment trials. In the future, studies will have to give more attention to these factors and to investigate the role they may have played in the present research. It is probable that the RBD's difficulties reflect a difficulty in the processing of semantically distant words. Such a possibility is consistent with the hypothesis put forth by Chiarello (1991) which claimed that the right hemisphere plays an important role in the activation of a broad set of related meanings in the course of word recognition. For the moment, one should be cautious in concluding that RBD subjects are less sensitive to co-hyponymic relationships than controls, because their problems are mainly apparent with two word pairs.

The tasks used in this study were in agreement with the methodology usually involved in neuropsychology and cognitive psychology in order to investigate the lexical-semantic abilities of normal or brain-damaged subjects (see Shallice 1988). However, it is clear that their validity calls for some cautiousness that must be kept in mind when interpreting the results. These results suggest that a lesion of the right hemisphere in a right-handed individual does not produce disturbances related to the automatic activation of lexical-semantic knowledge. Semantic associative relationships and the automatic access to semantic representations seem well preserved in the RBD patients who participated in this study. As the controlled aspect of the controlled priming task was not assured, the importance of the voluntary, effortful, conscious or strategic component of the lexical-semantic impairments of RBD subjects still remains to be shown. Within this study, the lexical-semantic difficulties of RBD right-handed subjects were observed exclusively in the semantic judgment task. However, this task may differ from both priming conditions with respect to the processes involved and the attentional resources it requires. Thus, impairments on this task do not provide clear information about their causes. Nevertheless, if one accepts that two of the three tasks used here were of the controlled type, the results of this study can be interpreted in the context of a continuum of attentional resources allocation rather than in the classical perspective of the "automatic-controlled" dichotomy. This means that RBD patients would have no problem at the automatic level and their semantic deficiencies would be related to the amount of resources needed by a given task. In this study, the semantic task would be the most effortful and, accordingly the most sensitive to semantic problems. Only such an approach would permit the exact evaluation of the levels of the use of lexical-semantic knowledge affected within these patients. Such a continuum should also be considered in the analysis and interpretation of the linguistic impairments found in other subject populations such as aphasics and demented patients.

Notes

1 However, they were not the first to refer to the automatic-non automatic dissociation in their attempt to explain the linguistic impairments observed in brain-damaged patients. Since Baillarger (1865, cited in Alajouanine 1960), the "dissociation automatico-volontaire" is well known in neuropsychology. Jackson (1878-1879) was probably the first to introduce this dissociation in a structured interpretation of language problems that can follow a lesion of the brain. For a discussion of this issue see Gagnon and Goulet (1992).

2 Part of this paper has been already presented in Gagnon et al. (1988, 1989).

References

Alajouanine, T. (1960): "Baillarger and Jackson: the principle of Baillarger-Jackson in aphasia". Journal of Neurology, Neurosurgery and Psychiatry 23, 191 – 193.

Anderson, J.R. (1976): Language, memory, and thought. New York: Halsted Press.

Baudot, J. (1970): Fréquence des mots en français. Montréal: Les Presses de l'Université de Montréal.

Béland, R. (1987): Le statut lexical des non-mots. Paper presented at Journée scientifique du centre de recherche du Centre hospitalier Côte-des-Neiges, Montréal.

Brownell, H. & R. Molly (1990): Lexical priming in right hemisphere brain-damaged patients. Paper presented at 28th Academy of Aphasia, Baltimore.

Brownell, H., H.H. Potter, D. Michelow & H. Gardner (1984): "Sensitivity to lexical denotation and connotation in brain-damaged patients: A double dissociation?" Brain and Language 22, 253 – 265.

Chertkow, H., D. Bub & M. Seidenberg (1989): "Priming and semantic memory loss in Alzheimer's disease". Brain and Language 36, 420 – 446.

Chiarello, C. (1991): Interpretation of word meaning by the cerebral hemispheres: one is not enough. In: P.J. Schwanenflugel, ed., The psychology of word meaning. Hillsdale, New Jersey: Lawrence Erlbaum Associates.

Chiarello, C. & L. Church (1986): "Lexical judgments after right-or left-hemisphere injury". Neuropsychologia 24, 623 – 630.

Collins, A.M. & E.F. Loftus (1975): "A spreading-activation theory of semantic processing". Psychological Review 82, 407 – 428.

Corbeil, J.C. (1986): Dictionnaire thématique visuel. Montréal: Québec-Amérique.

Favreau, M. & N. Segalowitz (1980): Semantic category norms for the English and French Québec Populations. Paper presented at Canadian Psychological Association, Calgary.

Fischler, I. (1977): "Associative facilitation without expectancy in a lexical decision task". Journal of Experimental Psychology: Human Perception and Performance 3, 18 – 26.

Fischler, I. & G.O. Goodman (1978): "Latency of associative activation in memory". Journal of Experimental Psychology: Human Perception and Performance 4, 455 – 470.

Gagnon, J. & P. Goulet (1992): "Des conceptions de Jackson aux modèles contemporains, l'opposition automatique-non automatique est-elle la même?" Revue de neuropsychologie 2, 117 – 150.
Gagnon, J., Y. Joanette, P. Goulet & B. Cardu (1988): "Automatic and controlled priming in right- and left-brain-damaged right-handers [Summary]". Abstracts. Academy of Aphasia 21, 5 – 6.
Gagnon, J., P. Goulet & Y. Joanette (1989): "Activation automatique et contrôlée du savoir lexico-sémantique chez les cérébrolésés droits". Langages 96, 95 – 111.
Gainotti, G., C. Caltagirone & G. Miceli (1979): "Semantic disorders of auditory language comprehension in right brain-damaged patients". Journal of Psycholinguistic Research 8, 13 – 20.
Gainotti, G., C. Caltagirone & G. Miceli (1983): "Selective impairment in semantic-lexical discrimination in right-brain-damaged patients". In: E. Perecman, ed., Cognitive processing in right hemisphere. New York: Academic Press.
Gainotti, G., C. Caltagirone, G. Miceli & C. Masullo (1981): "Selective semantic-lexical impairment of language comprehension in right-brain-damaged patients". Brain and Language 13, 201 – 211.
Hasher, L. & R.T. Zacks (1979): "Automatic and effortful processes in memory". Journal of Experimental Psychology: General 108, 356 – 388.
Jackson, J.-H. (1878-1879): "On affections of speech from disease of the brain". Brain 1, 304 – 330.
Joanette, Y. & P. Goulet (1986): "Criterion-specific reduction of verbal fluency in right-brain-damaged right-handers". Neuropsychologia 24, 875 – 879.
Joanette, Y., P. Goulet & D. Hannequin (1990): Right hemisphere and verbal communication. New York: Springer-Verlag.
Joanette, Y., P. Goulet & G. LeDorze (1988): "Impaired word naming in right-brain-damaged right-handers: error type and time-course analysis". Brain and Language 34, 54 – 64.
Laine, M. & J. Niemi (1988): "Word fluency production strategies of neurological patterns: semantic and phonological clustering". Journal of Clinical and Experimental Neuropsychology 10, 28.
Lesser, R. (1974): "Verbal comprehension in aphasia: an english version of three italian tests". Cortex 10, 247 – 263.
Meyer, D.E. & R.W. Schvaneveldt (1971): "Facilitation in recognizing pairs of words: evidence of a dependence between retrieval operations". Journal of Experimental Psychology 90, 227 – 234.
Milberg, W. & S.E. Blumstein (1981): "Lexical decision and aphasia: evidence for semantic processing". Brain and Language 14, 371 – 385.
Neely, J.H. (1977): "Semantic priming and retrieval from lexical memory: roles of inhibitionless spreading activation and limited-capacity attention". Journal of Experimental Psychology: General 106, 226 – 254.
Neely, J.H. (1991): "Semantic priming effects in visual word recognition: a selective review of current finding and theories". In: D. Besner & G.W. Humphreys, eds., Basic processes in reading visual word recognition. Hillsdale, New Jersey: Lawrence Erlbaum Associates.
Oldfield, O.D. (1971): "The assessment and analysis of handedness: the Edinburgh Inventory". Neuropsychologia 9, 97 – 113.
Posner, M.I. & C.R.R. Snyder (1975a): "Attention and cognitive control". In: R.L. Solso, ed., Information processing and cognition: The Loyola Symposium. Hillsdale, N.J.: Erlbaum.
Posner, M.I. & C.R.R. Snyder (1975b): "Facilitation and inhibition in processing of signals". In: P.M.A. Rabbitt & S. Dornic, eds., Attention and performance V. New York: Academic Press.
Psylab version 0.85 (1988): Montréal: Laboratoire Théophile-Alajouanine.
Quillian, M.R. (1962): "A revised design for an understanding machine". Mechanical translation 7, 17 – 29.

Schneider, W. & R.M. Shiffrin (1977): "Controlled and automatic human information processing: I. detection, search, and attention". Psychological Review 84, 1 – 66.

Shallice, T. (1988): From neuropsychology to mental structure. Cambridge: Cambridge University Press.

Shiffrin, R.M. & W. Schneider (1977): "Controlled and automatic human information processing: II. perceptual learning, automatic attending, and a general theory". Psychological Review 84, 127 – 190.

Tompkins, C.A. (1990): "Knowledge and strategies for processing lexical metaphor after right or left hemisphere brain damage". Journal of Speech and Hearing Research 33, 307 – 316.

Tweedy, J.R., R.H. Lapinski & R.W. Schvaneveldt (1977): "Semantic-context effects on word recognition: influence of varying the proportion items presented in an appropriate context". Memory and Cognition 5, 84 – 89.

Category-Specific Lexical Dissociations

Harold Goodglass, Boston

Introduction

Selective impairment or selective sparing of lexical categories is encountered repeatedly in the clinical examination of aphasic patients as well as in patients who have partially recovered from the effects of herpes encephalitis. These dissociations may affect a narrowly defined semantic category (e.g., body parts) or a broadly defined one (naturally occurring versus manmade objects). They may affect specific symbol systems (comprehension of letter-names or of number names), or psycholinguistically defined dimensions (particular parts of speech; proper vs common nouns, abstract versus concrete nouns). The dissociations observed in aphasic patients usually involve only a single modality (e.g., body part impairment only in auditory comprehension; grammatical morpheme impairment only in tasks of oral reading). Those observed in postencephalitic patients sometimes appear to span all aspects of semantic knowledge. The very disparity among these lexical dissociations suggests that they may arise from a number of different mechanisms. Other evidence indicates that certain subsets of dissociations arise from closely related mechanisms. For example, a given category (e.g., alphabet letters) may be selectively impaired in auditory comprehension testing, but selectively well preserved in naming. As a different example, impairments in the identification of animate objects are in complementary distribution with impairments in the identification of manmade ones. Such commonalities are suggestive as to where to look for underlying mechanisms. Nevertheless, most explanatory accounts to date are highly speculative. In some instances, empirical evidence relates the dissociations to anatomic regions of injury; in others, there may be selective impairment in the processing of critical semantic properties that are common to the members of a category. In this article I shall review the specific types of lexical category dissociations, imposing an organization that appears to me to be motivated by the likelihood of common underlying processes.

Aphasia-related dissociations

The lexical dissociations observed in aphasia have in common the fact that they are almost always confined to a single modality (e.g. auditory comprehension, or oral production, or oral reading, etc.) in any single patient, although a number of them appear most often as *deficits* in comprehension, but as *selectively spared categories* in oral production. Such opposite dissociations involving a particular category (e.g., alphabet letters) are occasionally, although rarely, observed in the same patient.

Letters of the alphabet

Goodglass, Klein, Carey & Jones (1966) first observed the fact that letters are most frequently the easiest category for an aphasic patient to name, but are also most frequently the hardest category for them to identify by pointing, on oral request. Goodglass, Wingfield, Hyde & Theurkauf (1986) found that these dissociations were primarily characteristic of fluent aphasics – i.e., those patients with lesions of the posterior speech zone. We have been able to demonstrate routinely that patients who fail to identify a letter in a multiple choice array, on hearing it named by the examiner, often point promptly when given a common word that begins with that letter, with a carrier phrase like "Which one is to write ..." (e.g., 'book', for the letter B). The latter phenomenon demonstrates that the failure involves the auditory appreciation of the letter name, rather than a failure to recognize it visually or even to associate the visually perceived letter to prior orthographic associations. In accounting for impaired letter name comprehension, I would suggest that the phonological information in a letter name is minimal, and its semantic information is virtually nil, so that there are few associative links to the letter form. The associative poverty of the letter name may be contrasted with the relative richness of the semantics of the spoken object name (e.g., 'book'), which has semantic and orthographic properties that are both familiar.
The frequent selective preservation of letter *naming* by aphasics, in contrast to their impaired letter name recognition is harder to explain. Further, there are also occasional patients who have a selective *loss* of letter name retrieval ('literal alexia' – Benson 1979). Literal alexia, better called 'anomia for letters', is usually found in patients with Broca's aphasia. Interestingly, these patients often misname the letter by producing a whole word that begins with the letter (e.g., saying "book" for 'B').

Numbers

In general, numbers are less often subject to selective impairment either for auditory comprehension or for naming, than is the case for letters of the alphabet. In fact, the naming of digits is regularly found to be preserved in patients who are severely impaired in the naming of objects, – particularly anomic aphasics. Auditory comprehension of number names has rarely been reported as a selectively impaired category. However, the patient of Goodglass & Budin (1988) was one who had this impairment, along with impairment in the comprehension of body parts, letters of the alphabet, and colors. For this individual, the deficit was confined to the auditory comprehension of these words; he continued to use a calculator to take care of the family finances. As with the category of body parts, he had no comprehension problem when the words were presented in writing.

Map locations – spared auditory comprehension

The success of globally aphasic patients in pointing on a map to named locations, such as cities, countries, and other geographical features was first reported by Wapner & Gardner (1979), and subsequently described by Goodglass & Butters (1989) and Goodglass & Wingfield (1993). This observation is striking because the patients involved may have little or no success in identifying common objects that are named for them. Goodglass and Wingfield found that selective sparing of geographic place names is also characteristic of many patients with Wernicke's aphasia – a disorder that impairs auditory comprehension of words. No other diagnostic categories of aphasics showed this pattern. Selectively *impaired* comprehension of map locations has never been reported, but spared naming of place names has been described by McKenna & Warrington (1980).

Body-part names – impaired auditory comprehension

The selective impairment of the auditory comprehension of body part names in aphasia has been described repeatedly (Goodglass et al. 1966; Dennis 1970; Assal & Buttet 1973; Semenza & Goodglass 1985; Goodglass & Budin 1988; Benedet & Goodglass 1989). At one time, it was common to refer to this disorder (incorrectly) as 'autotopagnosia' – defective awareness of the location of ones body parts, due to a disorder of the somatosensory representation of body image. Poeck & Orgass (1971) pointed out that most references to 'autotopagnosia' concerned only a failure to comprehend the spoken name. Assal & Buttet (1973) found that their patients could not point to named body parts but had no difficulty in locating where they wore various articles of clothing. Semenza & Goodglass (1985) showed that the impairment was not simply one of finding locations on ones body, because patients had similar problems in pointing to the locations on a drawn mannequin and in selecting cut-out drawings of body parts by multiple choice, when they were asked for by name. Even in the latter condition, errors were governed by their semantic relationship to the target word – i.e., pointing to a distractor picture that had an analogous function (eye for ear; wrist for ankle) or to one that was located on the same limb as the target. Goodglass & Budin's (1988) patient (Mr. A.) was an excellent reader and instantly responded to the written names of body parts that he could not understand orally. As in the case of Assal and Buttet's patient, Mr. A. could point fairly accurately to the location on his body of articles of clothing. His comprehension impairment extended to parts of animals, but not to parts of a bicycle. Mr. A. differed from most aphasic patients who have impaired comprehension of body parts, because his auditory comprehension of words was flawless, except for those that were within closely defined sets: – body parts, letters, of the alphabet, numbers and colors. Goodglass & Wingfield (in press) found that almost all instances of impaired body part comprehension occur in patients with reduced comprehension for object names in general – i.e., global aphasics and Wernicke's aphasics. These patients are simply more severely impaired on body parts. While this observation suggests that the temporal lobe may be implicated in this selective impairment, there is no finer localization suggested, nor is any particular structure suggested as the basis for it.

A curious clinical observation that we have found replicable in patient after patient is that the words 'hair' and 'teeth' are usually well understood by patients who cannot even show 'nose' or 'eye'. This exemption from impairment has been found as well for 'moustache' and 'fingernails'. The suggestion has been made that these parts are distinguished by the fact that they can be removed and are not part of the body proper. Some patients also appear to do better in locating internal organs (heart, brain, lungs) than surface parts.

Goodglass & Wingfield (in press) have recently found that the comprehension of body part names is selectively preserved in anomic aphasics. This diagnostic group consists predominantly of patients with lesions near the junction of the temporal and parietal lobes, in the posterior portion of the language zone. Their general level of word comprehension was at the average (52nd percentile) for aphasic patients, but their comprehension of body part names was at the 75th percentile.

Dissociations involving color

Consistent reports of difficulty in both understanding and producing color names is associated with the condition of 'alexia without agraphia'. In the great majority of these cases, there is a lesion that destroys the left visual cortex and that extends to the posterior portion (or 'splenium') of the corpus callosum. Loss of ability to read, with preservation of the ability to write, speak, and understand has been attributed to the fact that visual input is confined to the right hemisphere by reason of the splenial lesion, and thus disconnected from the language area in the left hemisphere. Geschwind & Fusillo (1966), in their report of a case of pure alexia noted that like other patients with this disorder, their patient had great difficulty in associating a color with its name, both for purposes of naming and in identifying colors that had been named for him. They pointed out that in spite of a disconnection between visual input and the language zone, the patient was not handicapped in naming seen objects, but only colors. The explanation offered was that objects seen in the right hemisphere might activate somatosensory and other associates that could communicate with the left hemisphere through other portions of the corpus callosum, but that color is a purely visual experience and is therefore particularly vulnerable to the disconnection. Damasio & Damasio (1983) noted that color difficulties are present only in a subset of patients with pure alexia. They described a set of anatomic markers that appeared to predict whether difficulties in color language would accompany pure alexia or not.

Aside from instances of pure alexia, color name dissociations appear sporadically in aphasia, but most often in the form of selective sparing of the ability to name colors (Goodglass, Wingfield, Hyde & Theurkauf 1986). Such sparing is seen more often in fluent than in nonfluent aphasics.

Part-of-speech based dissociations

A number of syndromes of aphasia are expressed, in part, through performance dissociations, based on a part-of-speech hierarchy. In all but one of these syndromes the hierarchy is one in which nouns are handled most competently, while verbs, adverbs, and adjectives are processed at an intermediate level, with many more errors than occur with nouns. Grammatical functors – both free and bound, are severely impaired in these disorders.

Part-of-speech effects in agrammatism

Agrammatism is a disorder affecting sentence production, in which there is a marked reduction in the variety and complexity of syntactic forms, many omissions of grammatical morphemes, as well as incomplete and grammatically defective sentences. Impaired access to grammatical morphemes in free discourse is the salient symptom. A second feature, remarked on by almost all observers, is that the speech of most agrammatics is heavily loaded with substantives and lacking in main verbs. One-word utterances, chiefly nouns, are prominent in their output, and subject-object constructions, the verb being omitted, are used repeatedly by many of these patients. In addition to the relative dearth of verbs in free discourse, Miceli, Silveri, Villa & Caramazza (1984) showed that agrammatics are significantly inferior in their ability to name pictured *actions* than to name pictured objects. In most agrammatics the impairment in the use of grammatical morphemes extends to the spontaneous writing of sentences. The selective impairment in access to grammatical morphemes, is intimately related to their syntactic role within the sentence and intimately related to the underlying deficit in cases of agrammatism. For example, auxiliary verbs are more subject to omission in sentences than are articles; the possessive marking morpheme ['s] is more subject to omission than the plural marker [s]. One way of conceptualizing the defect in agrammatism is that the patient has lost access to the automatic activation of the syntactic framework that corresponds to the intent of his message. Garrett (1980) refers to this framework as the 'positional frame', which includes the activation of the grammatical morphemes in their appropriate positions. Thus, the activation of the grammatical morphemes for normal speech is linked with their position in the framework. In this way, they are unlike the lexical terms, which are retrieved as a result of the activation of their semantics. Lacking the *automatic* activation of grammatical morphemes, agrammatic patients cannot retrieve them as they retrieve lexical terms, – i.e., through the mediation of their semantics; grammatical morphemes have little or no semantic content. In this sense, the impairment in the use of grammatical morphemes is a type of word retrieval difficulty that is specific to certain parts of speech. As we shall see, the semantic emptiness of grammatical morphemes keeps recurring as an explanation for failures on these words in syndromes other than agrammatism, failures that may involve reading comprehension, oral reading, repetition, or writing to dictation. Impaired access to verbs dissociates from other agrammatic symptoms, because it is not present in all agrammatic patients. Further, Berndt (1991) has found that failed access to verbs in free discourse may appear in grammatically fluent patients. Thus it appears that, while impaired access to verbs is characteristic of many agrammatic patients, and while this impairment contributes to the deficiency of their sentence structures, it is probably not *caused by* the agrammatism.

Selective difficulty in accessing verbs in oral production may appear in dramatically extreme form. For example, Caramazza & Hillis (1991) describe a patient (HW) who could not retrieve verbs to say them aloud, although she could write them. They contrasted her with another patient (SJD) who could say verbs, but was unable to write them. On testing with words that were homonymous as nouns and verbs (e.g., 'crack') these patients could supply the words in a context that called for their use as nouns, but not in their role as verbs.

How are we to account for the greater vulnerability of verbs than nouns in these cases of retrieval difficulty? The fact that the isolated right cerebral hemisphere can demonstrate good comprehension of object names, but not of action words (Gazzaniga, Bogen & Sperry 1965) suggests that the processing of nouns, but not of verbs is within the capability of a primitive language system. However, the generalization that verbs are intrinsically more difficult than nouns is invalidated by the observation than anomic aphasics show the reverse pattern: they name actions much more successfully than they name objects (Goodglass, Klein, Carey & Jones 1966). I would suggest that the distinction is a more subtle one, that is not quite captured by the notion that nouns and verbs are 'different parts of speech'. Rather, that verbs represent the operation of *predicating* while nouns represent the operation of *naming*. I suggest that it is these two different functional approaches to the use of words that are dissociated by aphasia. Even when it appears to the examiner that his test is designed to elicit the verb as the *name of an action*, the fact that verbs have originally been acquired in a predicative context may intrude in and derail the patient's efforts to activate the verb form. Except for the case of word retrieval in anomic aphasia, we shall see that the nominal function has the advantage over the predicative one in almost all the part-of-speech dissociations in aphasia.

Part-of-speech effects in deep dyslexia

Deep dyslexia is a disorder in which activation of the phonology of written words is non-functional, but a form of oral reading is made possible through an imperfect activation of written word semantics, such that many words are misread by the substitution of words that are semantically related to the written target. (For a detailed review, see Coltheart, Marshall & Patterson 1980.) The words that are most likely to be verbalized accurately are concrete nouns. Semantically related errors are more likely to be produced with abstract nouns (e.g., 'product' → "factory") and still more likely with verbs (e.g. 'shining' → "sun"), while grammatical functors are almost never correct, but are either omitted or substituted with another unrelated functor (e.g., 'the' → "is"). An inspection of lists of errors (Coltheart et al. 1980) reveals that verbs are likely to be nominalized, as in the above example, but very few verb-for-noun substitutions are found. The imperfectly functioning link between semantics and word phonology thus obeys the familiar hierarchy of noun > verb > grammatical morpheme. In the case of deep dyslexia, there is an additional facilitating effect of noun concreteness, which is not always a factor in other instances of the part-of-speech-governed hierarchy.

Part-of-speech effects in deep dysphasia

Deep dysphasia is a fairly rare disorder that affects repetition, in a small subset of patients with temporal lobe lesions who have a fluent aphasia, and impaired auditory comprehension. It was first described by Michel & Andreewsky (1983), who named it by analogy with deep dyslexia. The distinctive feature of this condition is that patients produce semantically related errors, when asked to repeat words. E.g. Katz & Goodglass' (1990) patient was identified as having deep dysphasia when he replied "rug" on being asked to repeat 'carpet'. Deep dysphasics are more successful in repeating concrete than abstract nouns, they make many errors with verbs, and fail almost totally with grammatical function words. They are unable to repeat nonsense words at all. Katz and Goodglass' patient reported that the sound of the word he was given to repeat escaped him immediately; his repetition was guided by what he retained of the semantics of the target word.

Part-of-speech dissociations in writing

Dissociations in writing, that involve differential performance according to part of speech have been described less commonly than those affecting reading. However, well-described cases have been reported by Bub & Kertesz (1982) and by Baxter & Warrington (1987). Both of these patients made semantic substitutions when writing dictated words, making more errors on verbs than nouns and performing worst of all on grammatical functors. Nominalization of verbs was particularly notable in the errors made by Baxter and Warrington's patient. The present author has described (Goodglass 1993) a patient who had no speech and limited word-writing ability that was almost totally restricted to nouns. When asked to write 'sleep', he wrote 'bed', 'pillow', and 'cover'; for 'eat' he wrote 'breakfast'. He was quite unable to write any grammatical functor. Mild indications of dissociation of the same type can commonly be detected in the examination of patients with very limited ability to write from dictation. Such patients will show a distinct advantage for dictated nouns over verbs and a disadvantage in the writing of grammatical functors from dictation.

Dissociations affecting proper nouns

Proper nouns have been observed to be selectively facilitated for some patients but selectively impaired in others. McCarthy & Warrington (1985) described an aphasic patient who had remarkably well preserved naming of famous people and places. McKenna & Warrington (1978) reported on a patient who had relatively preserved ability to name countries and body parts in the presence of almost total anomia for objects, animals, and colors. Warrington & McCarthy's (1987) patient, who was severely aphasic, had selectively preserved ability to match spoken and written names of famous people and particular places, but was poor in identifying names that did not refer to a unique referent.

Selective impairment of proper nouns, following a pattern diametrically opposed to that of Warrington & McCarthy's (1987) patient, was described in a remarkable case by Semenza & Zettin (1989). This patient, following a head injury, was left with a minimal word finding difficulty, except that in the case of proper nouns of any kind his performance was almost a complete failure. This was true for famous people, cities, countries, and musical selections. He could recall particular peoples' names neither from pictures nor from descriptions For example, he could not provide the names of two actors, nor of two politicians, although he could give rich background information about them, when shown a picture, or when he was provided with a name by the examiner. He had no difficulty in providing lists of peoples' names, provided that he did not have to associate them with anyones identity. In exploring the psychological basis for this disorder, Semenza and Zettin found that the patient was unable to form any arbitrary association to a word, although he was easily able to learn word pairs that had some semantic link between them. The authors suggest that their patient's deficit can be designated as an inability to retrieve purely referential, nondescriptive terms.

Dissociations of broad and fine-grained semantic categories

While most of the instances of the foregoing category dissociations have been seen as manifestations of aphasia, another class of dissociations are observed primarily in patients suffering from the aftermath of herpes encephalitis. I have referred to them as entailing 'broad' semantic categories, because the best characterization of the selective criteria have been in such terms as 'manmade' versus 'naturally occurring' or 'animate' versus 'inanimate'. Some of the cases of this type have involved different subcategories within the 'naturally occurring' class.

The first category-specific dissociations to be reported came not from the domain of language but from that of visual perception. Nielsen (1946) described a patient who had greater difficulty in identifying inanimate objects by sight than living things. Another patient had precisely the opposite pattern of difficulty. Hécaen & Ajuriaguerra (1956) also published a report on a visual agnosia for inanimate objects.

The first report of a category-specific word comprehension failure of a broad semantic type was that of Yamadori & Albert (1973), and involved an aphasic patient. This patient was particularly baffled when asked to point to objects in the room, including furniture and structural features, such as the wall of the room. He did not show similar word comprehension problems for outside objects nor for small manipulable objects. Warrington (1975) recognized the relationship between category specific visual recognition problems and those involving language. Her subjects were three patients who had developed progressive memory loss and intellectual decline, along with a visual object agnosia, without agnosia for written words, colors, or faces. Their object agnosia was not markedly different for natural objects, as opposed to manmade ones. These subjects could demonstrate partial appreciation of the semantics of the objects in response to probe questions. They performed relatively well when offered a superordinate label, such as 'is it a bird?' but they performed very poorly when the questions related to attributes or associates of the target, such as 'is it bigger than a cat?' in relation to animals or 'is it found indoors?' in relation to objects. Although these patients were not aphasic, they had the same type of deficit when asked these probe questions about objects that were presented orally, as they had been asked about the corresponding pictures. That is, superordinate questions were more often answered correctly than were questions about attributes.

Warrington & McCarthy (1983) and Warrington & Shallice (1984) reported a series of patients who showed dissociations affecting object name comprehension. These dissociations had features that had previously been reported only for visual recognition: i.e. opposite effects for inanimate objects, as compared to certain classes of naturally occurring objects, including foods. Warrington & McCarthy's (1983) patient was aphasic and had little success in identifying common inanimate objects when they were named for her, but performed exceptionally well with natural objects such as flowers. Warrington & Shallice's (1984) patients, were post-encephalitic. They showed the reverse pattern of dissociations from that of Warrington & McCarthy's patient, in that inanimate objects were well identified, while animate objects and foods were relatively deficient. Again, dissociations in visual recognition paralleled those in verbal identification. But even more striking than the parallel between visual and verbal identification was the performance of two of these patients in giving definitions for object names, as compared to animal names. Characteristic of the excellent definitions of small objects is patient JBR's description of a 'torch' as a "small hand-held light", while his description of a 'snail' was "an insect animal".

Warrington & McCarthy (1987) in their evaluations of these dissociations, prefer to recast the 'manmade' vs 'naturally occurring' dichotomy into the polarity of referents that are known and conceptualized primarily through their physical features versus those known primarily through their function. The 'physical' dimension is relevant for most of the objects that would be considered naturally occurring, such as animals, flowers, and foods. These are the objects for which visual form, color, and texture characteristics are primary. The 'functional' dimension obviously applies to implements. In their study of aphasic patient YOT, Warrington & McCarthy observe groupings of objects that do not fall clearly into one category or another. For example, 'large manmade objects', for this patient, tended to be well preserved, much like animals and foods, but unlike manipulable objects.

Abstract versus concrete nouns

Warrington and her collaborators have demonstrated in a number of patients a paradoxical superiority in their appreciation of abstract, as compared to concrete nouns, both by matching words to pictorial representations (Warrington 1981) and by having patients give verbal definitions to abstract and concrete words (Warrington & Shallice 1984). Their patient SBY was particularly impressive in giving definitions to abstract words, such as, for 'malice': "to show bad will against somebody", while his definition of 'tobacco' was: "One of your foods you eat." One may speculate that the preservation of abstract words may be accounted for by the fact that their meaning is acquired entirely within the verbal system, requiring no link to either sensory experience nor experience with the manipulability of the referent.

Modality-specific, fine-grained semantic dissociations

In recent years, there have been case reports describing dissociations affecting one or the other of two specific superordinate classes: animals and fruits and vegetables. In each case, the deficit involved naming. Hart, Berndt & Caramazza (1985) reported on a patient who had recovered from aphasia only to have the continued complaint that he could not retrieve the names of most fruits and vegetables, either on visual confrontation or in response to descriptions. Nevertheless, he could identify them perfectly from multiple choice when given the object name as a stimulus. Arguin, Bub & Dudek (1993) describe a patient who had selective difficulty in the visual recognition of fruits and vegetables as well as in verbally reporting anything about the appearance of such items. On the basis of experimental analysis of his visual perceptual functions, they attribute the problem with fruits and vegetables to the fact that their patient had great difficulty in discriminating among rounded shapes that differed in more than one dimension. The patient's ability to associate vegetable names to their pictures could be predicted from the type of shape discrimination that was required. A more recent case, reported by Hart & Gordon (1992) was associated with an inability to name animals through visual presentation (optic aphasia for animals). In addition to her category-specific and modality-specific naming disorder, this patient was unable to answer any question that referred to the physical attributes of animals, although she was perfectly conversant with their non-visual characteristics, such as their habitat, behavior, and their suitability as pets.

Perhaps the most unusual of the category-specific and modality-specific naming disorders is one that prevents access to the labels for visually perceived facial emotions and, concurrently impairs the ability to select a facial expression from multiple choice, in response to the name of the emotion. This phenomenon, reported in two different cases by Rapcsak, Comer & Rubens (1993) and by Rapcsak, Kasniak & Rubens (1989) is also unique in having a well defined anatomical site that provides strong reinforcement of recent evidence concerning the representation of emotional expression in the right temporal lobe. Rapcsak's et al. (1993) patient, although he could not name or identify facial affect from hearing its name, was shown to be intact in his ability to perform visual-visual matches between pictured emotional situations and pictured facial emotions. He was also intact in his ability to supply the names of appropriate emotions in response to verbally described situations. The authors propose that the temporal lobe contains cell groups that respond selectively to the emotional content of visually perceived facial expressions, but do so at a pre-verbal level. The activity of these units makes it possible for the patient to make appropriate matches within the visual domain, where no naming is required. These visual, affect-sensitive units are thought to be disconnected from access to the verbal system. The semantics of emotional expression within the verbal domain are also intact, and appear to function independently of the visual domain.

Summary

In this survey, we have taken the concept of lexical dissociation in its broadest sense. We have examined the variety of conditions in which some categorical feature of particular kinds of words appears to determine whether certain patients will have a selective impairment in processing them or else a selective preservation for words of that category. I have deliberately chosen the nonspecific term 'processing' because some dissociations involve access for oral production; others involve auditory comprehension, still others are expressed only in oral reading, or in writing, or in repetition. We have seen that the dissociations most common in aphasic patients are often defined by the linguistic character of the affected words and are also most likely to be confined to a single modality. Consequently some dissociative patterns are related to diagnostic type: anomic aphasics access verbs more easily than nouns; agrammatic aphasics show the reverse pattern. Aphasic patients also have selective dissociations affecting limited, closely defined sets, such as letter, color, and number names, body parts, and map locations. These category-based dissociations do not have well defined lesion sites, but they affect a significant proportion of aphasic patients.

The latter portion of this summary was devoted to dissociations that are quite rare, but have recurred sufficiently so that they tell us something about the semantic structure of word meanings and its relation to the brain representation of object semantics. The rarety of these phenomena, however, justifies the caveat that the brain-language organizations that make some individuals susceptible to these dissociations may represent atypical patterns. The lesions that give rise to such rare dissociations as anomia for proper nouns, impaired responsiveness to the names of manmade objects, etc., are not necessarily rare lesions nor are they generally uniquely predictive of a particular dissociation. What these lesions do share is that they involve diffuse damage to the inferior temporal lobe, associated with herpes encephalitis. The case of anomia for emotional facial expressions (Rapcsak et al. 1993) is exceptional both in terms of lesion specificity and independent neurobehavioral evidence for the localization of the affected function. We have seen that, according to the analysis of Warrington and her associates, most of the broadly based semantic dissociations affect either objects that are known chiefly through their visual features or else objects that are known chiefly through manipulatory experience. This observation leads to the general inference that certain selected clusters of experiential features are particularly important in terms of the brain representation of object semantics. It would be misleading to suppose that dissociations along any type of semantic criterion are possible. In fact, the bases for such dissociations are extremely limited. In the case of fine-grained semantic dissociations the categories observed to date are limited to animals and fruits and vegetables – visual form characteristics being critical in these cases.

The dissociations affecting proper names appear to entail mechanisms that have little to do with the sensory channel involved, since the patients described fail both in response to pictures and in response to verbally defined characteristics of the referent. At this point we can do little better than accept Semenza and Zettin's characterization of the disorder as one that affects 'pure referring expressions'.

References

Arguin, M., D. Bub, D. & G. Dudek (1993): A shape feature integration impairment as an account of agnosia for biological kinds. Paper presented at the Academy of Aphasia, Tucson.

Assal, G. & J. Buttet (1973): "Troubles du schéma corporel lors des atteintes hémisphériques gauches". Praxis 62, 172 – 179.

Baxter, D.M. & E.K. Warrington (1987): "Category-specific phonological dysgraphia". Neuropsychologia 23, 653 – 666.

Benedet, M.J. & H. Goodglass (1989): "Body image and comprehension of body part names". Journal of Psycholinguistic Research 18, 485 – 496.

Benson, D.F. (1979): Aphasia, Alexia, and Agraphia. New York: Churchill Livingstone.

Berndt, R.S. (1991): "Sentence processing in aphasia". In: M.T. Sarno, ed., Acquired Aphasia. San Diego: Academic Press, 223 – 270.

Bub, D. & A. Kertesz (1982): "Deep agraphia". Brain and Language 17, 146 – 165.

Caramazza, A. & A. Hillis (1991): "Lexical organization of nouns and verbs in the brain". Nature 349, 788 – 790.

Coltheart M., K. Patterson & J.C. Marshall, eds. (1980): Deep Dyslexia, London: Routledge and Kegan Paul.

Damasio, A.R. & H. Damasio (1983): "The anatomic basis of pure alexia". Neurology 33, 1573 – 1583.

Dennis, M. (1976): "Dissociated naming and locating of body parts after left anterior temporal lobe resection. An experimental case study". Brain and Language 3, 472 – 482.

Garrett, M. (1980): "Levels of processing in sentence production". In: B. Butterworth, ed., Language Production, Volume 1, Speech and Talk. London: Academic Press, 177 – 220.

Gazzaniga, M., J.E. Bogen & R.W. Sperry (1965): "Observations on visual perception after disconnection of the cerebral hemispheres in man". Brain 88, 221 – 236.

Geschwind, N. & M. Fusillo (1966): "Color naming deficits in association with alexia". Archives of Neurology 15, 137 – 146.

Goodglass, H. (1993): Understanding Aphasia. San Diego: Academic Press.

Goodglass, H. & C. Budin (1988): "Category and modality-specific dissociations in word comprehension and concurrent phonological dyslexia: A case study". Neuropsychologia 26, 67 – 88.

Goodglass, H. & N. Butters (1989): "Psychobiology of cognitive processes". In: R.C. Atkinson, R.J. Herrnstein, G. Lindzey & E.D. Luce, eds., Stevens Handbook of Experimental Psychology, Second Edition. New York: Wiley Interscience.

Goodglass, H., B. Klein, P. Carey & K.J. Jones (1966): "Specific semantic word categories in aphasia". Cortex 2, 74 - 89.
Goodglass, H. & A. Wingfield (1993): Selective preservation of a lexical category in aphasia: Dissociations in comprehension of body parts and geographical place names. Memory 1, 313 - 328.
Goodglass, H., A. Wingfield, M.R. Hyde & J. Theurkauf (1986): "Category-specific dissociations in naming and recognition by aphasic patients". Cortex 22, 87 - 107.
Hart, J., R.S. Berndt & A. Caramazza (1985): "Category-specific naming defect following cerebral infarction". Nature 316, 439 - 440.
Hart, J. & B. Gordon (1992): "Neural subsystems for object knowledge". Nature 359, 60 - 64.
Hécaen, H. & J. Ajuriagurerra (1956): "Agnosie visuelle pour les objets inanimés par lésion unilatérale gauche". Revue Neurologique 94, 222 - 233.
Katz, R.B. & H. Goodglass (1990): "Deep dysphasia: Analysis of a rare form of repetition disorder". Brain and Language 39, 153 - 185.
McCarthy, R. & E.K. Warrington (1985): "Category specificity in an agrammatic patient: The relative impairment of verb retrieval and comprehension". Neuropsychologia 23, 709 - 727.
McKenna, P. & E.K. Warrington (1980): "Testing for nominal dysphasia". Journal of Neurology, Neurosurgery, and Psychiatry 43, 781 - 788.
Miceli, G., M.C. Silveri, G. Villa & A. Caramazza (1984): "On the basis of agrammatics' difficulty in producing main verbs". Cortex 20, 207 - 220.
Michel, F. & E. Andreewsky (1983): "Deep dysphasia: An analog of deep dyslexia in the auditory modality". Brain and Language 18, 212 - 223.
Nielsen, J.M. (1946): Agnosia, Apraxia, and Aphasia. New York: Hoeber.
Poeck, K. & B. Orgass (1971): "The concept of body schema: A critical review and some experimental results". Cortex 5, 254 - 277.
Rapcsak, S.Z., A.W. Kazniak & A.B. Rubens (1989): "Anomia for facial expressions: evidence for a visual-verbal disconnection syndrome". Neuropsychologia 27, 1031 - 1041.
Rapcsak, S.Z., J.F. Comer & A.B. Rubens (1993): "Anomia for facial expressions: Neuropsychological mechanisms and some anatomical correlates". Brain and Language 45, 233 - 252.
Semenza, C. & H. Goodglass (1985): "Identification of body parts in brain injured subjects". Neuropsychologia 23, 161 - 176.
Semenza, C. & M. Zettin (1989): "Evidence from aphasia for the role of proper names as pure referring expressions". Nature 342, 678 - 679.
Wapner, W. & H. Gardner (1979): "A note on patterns of comprehension and recovery in global aphasia". Journal of Speech and Hearing Research 29, 765 - 771.
Warrington, E.K. (1975): "The selective impairment of semantic memory". Quarterly Journal of Experimental Psychology 27, 635 - 657.
Warrington, E.K. (1981): "Concrete word dyslexia". British Journal of Psychology 72, 175 - 196.
Warrington, E.K. & R. McCarthy (1983): "Category-specific access dysphasia". Brain 106, 859 - 878.
Warrington, E.K. & R. McCarthy (1987): "Categories of knowledge: Further fractionation and an attempt at integration". Brain 110, 1273 - 1296.
Warrington, E.K. & T. Shallice (1984): "Category-specific semantic impairments". Brain 107, 829 - 853.
Yamadori, A. & M.L. Albert (1973): "Word category aphasia". Cortex 9, 112 - 125.

Selective Impairments of Action Naming: Arguments and a Case Study*

Helgard Kremin, Paris

1 Introduction

Clinical observation very early suggested that the "nature" of the words themselves had an influence on the ease with which aphasics can produce their verbal labels. Lotmar, in 1919, studying the response latencies and error pattern of a patient with word-finding difficulties, stated that the naming of abstract words was more error-prone than the naming of concrete words. Later Goldstein (1948) suggested that sensory factors influence naming performance per se and consequently claimed that aphasics always have more difficulties with abstract than with concrete nouns. In its initial form this claim does not hold since the reverse dissociation with abstract words being better preserved than concrete words has since then been documented (Warrington 1975 – case AB, 1981; Warrington & Shallice 1984 – case SBY). The latter studies indicate that abstract words are not necessarily "more difficult" than concrete ones. Concreteness vs. abstractness may thus be one of the organizing principles of semantic structure. However, because of the discovery of so many more dissociations within the semantic system, clinical observation today favors the view of category-specific sub-domains within the semantic/lexical system (see Goodglass, this volume).
Neurolinguistic research has focused on yet another aspect of category-specific naming impairments: the influence of grammatical class on picture naming (objects/nouns vs. actions/verbs). These studies are not so much concerned with the organization of semantic memory, but rather with the different "realizations" of a concept as "noun" or "verb". Today the investigation of possible dissociations with regard to the naming of object vs. action pictures is at the core of this line of research. Its aim is to establish that some component of the lexical system is organized by grammatical classes. This latter issue forms the focus of the following review and presentation.

* I would like to thank Douglas Burrington for editorial advice.

2 The naming of nouns and verbs

2.1 Some general remarks on nouns and verbs

The importance of the influence of grammatical class on the performance of aphasic subjects has initially been observed in agrammatism. Agrammatism is a complex disorder characterized by the omission of grammatical markers, by reduced phrase length and difficulties in producing verbs, which can be either omitted or nominalized. Later, studies concerning a newly-described syndrome of specific reading impairment called "deep dyslexia" (Marshall & Newcombe 1973) confirmed that nouns could be better preserved than verbs. With more cases being published (see Colheart, Patterson & Marshall 1980), it became evident indeed that the production of semantic paraphasias was not the only variable of the syndrome. Other variables, especially the part-of speech effect with nouns being preserved better than verbs which in turn are preserved better than function words – first described in GR (Marshall & Newcombe 1966, 1973), were associated with the reading impairment and subsequently confirmed for other cases.

Thus, one could ask whether differences between nouns and verbs go beyond their syntactic privileges. The answer is yes. Gentner (1981) enumerates some such differences: verbs are harder to remember, more broadly defined, more prone to be altered in meaning when conflict of meaning occurs, and less stable in translation between languages than nouns. Finally, production and comprehension of verbs are also slower to be acquired by children. According to Gentner (1981) not only is the mean number of word meanings greater for verbs than for nouns, at all frequency levels, but also "the frequency distribution is different from that of nouns. Nouns increase in number as frequency decreases – in classic open-class fashion, having large numbers of members at the low frequency end. Prepositions and function words show a pattern opposite to that of nouns. They are well represented at the highest frequency and their numbers drop to zero for all lower frequencies; this is the classic closed-class pattern. Verbs show an intermediate pattern. They are well represented in the highest category, and in the second-highest category; but after that their number decreases", in contrast to nouns (p. 165). This observation, among others, leads Gentner to question whether verbs are open-class items in the same way as nouns are.

However, the interesting differences cited between nouns and verbs cannot readily explain the performance differences with both word types in deep dyslexia (when the two word lists are controlled for item frequency). Nor can they explain the differential performance of object picture versus action picture naming observed in brain-damaged patients (see below).

2.2 Naming nouns and verbs: data on normal controls

In order to define pathological behavior it is necessary to establish norms of normal performance. A few studies can be mentioned which furnish some normative data concerning the naming of nouns and verbs by normal subjects.

2.2.1 Picture naming by adults

Miceli, Silveri, Villa & Caramazza (1984) compared the performances of ten adult controls on the Boston Naming Test (Kaplan & Goodglass 1976) and the Action-Naming Test (Obler & Albert 1979). They found that adults perform equally well on both tests. In 1988, Miceli, Silveri, Nocentini & Caramazza confirmed these results with another naming test controlling for frequency: normal (Italian speaking) subjects produced on the average 98.2 % correct responses to the Object-naming-test and 96.1 % correct responses to the Action-naming test. Zingeser & Berndt (1990) also stated that object and action pictures (controlled for frequency) are equally well named by (English speaking) normal subjects.
It thus seems reasonable to conclude that adults name nouns and verbs equally well when targets are presented as pictorial stimuli. (Note, however, that such findings may be due to a ceiling effect.).[1]

2.2.2 Picture naming during language acquisition

In spite of general agreement that the status of verbs is different from that of nouns and that they may be more "difficult" than nouns during language acquisition, to our knowledge, no normative data with respect to the naming of object vs. action pictures during language development are available in the published literature. We therefore briefly mention the first purely quantitative results of a study recently undertaken with French preschool children. In the frame of a project on language development we also studied the oral naming of 14 object and 14 action pictures by 1109 children aged 3 to 6 (Kremin & Dellatolas 1993, in press). The picture material (simple black and white drawings) was selected with respect to high name agreement in earlier studies with adults. The global results show highly significant effects of 'age' on the naming of object pictures and of action pictures whereas 'sex' and 'handedness' did not have any effect on naming performance. Task comparisons show that object naming is significantly better than action naming.[2] The difference is greater in younger than in older children but this difference is not age-dependent.
In reality, however, 64 % of the children named objects better than actions and 14 % of the children named actions better than objects. More detailed analyses of a subgroup of 301 children by Chéreau & Faure (1993) showed that in the youngest age group the difference between the naming scores is 1 to 9 items (out of 14) for objects > actions and 1 to 8 items (out of 14) for actions > objects. Such dissociations are at variance with Gentner's (1981) assumption that verbs are *per se* more difficult to treat than

nouns. Our results rather seem to suggest that some children have *normal but different cognitive performance strategies* in naming object and action pictures.[3]

2.3 Nouns and verbs: data from studies of aphasic subjects

2.3.1 Oral naming of action vs. object pictures

Miceli, Silveri, Villa & Caramazza (1984) studied the performance on action vs. object picture naming by two groups of patients clinically defined as agrammatic and anomic. As a group, agrammatic speakers (n = 5) performed better on nouns (mean: 64.6 % correct) than on verbs (mean: 57 % correct). By contrast, the group of anomic aphasics (n = 5) named correctly more verbs (mean: 72.3) than nouns (mean: 42.5 %). It should be stressed, however that the relative difference in performance is rather small and not homogeneous in agrammatic patients: one patient performs 21.4 % better on nouns whereas three other patients only show from 5.6 % to 8.3 % better performance on nouns. Finally, one patient shows the reverse tendency with slightly better action naming (plus 5.6 %). In contrast, the anomic patients show a homogeneous pattern of better object vs. action naming (ranging from plus 5.7 % to 48.6 %).
On the basis of the foregoing citations we do not quite agree with the authors' conclusion that their results "are unequivocal in one respect: agrammatic patients as a group present with a *marked* deficit in naming actions relative to their ability to name objects" (p. 216). Nor do we agree that "this result strongly suggests that agrammatic patients are *selectively* impaired in lexical processing and specifically in processing a particular subcategory of the lexicon-verbs" (p. 216).
Although two detailed case studies – one of an agrammatic patient (McCarthy & Warrington 1985) and one of an anomic patient (Zingeser & Berndt 1989) – are in line with Miceli et al.'s hypotheses, the data from other studies of aphasic patients are at variance with the authors' strong assertions with respect to the relationship between *selective* impairments in object vs. action picture naming and *precise* types of aphasic impairment.
Zingeser & Berndt (1990) studied object and action picture naming in a small group of aphasic subjects (5 agrammatics and 5 anomics). Their results confirm that agrammatic patients, as a group and individually, name nouns better than verbs (means of 25.6/30 and 17.2/30 respectively). In contrast, the anomic group performed equally well with both kinds of picture material (mean 24/30 correct). However, at the individual level of performance one anomic subject (HY) performed better on nouns, another anomic patient (JSt) better on verbs (17 vs. 21 and 22 vs. 16 respectively). In spite of these heterogeneous findings with regard to the individual patient's naming performance, the authors' discussion largely assumes – like Miceli and co-workers (1984) – a *double* dissociation to exist with regard to the production of nouns and verbs in relation to precise types of aphasic impairments, agrammatism and anomia. As already mentioned this general conclusion is not substantiated by the observed data.[4]
Basso, Razzano, Faglioni & Zanobio (1990) finally examined the influence of two situational contexts on naming performances of non-fluent (n = 30) and fluent (n = 29)

aphasic patients, and compared object naming and action naming in the same groups. Here we refer only to the results for object picture vs. action picture naming. In both tasks, non-fluent patients seem to be more impaired (object naming: 61 % correct; action naming: 61 % correct) than fluent patients (75 % and 69 %), but the difference is significant only for noun naming. When the authors compared two selected subgroups (seven agrammatic and six anomic patients), they found a small, statistically non-significant difference in the direction expected from Miceli et al.'s (1984) aforementioned study: agrammatic patients were just better at object naming, and anomic patients at action naming. In fact, all seven clinically agrammatic patients showed preservation of nouns over actions, and three of the six anomic patients performed better at action-naming. However, two anomic patients showed the reverse pattern and, in one case, results were the same. These findings led Basso and co-workers to the conclusion that "single anomic patients may have equal difficulty in finding nouns and verbs" (p. 193). On the basis of the foregoing results and arguments, we think indeed that the data cited on group studies of aphasic patients do not justify the assertion of a direct relationship between precise types of aphasic syndrome and selective impairments in word production However, experimental evidence of *selective* impairments come from other studies that will be discussed in the next section.

2.3.2 Patterns of dissociation in the comprehension and production of nouns and verbs

McCarthy & Warrington (1985), studying the patient ROX, have shown that the ability to treat verbs may be dissociated from the ability to treat nouns. Indeed, the patient's inability to produce verbs (and to understand their meaning) contrasts with relatively good performance on nouns in various experimental tasks. These results were interpreted as support for the view that the mental lexicon is organized by form classes (nouns, verbs, etc.) and that these subcomponents of the mental lexicon may be selectively damaged. From this study it is not clear, however, whether such information is represented exclusively at a central level – and thus used for both comprehension and production – or whether form class information is also connected with the various input and output lexicons which, according to the information-processing approach, constitute functional components in the processes of recognition and production of words (see, for example, Morton 1980a, b). In such a view differential patterns of dissociations in the ability to process words of different form class should be observable in comprehension and in production.

In the latter perspective Miceli, Silveri, Nocentini & Caramazza (1988) undertook an experimental study concerning the comprehension and production of nouns and verbs in several aphasic patients. An object and an action picture naming test as well as comprehension tests of both word classes (by multiple choice of three pictures) were presented auditorily to twenty-five patients who displayed a wide range of language disturbances. Only seven of the original twenty-five patients showed category specific dissociations. Four of these patients (FDP, CS, FS, AM) presented with agrammatic speech, whereas the occurrence of anomia was the main characteristic for the three remaining patients (AA, SF, AE). The results show that four (agrammatic) patients named objects better than verbs (means: 84.9 % and 53.3 % respectively). The opposite pattern of results was obtained for three (anomic) patients who named 70.0 % of the actions correctly but only 47.9 % of the objects. The authors further observed that, for the seven patients under consideration, comprehension and naming abilities were not correlated. In spite of their relatively selective naming deficits three patients – two agrammatics, FS and AM, and one anomic, SF, – had normal comprehension of both nouns and verbs. Two patients (FDP and CS, both agrammatic) displayed normal comprehension of nouns but were impaired in the comprehension of verbs (as they were in the production of action names). One patient (AE, an anomic subject) was equally severely impaired in the comprehension of verbs and nouns (although nouns were better named than verbs), whereas another (anomic) patient (AA) showed normal comprehension of verbs but his comprehension of nouns was significantly impaired. Miceli et al.'s results thus demonstrate that the ability to comprehend nouns and verbs may be selectively damaged and, more importantly, that these dissociations can be independent of the nature of damage observed in word production. The authors state: "the presence of a specific form of impairment in naming did not predict whether or not a similar impairment was found in comprehension of nouns or verbs" (p. 357). Thus naming and comprehension disorders for nouns and verbs are, in principle, dissociable – the only constraint being that "if there is a dissociation in word comprehension for nouns and verbs then a similar dissociation obtains in word production" (p. 357).

Recently Caramazza & Hillis (1991) reported a double dissociation in the performance of tasks involving the oral and written production of verbs and nouns. Neither of the two patients they studied had any difficulty in the comprehension of verbs. However, one patient showed a selective deficit of verb name retrieval only in written production tasks (naming and dictation) whereas the other patient showed a selective deficit of verb name retrieval only in oral production tasks (naming and reading). In these two patients, the selective impairment affecting the class of verbs is therefore to be located at the level of the output lexicons (phonological in one case, orthographic in the other case) and/or access to them. These findings confirm the psychological reality of separate output lexicons for oral and written word production originally suggested by Morton (1980a).

2.3.3 There is no causal relationship between selective impairments on object vs. action picture naming and precise type(s) of aphasia

In spite of Miceli et al.'s (1984) initial hypotheses and notwithstanding the detailed case descriptions by McCarthy & Warrington (1985) and by Zingeser & Berndt (1988) – which seem to confirm them – we will argue that the relation between naming performance and precise type of aphasia is fortuitous and in no way causal in nature. Indeed, a recent study (see Kremin & De Agostini 1993) confirms Basso et al.'s (1990) finding that single anomic patients may have equal difficulty in finding nouns and verbs for picture naming. Moreover, and in contrast to HY (Zingeser & Berndt 1988), VED,

an Italian subject with pure amnestic aphasia, named object pictures as well as verbal definitions (84 % and 80 % respectively). Finally and in contrast to HY, VED's naming of object pictures did not differ from her naming of the same words in sentence completion (70 % in both cases). It thus follows that the dissociations observed in HY's performances (including the facilitation of the production of substantives by the task of sentence completion as compared to picture naming and/or verbal definitions) are not "typical" performance patterns of patients with the syndrome of amnestic aphasia. Rather they originate from HY's individual brain damage.
The following case study will further substantiate our view that there is no causal relationship between selective impairments on object vs. action picture naming and precise type(s) of aphasia.

3 Case GI: Selective deficit of verb retrieval in a fluent patient with sensory aphasia

3.1 Clinical case description

At the time of testing, GI, a right-handed (highly educated) 64 year old patient suffered from typical Wernicke's aphasia (after regression of initial jargonaphasia) due to a vascular accident of the left hemisphere. Neurological examination revealed no motor signs nor visual field defect. According to clinical language assessment, the patient showed no signs of anomia as regards visual and tactile object naming whereas word production was disturbed in repetition and writing from dictation. Reading was judged to be normal.

3.2 Special Testing of Language

In order to circumscribe the patient's language disorder in more detail we administered our protocols for language assessment. For the purpose of this presentation we only report on the patient's performances concerning the production of isolated words.

3.2.1 Reading, Repetition and Writing from dictation

Special testing of the patient's ability to produce isolated words in reading, writing and repetition included the parameters which are now standard in neurolinguistic research, that is frequency, meaningfulness, concreteness, word class and regularity. The patient's performances in reading, repetition and writing are represented in table 1. It is clear from table 1 that the patient's word reading was specifically disturbed since the reading of irregular words was error-prone. In contrast, none of the lexical variables (meaningfulness, concreteness, word class, frequency) played any role in

Table 1 Case GI: Reading, Writing and Repetition of words and nonwords

% correct	READING	WRITING	REPETITION
concrete nouns:	**95 %**	**75 %**	**47.5 %**
high frequency	95 % (19/20)	65 % (13/20)	50 % (10/20)
low frequency	95 % (19/20)	85 % (17/20)	45 % (9/20)
abstract nouns:	**92.5 %**	**25 %**	**27.5%**
high frequency	90 % (18/20)	10 % (2/20)	30 % (6/20)
low frequency	95 % (19/20)	40 % (8/20)	25 % (5/20)
verbs:	**95 %**	**20 %**	**35 %**
high frequency	95 % (19/20)	25 % (5/20)	40 % (8/20)
low frequency	NT	15 % (3/20)	30 % (6/20)
regular words*	**94 % (47/50)**	**58 % (29/50)**	**NT**
irregular words*	**56 % (23/50)**	**56 % (28/50)**	**NT**
open class words*	**100 % (25/25)**	**48 % (12/25)**	**48 % (12/25)**
closed class words*	**100 % (25/25)**	**8 % (2/25)**	**30 % (6/25)**
Nonwords	**100 % (50/50)**	**0 % (0/20)**	**10 % (5/50)**
Semantic errors	**NO**	**YES**	**YES**

* pairwise matched for frequency and number of letters

reading aloud. This pattern of dissociation is commonly called "surface dyslexia" (cf. Patterson, Marshall & Coltheart 1985) and reflects the use of a non-lexical production strategy where verbal output is obtained by means of phonological reading through grapheme/phoneme conversion. GI represents a rather pure form of the syndrome since his reading errors typically consisted in non lexical forms due to (correct) application of grapheme-to-phoneme correspondence rules.

Repetition and writing were also specifically disturbed. The patient could not reproduce meaningless stimuli. For word reproduction the patient relied on the semantic pathway in both tasks as shown by the presence of semantic errors and the influence of variables such as concreteness and word class. Such a pattern of performance has also been termed "deep dysphasia" with "deep dysgraphia" (cf. Morton 1980a, b).

In conclusion, GI suffers from a similar association of syndromes (but not from identical disturbances of word reproduction) as described for MK, the patient so carefully studied by Howard & Franklin (1988).

3.2.2 Picture naming

In order to study whether GI's apparently good confrontation naming was influenced by semantic category or by word class the patient was presented with a total of 120 objects pictures (taken from a French picture pool for children) and of 55 action pictures taken from McCarthy & Warrington (1985). The object pictures corresponded to 40 animal names and to 80 object names from various semantic categories. The results show that the oral and written naming of nouns was close to perfect (97 % and 95 % correct respectively). In contrast, the naming of verbs was selectively disturbed for both oral (45 %) and written (45 %) output.

3.3 Special testing of action picture naming

Since it cannot be ruled out that GI's problems in verb retrieval for repetition and for writing from dictation may, in fact, be due to artifacts of list composition (since the dimension of concreteness/imageability of the verb stimuli was not controlled) we decided further to investigate the patient's problems with verb retrieval exclusively in picture naming. Indeed, as regards naming the dimension of concreteness/imageability ought to play a minor role (or none at all) since pictorial stimuli (simple black and white drawings) are used.

3.3.1 The influence of word frequency on naming

The frequency of the target word being such a crucial variable in aphasiology we decided pairwise to match 30 object and 30 action names of pictures (list A) according to their frequency of occurrence in French (Julliand, Brodin & Davidovich 1970). We thus stated that the patient's selective problem with the production of verbs is not related to a possible artifact in terms of the frequency of the word to be produced. Verbs were still more difficult to name than nouns (60 % (18/30) and 100 % (30/30) correct respectively). Still, the impairment *itself* may be related to the frequency of the verbs to be retrieved. We therefore divided the SO action pictures (list B) from a standardized picture pool in French (Vignau-Barthélémy 1990) into frequent vs. less frequent words.[5] GI named 53 % (15/25) of the frequent verbs and 43 % (13/25) of the less frequent items. This suggests that the frequency of the word to be named has no explanatory power for the observed naming deficit.

3.3.2 The influence of visual redundancy on action picture naming

We also looked for the possible influence of visual redundancy on action picture naming. The naming of 30 items was solicited by presenting one single picture whereas another 25 action names were solicited by simultaneous presentation of two different drawings depicting the same verb.[6] Like McCarthy & Warrington (1985) we wanted to study whether the patient's verb naming would benefit from redundancy of visual input in the condition of simultaneous action picture presentation. This was not the case. With single picture presentation GI scored 50 % (15/30) correct and in the two-picture condition his naming of verbs was 40 % (10/25) correct.

3.3.3 The influence of name agreement

One of our students, Florence Vignau-Barthélémy, undertook a study of action picture naming by 120 normal controls (Vignau-Barthélémy 1990). These fifty pictures (which overlap with the McCarthy & Warrington's (1985) picture pool without being identical) were presented to GI for oral naming. The patient's naming was scored correct if it corresponded to either the dominant response or to *any* of the non-dominant response given by normal controls.[7] According to this scoring criterion the patient's action naming was still selectively disturbed (56 % correct).

It is still possible, however, that the variable of name agreement – in terms of a more or less unique link between picture and name – accounts for the observed naming deficit. According to Barthélémy's standardization study 26/50 action pictures obtain 80 % to 100 % name agreement by all subjects, whereas 24/50 action pictures obtain less than 80 % name agreement with regard to the dominant response. Patient GI names 65 % (17/26) of the pictures with high name agreement as compared to 45 % (11/24) of the pictures with weak name agreement. The patient seems indeed slightly to benefit from the incidence of high name agreement. However, this variable does not *explain* the patient's naming performances.

3.4 Comprehension of object and action picture names

We investigated the patient's auditory comprehension of nouns and verbs by means of pictorial multiple choice tasks. One array of four pictures (set 1) consisted of the target picture (n = 50), a picture with a semantically related name, a picture with a phonologically related name and one with visual similarity. Another four picture array (set 2) consisted of the target picture (n = 25) with three semantically related foils. The patient's auditory comprehension of both nouns and verbs was equally well preserved in the two comprehension tasks. In set 1 the patient performed 94 % and 92 % correct respectively; in set 2 the patient performed 88 % correct for both nouns and verbs.

This performance pattern contrasts with the one observed with the (agrammatic) patient described by McCarthy & Warrington (1985), who suffered from both difficulties of verb retrieval and impaired comprehension of verbs. In contrast to ROX, GI exhibited no substantial impairments at the central level. His main difficulty consisted in accessing both output lexicons for verb retrieval.

3.5 Naming and repetition of same words (action picture names)

If the patient's pattern in word repetition – which corresponds to the syndrome of deep dysphasia, including problems with verb retrieval – is *not* due to problems of *accessing* meaning, given auditory input, then (given his relatively preserved auditory comprehension in word/picture matching – see paragraph 3.4) the performances in oral picture naming and repetition of (same) action picture names should parallel one another since both deficits ought to originate from a *post-semantic* word retrieval problem. This is indeed the case. The patient named 28/50 (56 %) of the action pictures of list B (see 3.3) and repeated 32/50 (64 %) of the corresponding action picture names. With the words of list A (see 3.3) the patient's performance pattern is similar: GI names 60 % (18/30) action pictures and repeats 70 % (21/30) of the corresponding action picture names.

3.6 Verb retrieval in other production tasks

We studied the patient's ability to retrieve verbs in other production tasks. They were administered for *written* production in order to prevent the patient from continuously commenting on his problems of verb retrieval.

3.6.1 Description of Cookie Theft Picture

The patient's written description of the Cookie Theft Picture from the BDAE (Goodglass & Kaplan 1983) consists of a total of 53 words. All words are written without orthographic errors. The text (which contains syntactic errors) decomposes into the production of 19 articles, 20 nouns, 1 adjective, 2 verbs, 10 prepositions and 1 conjunction. The 20 noun types correspond to 17 different tokens whereas the 2 instances of verb production correspond to the same lexical entry. Notwithstanding the lack of data from control subjects it is evident that the patient's verb retrieval in written picture description is extremely poor and contrasts which his ability to produce numerous precise labels for objects/nouns.

3.6.2 Production of antonyms

We investigated the patient's ability to generate antonyms for various word classes. The list included nouns (e.g. *père/father*), adjectives (*beau/beautiful*), verbs (*entrer/to enter*) and function words (*devant/in front of*). GI correctly produced 12/15 (80 %) noun pairs, 8/15 (53 %) adjective pairs, 4/15 (27 %) verb pairs and no antonym for function words. Only for verbs did GI produce non-lexical forms which are probably obtained by morphological derivation from existing nouns, e.g. (*freiner/to brake*) > *accélérater (derived from *accélérateur*?)

3.6.3 Verbal fluency

We asked the patient to write as many nouns as possible within 4 minutes. GI produced 37 items including two minor dysorthographies (*le véhicule, la voiture, les pneus, la brise pare (= pare brise?), la jante, l'assiette, torchon, fourchette, soupe, tasse, bouteille, scie, tournevis, sabot, bateau, embarque (= embarquement?), nage, route, sentier, pic, rocher, volée, avoine, maïs, usine, vallée, ruisseau, rivière, fleuve, mer, océan, lac, bureau, machine à écrire, téléphone, magnétoscope, photographie).*
When asked to produce as many verbs as possible within the same time limit, the patient produced 20 verbs *(téléphoner, télégraphier, marcher, courir, grimper, se laver, jardiner, scier, peller, conduire, nager, écrire, cuisiner, machiner, radiographier, examiner, golfer, conter, manger, boire)* and 3 neologisms *(*bicycletter, *mécanicier, *dentister)* which are probably derived from existing nouns (e.g. bicyclette, mécanicien, dentiste). These results suggest that in a free production task like verbal fluency the patient's lexicalization of verbs does not seem to be dramatically hampered. On the contrary, he often produces extremely rare verb forms. It is striking, however, that the produced verbs typically have a morphological relation to existing nouns (e.g. peller – la pelle, golfer – le golf, etc.). Indeed, GI did not produce any verb, even among the most frequent ones, without such morphological component.

3.6.4 Writing from dictation of compound nouns

Since the patient's success in writing from dictation was not influenced by word frequency (cf. table 1) we decided to test GI's writing from dictation of compound nouns. Two lists of 20 items each were constituted: one list (N+N) refers to compound nouns which contain two nouns (e.g. stylo plume, lampe de chevet, etc.) whereas the other list (V+N) contains compound nouns which are composed of a verb plus noun (e.g. porte-plume, pèse-bébé, etc.). The patient correctly wrote 13 of the N+N compounds including two minor errors (75 %) but he wrote only 4 of the V+N compounds including two minor errors (40 %). Although compound nouns have an unambiguous lexical entry as a noun it would thus seem that, in the case of V+N compounds, there is a "cognitive souvenir" of the composite elements in terms of word class.[8] As a consequence GI's general problems with verb retrieval even show up in this dicatation task of substantives.

3.7 Qualitative analysis of errors in action picture naming

On the standardized list for action picture naming (list B mentioned under 3.3) GI committed 44 % (22/50) errors in oral naming, five of which were self-corrected (see appendix). Our scoring counts non-dominant responses as correct as well as rare but acceptable naming responses which were not found among the non-dominant responses of normal controls. Qualitative analysis shows that the initial naming errors correspond to 13 'changes of word class' (that is the production of a noun instead of a verb), 4 responses were classified as true 'semantic paraphasias', two responses corresponded to 'pronomilizations', two to 'perseverations', one was a 'phonemic paraphasia' and another one was classified as 'comment'. The majority of GI's naming errors in action picture naming thus consists of the production of a noun instead of a verb.

In order tentatively to circumscribe the patient's nominalization strategy we identified 12 items among the 50 pictures of list B where the verb and the object related to the action have the root morpheme in common (e.g. *scier* avec une scie; *peindre* une peinture; *lire* un livre). Our question was of course whether these items are more easily named than those where such morphological relation is absent (e.g. *se regarder* dans une glace; *écrire* une lettre/avec un crayon, etc.). The patient seems indeed to benefit from such relations since he named 66 % (8/12) of the morphologically related items as compared to 47 % (17/38) of the unrelated items. But the advantage cannot be considered important.

Still, as regards nominalization a closer look at the patient's performances (see appendix) reveals that he often (in 9/13 instances of nominalization) produces a noun sharing the root morpheme with the target word. But this noun does not necessarily have an object/agent relation with the target word and it may be rather infrequent or even abstract, e.g. (écrire) > ecriture/ekri(= écrit?)//ekrit(= écrite?)//ekritwar(= *écritoir)/. It seems clear from the example cited that the morpho-lexical strategy – which is spontaneously employed by the patient to overcome his problems of post-semantic response-blocking in the case of oral and written output exclusively for the class of verbs – corresponds to something like "Look for a noun candidate and try to make it a verb by adding the infinitive affixes -ER, -IR or -OIR".

It should be underlined that the patient's morpho-lexical strategy does not necessarily result in final naming success: only 3/9 items of list B are self-corrected. Sometimes his attempts at verb lexicalization are hampered by apparently minor but in fact dramatic production difficulties. In this context let us cite an example from written naming (see appendix). It concerns an item which was presented twice on different sessions:

1 – balayer/to sweep > Before writing the patients comments "... balai mais... j'ai pas le verbe.../ba/balader non!... balai... *balaisez non".[9] He then writes: BALAI + ER?... BALAI + DER?

2 – balayer/to sweep > Before writing the patient comments "le balai... la dernière fois j'ai pas trouvé le verbe... balader... c'est bon ça? non... balader... balader... non... je sais pas.... balai... B.A.L.L.E.R. non...."[10] He then writes the following neologisms: *BAILLER, *BALAIDER, *BALAITER... BALAI +?.

Indeed, for GI the morpho-lexical strategy seems to be the dominant production strategy to "obtain" verbs since the patient employs the strategy of noun-to-verb derivation even in the absence of lexical similarity between both classes of words. Therefore many of his productions are totally neologistic, for example, written naming of the picture *pleurer/to cry* results in *LARMER which is supposedly derived from la *larme*/the tear. As another striking example we can cite GI's written naming of *cueillir/to pick* (the picture shows a girl picking fruit). On one occasion the patient's

response is *FRAISER which is supposedly derived from *les fraises*/strawberries; on another occasion he names it *GROSEILLER which is supposedly derived from *les groseilles*/red-currants.
As a consequence of the morpho-lexical strategy the patient's written naming may also result in existing words which are however inadequate derivations from the object/noun represented on the action picture. Let us take the example of *souffler/to blow* depicting a girl blowing out the candles of her birthday cake. The patient names this picture > BOUGER/to move. This verb does have a lexical entry. In the light of the patient's morpho-lexical production strategy it seems more probable, however, that the produced verb is derived – in a "neologistic manner" – from *la bougie*/the candle and that the correspondence with an existing lexical entry is rather fortuitous.
More examples of GI's attempts at verb formation can be found among the naming responses which are reproduced in the appendix. Unfortunately they can be fully appreciated only by French-speaking subjects.

3.8 Discussion

The case under study, GI, suffered from a disturbance of verb retrieval for both oral and written production. Notwithstanding Geschwind's (1967) earlier claim that written production is dependent upon oral output, the parallel of the observed production deficits is not causal in nature. Indeed, independent output lexicons are not only a theoretical claim in the frame of information-processing models (Morton 1980; Ellis 1982). The view that access to the phonological and to the graphemic output lexicon is separate has also been experimentally substantiated by numerous case studies reporting on dissociations between oral and written naming (Bub & Kertesz 1982; Caramazza & Hillis 1991; Hier & Mohr 1977; Lhermitte & Dérouesné 1974; Michel 1979).
GI's naming deficit for action pictures is not due to a central disturbance but is located at the output lexicons and/or access to them. Indeed, the level of picture/word comprehension is equally preserved for verbs and nouns. Nonetheless the naming of action pictures is selectively disturbed. Similar post-semantic action naming deficits were described by Caramazza & Hillis (1991) – see also Miceli et al. (1988).
In agreement with the specialized literature (cf. Miceli et al. 1984) GI's disturbed action picture naming resulted in numerous spontaneous nominalizations. We tried further to specify GI's action naming. Qualitative rather than quantitative error analysis suggests that the patient, in addition to nominalization, employs another compensatory strategy which we termed the 'morpho-lexical strategy'. It consists of (more or less arbitrary) derivation of verb form from existing nouns in order to obtain output for the "lesioned" word class of verbs. In this context one may refer to Gentner's (1981) view that differences between nouns and verbs stem in part from a basic cognitive distinction that is correlated with the noun-verb distinction: the distinction between object reference concepts and relational concepts. In this view object-reference concepts are typically lexicalized as concrete nouns (such *as dog)* whereas relational concepts from the same concrete level are typically lexicalized as verbs (such as *bark*). Some concepts can even

be lexicalized either as nouns or verbs, e.g. *He put a cover on it = He covers it.* It seems as though GI uses this principle as a strategy in order to overcome his severe action naming deficit. Unfortunately this principle is not a general one and therefore the patient's verb retrieval often goes wrong, resulting in faulty lexicalizations.

With regard to GI's problems of verb retrieval we would like briefly to discuss another point. As in Caramazza & Hillis' (1991) observations, our patient's problems with action names were not specific to the task of picture naming but extended to virtually all tasks where verbal output was obtained via semantic treatment, such as word repetition and dictation, picture description, etc. Indeed, action picture naming and repetition of the same action picture names resulted in similar performance patterns. The effect regarding verbs observed in GI's "deep dysphasic" pattern of word production (in repetition as well as in writing) is thus a true word class effect and not due to artifacts of list composition.

It is however open to question whether the word class effect concerning verbs is part of a deep pattern of performance *per se*. Marshall & Newcombe (1966, 1973) were the first to observe an overall word class effect with nouns > adjectives > verbs > functors with their patient GR who was a deep dyslexic. Subsequently such word class effects were confirmed for several other cases. However, Allport & Funnel (1981) provided suggestive experimental evidence for the notion that the part-of speech effect between nouns and verbs – (in the deep dyslexic reading of five patients) – may be due to uncontrolled imageability values of the presented stimuli. On the other hand, Howard & Franklin (1988) found that MK's deep dysgraphic writing from dictation does not demonstrate that there is a difference in performance either between nouns and verbs or between content and function words, once imageability is controlled. In this context note also that for at least one patient with deep dyslexia (Coslett, Rothi & Heilman 1985) the oral reading of concrete as opposed to abstract words is not statistically significant. Similarly, for patient HW (Caramazza & Hillis 1990) the difference of errors in reading abstract words as compared to concrete words is minor (86 % vs. 81 % respectively). (However, the patient produced numerous semantic errors in oral reading, which was also clearly affected by a word's grammatical class and he was unable to read non-words.)

Such state of affairs suggests that "deep dyslexic" reading, as well as "deep dysphasic" repetition and "deep dysgraphic" writing are indeed 'multi-component syndromes' (see Shallice & Warrington 1980) – in an even broader sense, however, than is usually indicated. In any case, such variation precludes "unitary accounts" of the "deep" syndromes (see Kremin, in press, for more detailed discussion of this topic).

4 General conclusion

We described the case of an aphasic patient suffering from a rather selective deficit of action picture naming. From a clinical point of view it is important to stress that this patient was of the fluent type corresponding to Wernicke's aphasia after regression of initial jargonaphasia. In line with the arguments spelled out in the reviewing section of this paper the case study presented furnishes further experimental evidence for our claim (see also Kremin & Basso 1993) that there is no causal relationship between selective impairments on object vs. action picture naming and precise type(s) of aphasia. Aphasia syndromes are mostly the result of the pattern of vascularization of the brain whereas the dissociation between different word classes (nouns and verbs) is a principle of language organization. It should come as no surprise that these two levels do not coincide.

Appendix

GI's oral naming of 50 action pictures

1 traire (to milk): +
2 frapper (to knock): +
3 manger (to eat): +
4 skier (to ski): +
5 taper ...à la machine (to typewrite): c'est une dactylo... machine à écrire... frapper oui frapper
6 souffler (to blow): ... *(patient blows)* +
7 jouer... aux cartes (to play cards): des cartes... des jeux... de cartes
8 cueillir (to pluck): ici c'est des fruits... *(what does the person do?)* demander des... des fruits alors comment donc je regarde chez moi avec des fraises... qu'est-ce que fais?... ben rien sans doute je sais pas
9 jongler (to juggle): +
10 embrasser (to kiss): baiser mais... il y a la mère
11 boire (to drink): +
12 marcher (to walk): manger... marcher pardon
13 arroser (to water flowers): arrosoir... ah! euh..../arwa/.. je ne sais pas comment on dit le verbe
14 cirer (to polish shoes): glissant... pardon... polir
15 se raser (to shave): + (raser)
16 caresser (to caress): une caresse... caresser
17 sortir (to go out): +
18 perdre (to lose): se jeter
19 croquer (to eat an apple): marcher euh!... marcher... si vous entendez... enfin c'est manger mais pour une pomme c'est pas tout à fait ça
20 saluer (to salute): c'est le.... saluer... militaire
21 se regarder (to look into the mirror): se mirer... mi- mirer c'est bien ça? c'est curieux autrefois...il y a une fable sur regarder et sur une flaque d'eau oh je sais plus
22 éplucher (to peal): peler
23 balayer (to sweep): +
24 jouer d'un strument (to play an instrument): souffler... ah je suis d'accord mais on peut souffler dans plein de choses... qu'est-ce qu'il fait... une histoire de musique... je sais pas
25 applaudir (to applaud): c'est un applaudissement donc... applaudir
26 pleurer (to cry): des pleurs... pleur... pleurer
27 nager (to swim): +
28 sentir (to smell): ouir... bon c'est pas bon ah ben oui si c'est ça parce que c'est dans l'oreille (*what is the name* of the *word you are looking* for?)... sentir
29 peindre (to paint): +
30 opérer (to operate): chirurgie ou plomberie c'est pareil... euh opération... mais je sais pas
31 téléphoner (to telephone): +

32 se moucher (to blow one's nose): mouchoir je ne sais plus le verbe...(*try to find* it) je sais pas
33 tricoter (to knit):/*tricon/.../*tricone/... tricoter
34 pousser (to push): +
35 fumer (to smoke): +
36 voler (to fly): +
37 danser (to danse): +
38 écrire (to write): écriture/ekri//ekrit//*ekritwar/
39 porter (to carry): histoire de vendange... vendanger
40 se laver (to wash): + (laver)
41 tirer (to pull): grimper
42 lire (to read): +
43 dormir (to sleep): s'endormir... euh coucher c'est pas tout a fait ça
44 courir (to run): +
45 verser (to pour): qu'est-ce je fais je prends une carafe... je sais pas il y a un verre mais....
46 scier (to saw): +
47 repasser (to iron): +
48 plonger (to dive): +
49 escalader (to climb): histoire d'alpinisme.... grimper
50 se balancer (to swing): c'est un.... une histoire de balançoire

GI's written naming of the same pictures on various occasions:

1 traire: +
2 frapper: 1/HACHER; 2/POINDRE; 3/CASSER; 4/+
3 manger: +
4 skier: +
5 taper: +
6 souffler: 1/BOUGER; 2/+
7 jouer: +
8 cueillir: 1/(omission); 2/FRAISER; 3/GROSEILLER; 4/(omission)
9 jongler: +
10 embrasser: 1/BAISER; 2/BAISER; 3/+ (s'embrasser)
11 boire: +
12 marcher: +
13 arroser: 1/(omission); 2/S'ARRIVER
14 cirer: 1/BRILLER; 2/BROSSER; 3/+
15 se raser: +
16 caresser: 1/(omission); 2/(omission)
17 sortir: 1/SE PRFSENTER; 2/S'INFORMER .. PORTER
18 perdre: SE PERDRE
19 croquer: MANGER ... SE CROCHER ... CROQUER
20 saluer: 1/GARDER; 2/S'ECARTER?; 3/CONDUCTER ... RIRE... SE REGARDER
21 se regarder: 1/(omission); 2/S'ENT.....
22 éplucher: 1/COUPER; 2/S'EPLUCHER
23 balayer: 1/BALAI+ ER?... BALAI+DER?; 2/BALAIDER... BALAITER... BALAI+?
24 jouer d'un instrument: 1/CONTINUER; 2/+
25 applaudir: 1/BRAVISSER; 2/S'APPLAUDIR
26 pleurer: 1/LARMER; 2/+

27 nager: +
28 sentir: 1/(omission); 2/ODORER
29 peindre: 1/PEINTRER; 2/+
30 operer: S'OPERER
31 téléphoner: +
32 se moucher: SE MOUCHOIR
33 tricoter: +
34 pousser: 1/(omission); 2/OUVRIR
35 fumer: +
36 voler: 1/(omission); 2/PLANER
37 danser: 1/SE D'ANSER; 2/+
38 écrire: 1/ALPHATHISER; 2/S'ECRITURER; 3/+
39 porter: 1/(omission); 2/+
40 se laver: 1/S'ETTOYER; 2/+
41 tirer (une corde): 1/CORDER; 2/GLISSER
42 lire: 1/LIRER; 2/+
43 dormir: 1/S 'END?; 2/+
44 courir: 1/GALOPER; 2/MARCHER; 3/+
45 verser: 1/EPROUVER; 2/S'ENTROUVER?
46 scier: +
47 repasser: +
48 plonger: 1/PLONGEON; 2/PLONGEON... PLONGER
49 escalader: 1/MONTER ...SE GRIMPER; 2/+
50 se balancer: S'ENDOR?

And also: Written naming of non standardized actions, mainly from the picture pool of McCarthy & Warrington (1985)

naviguer: VOILER ... REGATER; donner: REMISER; bailler: LARM... BAILLIR; patauger: S'ECHAUFFER; clouer: CASSER; attraper (un ballon): 1/BALLER; 2/S'ENTROUVER; tomber: S'ENFONDRER; attaquer: 1/SE PIQUER; 2/VOLER; bruler: 1/CONSUMER; 2/ATTISER; 3/BRULER; montrer (avec le doigt): 1/SIGNALER; 2/SE POINTER; hisser un poids (avec une grue): 1/MONTER; 2/HISSER; 3/GRUE+TER... GRUTER; empaqueter: 1/PAQUETTER ... FICELLER; 2/S'INFICELER; creuser: 1/BECHER; 2/PELLER; 3/JARDINER; tomber: 1/(omission); 2/S'ENFRONDRER; soulever un poids (en gymnase): 1/MUSCLER; 2/GYMNASTER.

Notes

1 In this context, note that performance differences may emerge when some metalinguistic task has to be performed on the noun and verb stimuli as in the "synonym generation" and "sentence generation" paradigms employed by Kohn, Lorch & Pearson (1989). In this case verbs may be more vulnerable. With respect to our working hypothesis (see 2.3.3) note also that the authors stated that "whether an aphasic was fluent or nonfluent did not help account for the data" (p. 65) from pathology.
2 It was also observed that pointing to object pictures is easier than pointing to action pictures in a multiple choice paradigm with controlled distractors.

3 In the absence of follow-up studies of the individual children one must be cautious, of course, since it is also possible (but, in our view, not probable) that the score differences in naming nouns and verbs reflect in fact "pathological" dissociations in normally developing children. As we will see later such dissociations characteristically occur in brain damaged adults with specific naming disturbances.
4 It is probably due to an overinterpretation of a second experimental finding which concerns the naming of nouns and verbs from verbal definitions. In the latter task the group of anomic aphasics did indeed produce verbs more easily than nouns (85 % vs. 67 % correct respectively).
5 They correspond to items with a frequency range of > 4000 vs. < 4000 according to Imbs (1971).
6 These pictures are identical to those used by McCarthy & Warrington (1985). We thank them for so kindly lending us their drawings of actions.
7 For example, the picture "boire/to drink" elicits only the dominant response BOIRE/to drink. In contrast, the picture "marcher/to walk" elicits the dominant response MARCHER and the following non dominant responses: *déambuler, s'en aller, promener, se promener, aller se promener, partir, revenir, voyager, se balader, se presser, partir en voyage.*
8 Some colleagues have the impression that a similar phenomenon can be observed during language acquisition. But no experimental data seem to be available from the published literature.
9 "broom but... I do not have the verb.../ba/to walk no!... broom... (production of the neologism:) *balaiser no..."
10 "the broom... the last time I didn't find the verb.... to walk... that is right? No... to walk... to walk... no... I don't know... broom... (spells:) B.A.L.L.E.R. no..."

References

Allport, A. & E. Funnell (1981): "Components of the mental lexicon". Philosophical Transactions of the Royal Society of London B295, 397 – 410.

Basso, A., C. Razzano, P. Faglioni & E. Zanobio (1990): "Confrontation naming, picture description and action naming in aphasic patients". Aphasiology 4, 185 – 195.

Bub, D. & A. Kertesz (1982): "Evidence for lexicographic processing in a patient with preserved written over oral single word naming". Brain 105, 697 – 717.

Caramazza, A. & A.E. Hillis (1991): "Lexical organization of nouns and verbs in the brain". Nature 349, 788 – 790.

Chéreau, C. & L. Faure (1993): Etude quantitative et qualitative de l'acquisition du langage chez l'enfant de 3 à 6 ans au travers d'épreuves de répétition et de dénomination. Mémoire d'Orthophonie. Université Paris VI.

Coltheart, M., K.E. Patterson & J.C. Marshal, eds. (1980): Deep Dyslexia. London: Routledge and Kegan Paul.

Coslett, H.B., L.G. Rothi & K.M. Heilman (1985): "Reading: Dissociation of the lexical and phonologic mechanisms". Brain and Language 24, 20 – 35.

Ellis, A.W. (1982): "Spelling and writing (and reading and speaking)". In: A.W. Ellis, ed., Normality and Pathology in Cognitive Functions. London: Academic Press, 113 – 146.

Gentner, D. (1981): "Some interesting differences between verbs and nouns". Cognition and Brain Theory 4, 161 – 178.

Geschwind, N. (1967): "The varieties of naming errors". Cortex 3, 97 – 112.

Goldstein, K. (1948): Language and Language Disturbances. New York: Grune and Stratton.

Goodglass, H. & E. Kaplan (1983): The Assessment of Aphasia and related disorders, second edition. Philadelphia: Lea and Fibiger.
Hier, D.B. & J.F. Mohr (1977): "Incongruous oral and written naming". Brain and Language 4, 115 - 125.
Howard, D. & S. Franklin (1988): Missing the Meaning? A Cognitive Neuropsychological Study of Processing of Words by an Aphasic Patient. Cambridge, Massachusetts: M.I.T. Press.
Imbs, P. (1971): Dictionnaire des Fréquences. Paris: Klincksieck.
Julliand, A., D. Brodin & C. Davidovich (1970): The frequency dictionary of French words. The Hague: Mouton.
Kaplan, E. & H. Goodglas (1976): Boston Naming Test. Boston: Boston University School of Medicine. Now: Kaplan, E., H. Goodglas & S. Weintraub (1983): The Boston Naming Test. Philadelphia: Lea & Febiger.
Kohn, S., M.P. Lorch & D.M. Pearson (1989): "Verb finding in aphasia". Cortex 25, 57 - 69.
Kremin, H. (in press): "Apropos imageability". In: M. Joshi & C.K. Leong, eds., Developmental and acquired Dyslexia: Neuropsychological and Neurolinguistic Perspectives. Dordrecht: Kluwer Academic Publishers.
Kremin, H. & M. Agostini (1993): "A propos d'aphasie amnésique pure: étude d'un sujet trilingue". Revue de Neuropsychologie 3, 118 - 119.
Kremin H. & G. Dellatolas (1993): "Access the lexicon during language acquisition: repetition (word/nonwords), picture naming, and pointing (objects/actions) in preschool children (aged 3 to 6)". Eleventh European Workshop on Cognitive Neuropsychology, Bressanone (Italy), 24 - 29 January.
Kremin, H. & A. Basso (1993): "Apropos the mental lexicon: nouns and verbs". In: F.J. Stachowiak, ed., Development in the Assessment and Rehabilitation of Brain-Damaged Patients: Perspectives from a European Concerted Action. Tübingen: Narr, 233 - 242.
Kremin, H. & G. Delllatolas (in press): "L'accès au lexique: une étude de standardisation chez l'enfant d'âge pré-scolaire". Pour un numéro spécial sur les difficultés d'acquisition du langage édité par M. T. Le Normand: Les cahiers du Centre Technique National d'Etudes et de Recherches sur les Handicaps et les Inadaptions.
Lhermitte, F. & J. Derouesné (1974): "Paraphasies et jargonaphasie dans le langage oral avec conversation du langage écrit". Revue Neurologique 130, 21 - 38.
Lotmar, F. (1919): "Zur Kenntnis der erschwerten Wortfindung und ihrer Bedeutung für das Denken des Aphasischen". Schweizer Archiv für Neurologie und Psychiatrie 5, 206 - 239; 6, 3 - 36.
McCarthy, R. & E.K. Warrington (1985): "Category specificity in an agrammatic patient: the relative impairment of verb retrieval and comprehension". Neuropsychologia 23, 709 - 727.
Marshall, J.C. & F. Newcombe (1966): "Semantic and syntactic errors in paralexia". Neuropsychologia 4, 169 - 176.
Marshall, J.C. & F. Newcombe (1973): "Pattern of paralexia: A psycholinguistic approach". Journal of Psycholinguistic Research 2, 175 - 199.
Miceli, G., C. Silveri, G. Villa & A. Caramazza (1984): "On the basis for the agrammtic's difficulty in producing main verbs". Cortex 20, 207 - 220.
Miceli, G., C. Silveri, U. Nocentini & A. Caramazza (1988): "Patterns of dissociation in comprehension and production of nouns and verbs". Aphasiology 2, 351 - 358.
Michel, F. (1979): "Préservation du langage écrit malgré un déficit majeur du langage oral". Lyon Medical 241, 141 - 149.
Morton, J. (1980a): "The logogen model and orthographic structure". In: U. Frith, ed., Cognitive Processes in Spelling. London: Academic Press, 117 - 134.
Morton, J. (1980b): "Two auditory parallels to deep dyslexia". In: M. Coltheart, K.E. Patterson & J.C. Marshall, eds., Deep Dyslexia. London: Routledge and Kegan Paul, 189 - 196.

Patterson, K.E., J.C. Marshall & M. Coltheart, eds. (1985): Surface Dyslexia. Neuropsychological and Cognitive Studies of Phonological Reading. London: Lawrence Erlbaum.
Obler, L.K. & M. Albert (1979): Action Naming Test. Unpublished Experimental Version. Boston.
Shallice, T. & E.K. Warrington (1980): "Single and multiple component central dyslexia syndromes". In: M. Coltheart, K.E. Patterson & J.C. Marshall, eds., Deep Dyslexia. London: Routledge and Kegan Paul, 119 – 145.
Vignau-Barthélémy, F. (1990): La dénomination orale d'images d'actions chez le sujet normal et chez le sujet aphasique. Tours: Mémoire d'Orthophonie.
Warrington, E.K. (1975): "The selective impairment of semantic memory". Quarterly Journal of Experimental Psychology 27, 635 – 657.
Warrington, E.K. (1981): "Concrete word dyslexia". British Journal of Psychology 72, 175 – 196.
Warrington, E.K. & T. Shallice (1984): "Category specific semantic impairments". Brain 107, 829 – 854.
Zingeser, L.B. & R.S. Berndt (1988): "Grammatical class and context effects in a case of pure anomia: implications for models of language production". Cognitive Neuropsychology 5, 473 – 516.
Zingeser, L.B. & R.S. Berndt (1990): "Retrieval of nouns and verbs in agrammatism and anomia". Brain and Language 39, 14 – 32.

Some Remarks on Representational Aspects of Language Production*

Helen Leuninger, Jörg Keller, Frankfurt

Introduction

In 1847 something rather curious happened to some person about to prepare the printing of the 2-Pence-stamp for Mauritius:

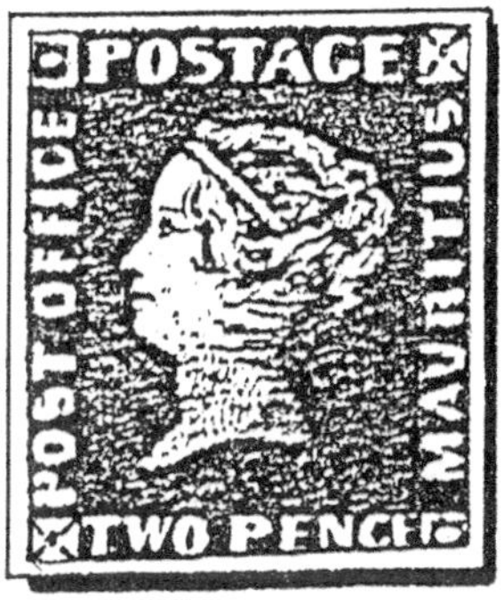

Instead of *post paid* he put *post office* as the imprint. Possibly, the man was distracted during his work, so his language planning system, say lexical access, was in an unstable state and therefore the more frequent lexical item, *post office*, interfered. In any case, this error yielded unexpected consequences – as surely everyone knows.

Yet the language errors of everyday life are just as precious as this stamp and the same applies to speech errors of aphasic speakers. These mistakes are especially apt to help us answer questions about processing stages and units because of their selective character that allows psycho- and neurolinguistic research to focus on crucial aspects of linguistic processing.

In this paper, it is those errors which have implications for the psycholinguistic and linguistic properties of the lexicon that we will concentrate on. We will show that they have structural properties not systematically investigated either by traditional top-down approaches nor by interactionist or even connectionist approaches. We consider this a theoretical and empirical gap which **has** to be filled if one takes the data serious.

* We thank Gerda Lauerbach for correcting our English and Thomas Berg, Jürgen Dittmann and Ulrich Schade for their last-minute remarks which we unfortunately are not able to discuss in this paper.

We classify the errors according to a slightly modified top-down language production model devised by Garrett (Garrett 1975, 1976, 1988; Keller & Leuninger 1993):

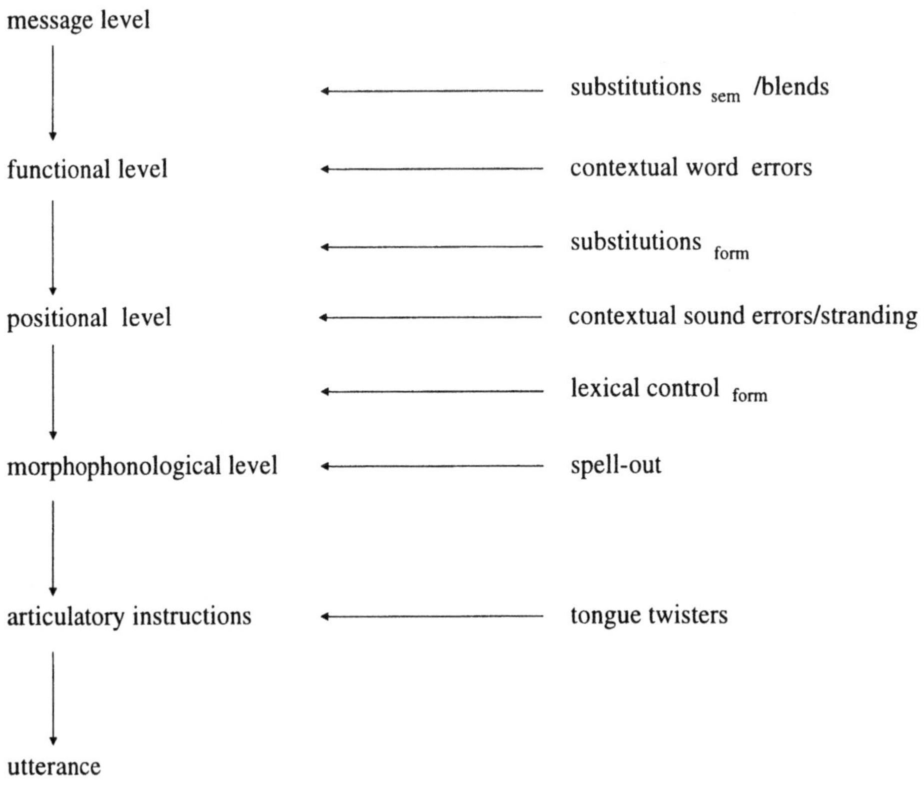

This model has diverse implications concerning representational and procedural aspects of language processing. In fact, we have to consider three aspects of psycholinguistic modelling which should be kept apart; each of these refers to an autonomous bundle of methodological and empirical questions:

1. Representation
2. Processing
3. Implementation

Representation subsumes the structural constituency ("granularity") and the boundaries of language planning units (segments, syllables, words, phrases, sentences). By **processing** we mean any sort of computation the language processing system can perform, e.g. lexical access, translation operations mapping one level onto another, including spell-out mechanisms specifying the phonetic content of grammatical information delivered to the next higher level. **Implementation** includes all sorts of procedural implementations, e.g. activation patterns as well as the material substrate of the system.

In the following, we will concentrate on the relation between the first two aspects, thereby following Fodor's (1975) premiss: "No computation without representation".

1 Representation: Part One

In both fields of cognitive science investigating language production, viz. the traditional symbolic and the connectionist approach (a distinction due to Fodor & Pylyshyn 1988), the question of how "deep", that is how detailed, the production system computes linguistic material, has not been systematically explored.[1]

Take for instance Fodor's (1983) modularity thesis. According to this thesis, the language input system essentially has only one general task, namely, to map utterance tokens onto utterance types. The perceptual analysis merely yields rather "shallow" structures. To Fodor, this is a natural consequence of the restrictions due to on-line processing.

One can find analogous argumentation with respect to language production. Garrett (1975: 135 f.) puts it this way: It is an open question how the planning system processes e.g. the morphological structure of words. While the morphological theory analyzes *bigger* as being composed out of a free and a bound morpheme, it is not at all clear that the processing vocabulary has independent command of a functional unit realizing "comparative-*er*".

In contrast to this, we want to show that errors involving morphological structure require a processing vocabulary which includes very detailed structural information. Otherwise, these utterances could not have been adequately computed.

There has been an interesting discussion of the question of what structural shape the syllable may have in on-line language processing for some time. It seems to be uncontroversial nowadays that the syllable is a relevant psycholinguistic unit, especially since the findings of the well-known shadowing experiments which evidenced the syllable as the first accessible unit (Marslen-Wilson & Tyler 1980).

Moreover, one gets the right partition of aphasic and normal speech errors by comparing the syllable structure of error and intended item. Klein & Leuninger (1990) were able to show that the relevant distinction between these two types of data is not on the segmental level, but on the CV-level of words. Aphasics' phonological paraphasias seem to disturb the CV-level (and extrasyllabic positions) more often than non-disturbed speakers do in producing segmental errors:

(1) (a) tanteshors ← Krankenhaus (Wernicke)
(b) krak[e:]rin ← Sekretärin (Global)
(c) sch[a:]pfaller ← Staubsauger (Broca)

By substituting *kr* with *t* in (1a) one C-position at the CV-level is deleted; the other segmental modifications do not affect the CV-structure. In (1b) the number of syllables is reduced, and in (1c) the extrasyllabic position dominating š disappears by deleting the segment *t*. Here again, all other segmental substitutions do not change the CV-structure of the intended item.

Apart from the assumption of extrasyllabic positions such as in (1c), the distribution of the data is neutral with respect to the underlying syllable model. In their investigation, Klein & Leuninger (1988, 1990) used the shallow syllable structure which Wiese (1988, 1991) devised for German, i.e. the syllable node only dominates CV-positions, but no hierarchically higher constituents, such as e.g. onset, rime, peak, and coda. The distinction between phonological paraphasias and phonological speech errors can thus be explained by a modular approach: The segmental error type is the same for both groups of speakers, though one finds more tokens, that is, more segmental modifications within one word, in phonological paraphasias. In contrast, the type of CV-errors differentiates both classes of data. Lexical syllabification is weakened in aphasic language production, but not in non-disturbed language processing. As we will show later, phonological paraphasias must be located in the lexicon on all levels of lexical derivation (cf. Dittmann 1991).

This characterization leaves open the question of the granularity of syllabic structure. A closer inspection of the strings might require the assumption of more structure in this psycholinguistic unit. Treiman (1989) for instance argues for a maximally structured syllable, i.e. one in which the syllable node dominates onset and rime, and the rime constituent dominates peak and coda (cf. Selkirk 1982 vs. Clements & Keyser 1983). Her evidence are speech errors, language games, and experimentally induced memory errors. In memory experiments with nonwords, subjects tended to remember the onset or the rime, but only seldom remembered peak and coda sequences.

Questioning Treiman's assumptions, Laubstein (1987) shows that language production processes merely affect onsets, peaks, and codas, arguing on distributional regularities in a corpus of natural speech errors. Therefore, this discussion is directly relevant to the question of what degree of elaboration language processing must have. We may thus assume that syllables consist of a tripartite structure of onset, peak, and coda as language planning units (cf. Grinberg Pla 1994).

To illustrate the need for deep representations, let us have a brief look at the following errors.[2]

Blend

(2) (a) Laßt uns auf das Wohl des *Säuflings* trinken ← Säuglings/Täuflings
(b) Die Transsexualität war vor der *Pubertätheit* da ← Pubertät/Kindheit
(c) Das sollten wir *eräutern* ← erörtern/erläutern
(d) Die muß man *mit rohen Handschuhen anfassen* ← wie ein rohes Ei behandeln/mit Samthandschuhen anfassen

Substitution

(3) Da gibt's doch so'n *fliegenden Spruch* ← geflügeltes Wort

Stranding

(4) Ich möchte meine *Gitter verfenstern* ← Fenster vergittern

Anticipation

(5) (a) Wird das mit *Bindeschrift* geschrieben? ← Bindestrich
(b) Weil auch dieser Treffer die *Decken* in der 96er Abwehr aufdeckt ← Lücken

Errors such as in (2a)-(2c) may only require a shallow analysis, such as a break after the first segment in (2a), a break after the stem in (2b), or a break in the second syllable

after first segment in (2c). Such a surface analysis seems inappropriate for the other errors however, e.g. (2d).
If language errors are motivated by the organization of the processing system – an assumption which seems well-grounded – then one needs considerably finer granular structures underlying at least (2d), (3), (5) than a pure surface oriented parsing would allow. Therefore, investigation of language production data will result in the formulation of lower and upper boundaries of granularity.

2 The lexicon

The analysis of our language production data suggests the following three different functions of the lexicon during the language production process:

I. Semantic-conceptual grouping of lexical items
II. Form-based grouping of lexical items
III. Form-based control processes

We will look at each one in turn.

I. Semantically based substitution errors as in (6) are evidence for some sort of semantic/conceptual groupings of lexical items:

(6) (a) ich muß mir noch die Haare *putzen* ← waschen
(b) die Spontansprache des *Angeklagten* ← Patienten
(c) das geht allen ganz schön an die *Leber* ← Nieren
(d) damit kommst du auf keinen grünen *Baum* ← Zweig
(e) dann brauchen wir vorläufig den *Mitgliederpreis* nicht zu erhöhen ← Mitgliedsbeitrag
(f) mein Gott, ich kann das kleine *ABC* nicht mehr ← Ein-mal-Eins

During the last 30 years much work has been done in this area (cf. Garrett 1992; Hillert 1994b; Hotopf 1980; Huber 1981; Levelt 1989; Stachowiak 1979, 1982; for a critical overview see also Hillert 1992). A large number of organizational parameters have been proposed, especially in neurolinguistic, language acquisition, and other psycholinguistic research. Whether such relational parameters are psychologically real depends on an intricated set of methodological and empirical aspects, i.e. aspects concerning the status of semantic theory in general, the status of such distinctions as e.g. classificational and associative dependencies, the amount of subjective portions in the lexicon and so forth (cf. Fodor et al. 1980; Leuninger 1989). Whatever the outcome of these discussions may be, errors like those listed above point to a semantically based grouping of lexical items. It is this organization that makes rapid lexical access possible (cf. Hillert 1994b). Furthermore, errors like (6d) show that even in idiomatic expressions or collocations lexical relations are so stable that otherwise not decomposable expressions can be broken up, i.e. syntactically computed. Even in so-called contextual errors (Harley 1984) such lexical relations are used, as in:

(7) und wenn ich es auf den Anrufbeantworter *schreibe* ← spreche
(situation: writing of a paper)

Note by the way: While the central systems may process a huge domain of ideas, beliefs etc., the language production system modularizes them according to presumably narrow options.
Therefore, the first relevant function of the lexicon in on-line language processing is to provide as rapid as necessary a set of items, to make a rich offer to the planning system. This definitely is a psycholinguistic function, which consists of two components, however:

- semantic representation
- lexical processes, viz. access routines etc.

II. Form-based substitution errors such as in (8) are evidence for another set of organizational principles, namely, grouping of lexical items along some sort of similarity metric, e.g. same syllable constituency or syllable structure (including metrical structure), sound or feature similarities, same first portion, same morphological construal of the processed items and so forth (cf. Fay & Cutler 1977).

(8) (a) Kampfpanzer *Leopold* ← Leopard
(b) ich werde mir mal diese *Lohnsteuertabletten* anschauen ← Lohnsteuer-tabellen
(c) da kann ich den schönsten *Hund* auf dem Kopf haben ← Hut
(d) ich muß noch mein *Pils* verlängern ← meinen Paß

As with the aforementioned semantic organization principles according to a semantic similarity metric, the precise character of the formal similarity metric is not yet known and may be rather vague. It is not even clear how deep into the morphophonological constituency the processes may go (cf. Stemberger 1983, 1985). Nevertheless, we need such a metric to explain formal substitutions because they are motivated by the form of the respective items.[3]
Here too, contextually induced errors show those form principles at work.

(9) (a) ich möchte mich nur etwas *umsitzen* ← umsehen
(while walking through a furniture shop)
(b) da habe ich einen tollen *Auspuff* geprägt ← Ausdruck
(after having sold a car)

As is the case in other naturally produced utterances, some of these formal substitutions seem to show rather global estimations of formal similarity, as e.g. *tabletten* in (8b). In this case, a precise similarity metric may be difficult to formulate.
With respect to the components needed to characterize formal substitutions, again two different ones are required:

- representation of the morphophonological form
- similarity metric which computes this form and a formal similarity based lexical access (see fn. 3).

III. Whereas the first two lexical functions discussed may permit analyses rather close to surface constituency, the third function of the lexicon we will consider is the most significant for answering the question: What structural depth does the processing system have to cope with in principle? Pertaining to this question are firstly data which cannot naturally be explained by shallow structure and secondly the details of lexical analysis on which the production data is based.
But before we will consider this question, let us have a look at a very interesting type of procedural error, one which cannot easily be explained by merely one planning failure.

3 Control processes

By and large, linguistic errors, at least those produced by unimpaired speakers, originate from exactly one processing failure. By this, we mean one type of failure, be it caused by form or by content.
Apparently, accommodations are an exception to this. But those processes, which we call spell-out processes, are cost-free adaptations of linguistic errors to grammatical/phonological well-formedness restrictions. The following blend illustrates the result of such a spell-out mechanism:

(10) Als *graues Mauerblümchen* wurde er in die Welt geschickt ← graue Maus/Mauerblümchen

Check and subsequent matching of the gender feature to the head of the NP (*Mauerblümchen)* can only happen after the fusion because the phonetics of the gender morpheme is not present in one of the alternatives. Blends containing stranding (cf. Wiegand, in prep.) may be less clear, for in this type of blending one of the competing constructions contains the respective morphophonological information as in *das ist wirklich ein dickes Stück* ← stark-***es*** *Stück/dick-er Hund.* In spite of this, many errors show accommodations and must therefore be characterized by spell-out which is some sort of grammatical control mechanism. Therefore, accommodation is no exception to the general tendency: one error, one type of processing failure.

3.1 Lexical control

The following errors seem to contradict this "rule":

(11) (a) 'nen kleinen *Stinkspruch* ← Trinkspruch
(b) *Schattenspieler* ← Plattenspieler
(c) durch die *Kutsche* latschen ← Küche
(d) und die macht keinen *Kummer*, keinen Finger krumm

(12) (a) *Platztante* ← Tanzplatte
(b) *buddhistisches Standesamt* ← statistisches Bundesamt

(13) (a) Er wohnt in Berlin und studiert *Benzin* ← Medizin
(b) Das Silbenschema muß halt *spinnen* ← stimmen

Everything we know about form, motivation and restrictions of linguistic errors suggests that (11)-(13) are phonological misplannings. Their results do not surface, however:

Anticipation: *Strinkspruch*; *Schlattenspieler*; *Kütsche*; *Krummer*
Exchange: *Planztatte*; *bundistisches Statesamt*
Perseveration: *Bedizin*, *spimmen*

These "internal" forms could have arisen, as all of them accord with the phonotactic restrictions of German. It is because of these restrictions that "internally" *spimmen* is computed. The devoicing of the labial obstruent is a cost-free phonological adaptation. But why do we analyze errors such as (11)-(13) as phonological errors at all? Wouldn't it suffice to subsume them under the class of form substitutions like (8) or like the following?:

(14) (a) Kontaminationen und die Struktur des *Sprachprofessors* ← Sprachprozessors
(b) *Projekthüllen* ← Prospekthüllen

As we argued above, formal substitutions (including malapropisms such as (9)) arise by computing two lexical entries along a similarity metric, that is, they are word-bound. They show no intrusion effects of the surrounding segmental material and occur in one computational step.
Contrary to this, the errors in (11)-(13) which we label lexically controlled errors, involve two computational steps:

1. contextually induced segmental errors
2. match with a lexical entry along a similarity metric

The second step, namely lexical control, is therefore of the type of a formal substitution. This really is a second operation, which, contrary to the aforementioned grammatical/ phonological control presumably is not cost-free.
As far as we know, this assumption of a two-step error was first formulated by Meringer (Meringer & Mayer 1895: 22 f.). Meringer classifies (15) as sound exchanges:

(15) (a) *Schimmelsenkel* ← Schinkensemmel
(b) *begreiflich* ← gebräuchlich

With respect to (15a) the predicted form *schimmen* is adapted to the more frequent form *Schimmel*, and with respect to (15b) the more frequent lexical entry *begreiflich* interferes and replaces the expected exchange *begräuchlich*. In our opinion, frequency is not the crucial factor here, as e.g. (11c) illustrates. *Kutsche* is not an item of high frequency, but is formally similar to *Kütsche*. Strictly speaking, one cannot allude to frequency when comparing non existing with existing items. Anyway, Meringer had already devised two steps for these types of errors.

Recently, Laubstein (1987) made an analogous proposal in her analysis of phonological exchange errors. As already mentioned above, Laubstein argues for a "semi-shallow" syllable which excludes the rime as a psychologically real syllable constituent. Errors which involve peak-coda-sequences pose a problem to this hypothesis, because they apparently constitute evidence for a rime constituent:

(16) *Sake Lalt* City ← Salt Lake City

How does Laubstein's model cope with such data? Errors like (16) occur very rarely in Laubstein's corpus. The same observation holds with respect to our corpus. Peak-coda-movements such as (17) are extremely rare:

(17) (a) Die *Brie*, äh, *quä*, äh, die Bremsen quietschen
(b) Echt *steil gark* ← echt geil stark

Because of their low probability, Laubstein proposes a two-step analysis for errors like (16):[4]

i. Morpheme exchange → Lake Salt
ii. Onset exchange → Sake Lalt

Further confirmation for our idea of lexical control derives from the observation that agrammatic speakers have intact morphological capacities. In one of the first explanations of the deficit patterns found in agrammatism which had a methodologically well motivated background, Kean (1977, 1981) showed that morphological relations between lexical entries are retained in agrammatism. This spared capacity is responsible for reductions like *definiteness* → *definite*, but also *definitive* → *definite*. Otherwise, the last reduction would remain unexplained as the deletion of *-ive* changes the stress pattern of the word (as well as the connotation) and therefore is not expected. The strategy used by Broca aphasics is a performance strategy also operative in non-disturbed linguistic behavior which Kean labels "lexical construal":

(18) My *frozers are shoulden* ← my shoulders are frozen

Obviously, the processor temporarily misanalyzes *shoulder* as a morphologically complex noun, derived by *er*-nominalization, as e.g. *roller*. Because of lexical construal (18) is a "normal" stranding error, perhaps comparable to (19):

(19) mein *Stirbchen bäumt* ← Bäumchen stirbt

Here too, *stirb* is misanalyzed as a word stem so that stranding can take place.

3.2 Relexicalizations

Another type of neurolinguistic evidence for the concept of lexical control are relexicalizations. In order to test the capacity of aphasic speakers for phoneme-grapheme-conversions, the processing of non-words can be tested. While it is clear that the orthographic lexicon must be entered in other writing conditions to sort out the conversion independent irregularities of spelling as in *Bus* [bus] vs. *Mus* [mu:s] or *Kuss* [kus] vs. *Fuss* [fu:s], this is not evident in the processing of non-words.
Still, when patients with disturbed or blocked form routes occasionally relexicalize non-words and paragraphias arise as in (20) (examples from Blanken 1992b), they must have accessed phonological and orthographic information of the lexicon.

(20) (a) Geuge (target: non-word) → *Geige* (relexicalized: word)
(b) Hond → *Hund*
(c) Burt → *Boot/Burg//Schiff* (via *Boot*)
(d) Zenge → *Ziege*
(e) Kirb → *Markt* (via *Korb*)

(20c) and (20e) are of major relevance for our hypothesis because these paragraphias can only be explained by assuming an internal control mechanism (lexical control). Without lexical control, namely, *Boot*, *Schiff* would be unmotivated. The same holds for *Markt*, a semantic paraphasia of the internally generated *Korb* accessed in a second step. Thus, relexicalizations constitute another piece of independent evidence for lexical control.

3.3 The status of writing errors

One might object that relexicalization is of no relevance to speech processing as it is an off-line phenomenon. Furthermore, processing models adhering to some variety of the logogen model (e.g. Morton 1980, 1984; Ellis & Young 1988) apparently show there to be different subsystems for e.g. word, grapheme, or phoneme processing. Does this mean that we need as many processors as there are subsystems? We doubt this because it is only the representational substance that changes, whereas the formal characteristics of the processing is the same.
There is evidence that makes us believe that the off-line vs. on-line distinction itself is not relevant for processing errors. Slips of the pen or ear, the latter hard to sample, show that different representational substances may still be equivalent for the processor. Think of slips of the hand, which are acknowledged to have the same properties as slips of the tongue (cf. Newkirk et al. 1980). They make it necessary to postulate a distinct set of features, e.g. movements, hand forms, features etc., that are subject to processing errors and that for this very reason must be part of some representation. Thus distinct representations may not necessarily demand distinct processors, and at any rate will not demand different capabilities of these/this device/s. Of course this reminds us of the simple homogenous processing units in connectionist modelling. For

the sake of simplicity and because it will not affect the point of our analysis we will not take a position here, that is, we will abstract away from neuronal modelling. Any model with separate processors for separate representations seems to be overloaded for the time being. Only evidence to the contrary, i.e. necessity, should force us to extend the intrinsic power or number of our processing mechanisms.

Because of slips of the hand, we already know that a particular representational content is no prerequisite for processing.[5] In bimodal bilingualism, i.e. simultaneous acquisition of signed and spoken language, both representations must be present simultaneously. Therefore, we do not actually have to present evidence that bears on representational differences. Yet, to pinpoint the question of on-line/off-line differences a short sample of another representational format may be informative.

In slips of the pen recorded on handwriting, some of which are given in (21)-(23), we find the same properties as in speech errors, e.g. anticipation (21a,b), perseveration (21c,d), addition (22a), deletion (22b), exchange (23ab):

(21) (a) *obljga* ← obligatorisch (feature: down)
(b) es sei eine große Anzahl Waffen *fonfisziert* worden ← konfisziert (grapheme)
(c) vor *alemm* ← vor allem (feature: double)
(d) ich fühle mich nicht *nicht* geneigt ← nicht geneigt (word)

(22) (a) *Segement* ← Segment (grapheme)
(b) *Schmikpinsel* ← Schminkpinsel (grapheme)

(23) (a) die *Sible* ← die Silbe (grapheme)
(b) *Btee* ← Bett (grapheme with feature stranding)

Of course, most errors on the word level may easily be accounted for by errors in early processing and don't need to be attributed to some error in the writing process. We have therefore only given one example in (21d). Let us assume for the moment that they are irrelevant then.

Nevertheless, there are errors that remain unexplained in terms of our present conception of language processing. The most revealing of these are errors that point to a feature decomposition of graphemes, two of which are doubling or directed movements (up, down, forth, back). Both have no representational status in any present framework, but still seem to be accessed and may be disturbed by some process. As there is no processing and no processing error respectively without representation, we are led to believe that there must be more than just a phonological feature matrix.

Applying the same line of reasoning as above to grapheme errors will not work, but there is another aspect that will. Note that slips of the pen may result in forms that would be pronounced differently (21c) and even in non-word or non-syllable forms as in *Btee*. What do you make of such errors, if there is no independent feature or grapheme level in processing? Any phonological processing would reject it as incompatible with the phonotactic rules of German or adjust it.

Due to the finding that write-out errors are akin to speech errors in some respects we readily expect them to be similar in others as well. Above we have refused to simply

attribute write-out errors on the word level to genuine write-out representations as they may just as well be explained by errors that occurred earlier in production. This will apply to many write-out errors on the word level, so they would seldom be identified. (21d) may as such be a rare example that will not easily fit into this line of reasoning as the landing site of the perseverated *nicht* is in no apparent structural slot. This is not to deny, however, that the evidence for word-level writing errors is still unconvincing. So this implies firstly that we need to have an extra grapheme and feature representation, secondly that spelling processes do not simply consist of conversion rules and lexical matching of irregular forms, thirdly that writing errors could in principle be handled by the same processing facilities as speech or signing errors, forthly that the processing of writing must be serially after or parallel to the processing of phonological information (no interaction could explain the facts), and last that the distinction between on-line and off-line processing is of no central concern here. Recall that we started out by saying that relexicalizations support our view of a formal lexical control mode in production. We now have established that the possibly off-line or possibly late mode of write-out (spell-out) is not spared of errors. We conclude: The lexicon may optionally be accessed from any stage of production. Relexicalization of non-words supports the lexical control hypothesis and cannot be explained away merely by an appeal to off-line or early processing, but must be due to form bound access routines.
It may look as if that view is to some extent contradicted by the facts about writing errors just adduced, but note that two options remain: We need not limit lexical control to accessing formal information of the phonological type by applying to intermediate conversion rules to give way to the phonological representation formats in writing errors. Errors that are repaired this way would forever fit other production errors.
We only have to add some compositional visual/orthographic information to lexical entries, a solution that is called for independently for representations of sign language. This would mean that lexical control may still be a one-type-of-information-retrieval. Whatever form this information has, the retrieval process will be less accurate in a later stage of production than with multiply specified entries. And it will explain how someone can speak out correctly while producing an error in simultaneous writing.
Lexical control, then, seems to be a strategy exploited by normals and aphasic disturbed speakers which makes it a good candidate for a functional processing mechanism.

3.4 Locality

In computing the form of lexical items in one or two steps, the processor is insensitive to the overall semantic plausibility of the utterance in general. This does not mean that meaning is irrelevant, but lexical control is clearly not capable of reorganizing the entire proposition; only single items can be matched. In our opinion this empirically grounded observation is a rather compelling piece of evidence against interactionist production models. At the point at which form is computed, content is not accessible (see e.g. Forster's (1979) distinction between perceptual and postperceptual language processing).

Therefore, internal control operations normally do not result in utterances principally able to express messages. Obviously, it could happen, but only by chance. This is in contrast to many, but not all, external corrections which seem to be guided by the principle "be message adequate".
Thus, lexical control is a quite clear indicator for the locality of lexical access. Not the overall meaning is checked, but only **one** item caused by a phonological (i.e. formal) planning failure is compared with another item, namely a lexical entry, along the above mentioned similarity metric.
Further evidence confirming the strict locality of form-based lexical access comes from the following written errors, caused perhaps by hearing errors and reading errors, respectively (cf. Browman 1980):

Writing

(24) (a) Herr X. ist bei den *Sieben Zwergen* angestellt (written) ← Siemens-Werken
(b) Frau M. wurde als *Türkin* bestellt (written) ← Bürgin

Reading

(25) (a) die *erklärungsbedingte* Nasalität (read) ← erkältungsbedingte
(Preceding verbal context: nasality due to a cold)
(b) *Ladendiebstahl* wurde zu einem verbreiteten Delikt (read) ← Leichen-diebstahl
(Preceding verbal context: Experiments with corpses)

It seems obvious that these errors can only have arisen out of the strictly local access to a single lexical item. The meaning of the preceding verbal context already computed is not strong enough to suppress form-based lexical substitution. In (25b) e.g. the higher frequency of *Ladendiebstahl* was the crucial factor inducing the error, therefore (25b) is of the "Blue Mauritius-type".
Even an immediately preceding item in a dialogue can be "modified" by a malapropism:

(26) A: ... Familienduell
B: ... Also ich finde die Sendung *Familienmodell* langweilig.

3.5 Corrections

We said above that lexical control is a sort of internal correction. Nevertheless lexical control has to be distinguished from "normal" corrections which usually involve some conscious processes (cf. Levelt 1983). Because of the participation of central systems, corrections may be only partially relevant for testing lexical organization processes of the language production module. In our corpus one finds, however, corrections suggesting unconscious access rather than conscious command of the language system:

(27) sie haben sich an der Ente *unschädlich getan, gemacht*, gehalten ← schadlos gehalten

This type of correction contains no perceptible metalinguistic markers indicating search procedures which normally interrupt those utterances. This may be another type of evidence rendering a clear cut distinction between on- and off-line processes unplausible. But apart from this, it illustrates locality rather clearly. The correction doesn't affect the complete verbal expression, but only one constituent and leaves the first one unmodified.
That the correction weakens the system of lexical access routines up to a "break down" is perhaps due to factors not very well understood and close to anomic patterns in aphasic speech.

3.6 Statistics

As already pointed out, formal substitutions show a high degree of similarity to the intended item. The same holds for lexically controlled errors. But while we take formal substitutions to occur as an one-step error induced by similarity of word-form, we take a lexical control error to be a two-step error. The first step is induced contextually and will lead to some intermediary non-realized form, usually a non-word. The presumably not cost-free second step – lexical control – is local and will suit this intermediary non-word-representation by means of a purely formal similarity to some existing word-entry. Under the premiss that lexical entries are accessed from left to right, this adaption should also be from left to right (cf. Garrett 1988).
Therefore, substitution and lexical control errors resemble each other in some aspects, but not in others. In lexical control, the starting point is a erroneous non-word, the processing product an erroneous word, so category identity may not really be calculated. We have still indicated it, as there may be cases where the errors have occurred at a stage where categorial status is given. Stress pattern, on the other hand, was not counted, since intermediary non-words were predominantly one syllable morphemes. Future work has to be done here.
The question at stake then is: Could these errors be of the same type, namely formal substitutions, – i.e. are there only formal substitutions and no lexical control errors? To our belief, the following figures evidence lexical control as an independent routine. Our predictions are:

1. Two-step lexical control errors are less frequent than one-step errors.[6]
This remains a relatively trivial prediction as long as we don't exactly know the relative frequency of occurrence of speech errors of specific types in general. As soon as we know, a calculation of the costs of lexical control will be possible. We must also admit that we have not yet differentiated between the types of segmental errors that elicit lexical control. Therefore, the statistics presented below may have to be changed in the course of further inquiry.

Table 1 Distribution of error types and affected units in the Frankfurter Versprecher Corpus

(N = 2100)	absolute frequency	relative frequency
error types:		
Substitutions	24 %	
Anticipations	19 %	
Perseverations	17 %	
Exchanges	15 %	
Blends	21 %	
affected units:		
segments	36 % (N = 747)	
words	30 % (N = 623)	
Formal substitutions	8 % (N = 167)	27 % of word errors
Lexical control	2 % (N = 39)	5 % of segmental errors

Word errors will not serve as an input to lexical control, but at least one third of all remaining errors, e.g. of the segmental type, will. As only 5 % of the segmental errors are lexically controlled, but 27 % of the word errors are formal substitutions, lexical control seems to be costly.
A rough example may be helpful. Suppose for instance, a speech error occurred at an average rate of 0,1 %, i.e. every 1000th word. Then, in around every 3000 words one finds one word-type error, and in about every 11000 words one finds a formal word substitution. One also finds about one segmental-type error in every 3000 words, but one would only detect one lexical control error in every 60000 words.

2. Formal substitutions and lexical control errors vary with respect to similarity of target and erroneous word, because of the contextually induced first step in lexical control.
For formal substitutions, Fay & Cutler (1977) observed a high formal similarity between error and target word. This was consistently found in surveys of different corpora (e.g. Dell & Reich 1981).
Table 2 shows the formal relations between 167 formal substitutions and their target words observed for German in the Frankfurter Versprecher Corpus and for English and compares these to the similarities between target and lexically controlled item. The German data nearly reproduce the results found in English corpora with respect to formal substitutions in stress pattern, category identity and number of syllables. There is also a comparable, but weaker tendency for onset and rime identity.
Lexically controlled items and target words show a significant difference in onset and coda identity. Therefore, form-based substitutions and lexical control are distinct processes. This also explains the relatively larger amount of categorial change as a result to be attributed to later lexical processing.

Table 2 Comparison of similarity between formal substitutions in German and English with similarity of target and lexically controlled item

	formal substit.		target/lex. control German (N = 39)
	German	English	
category identity	98 %	99 %	92 %
number of syllables	80 %	87 %	87 %
stress pattern	93 %	98 %	90 %
onset identity	67 %	87 %	15 %
peak			82 %
coda identity	70 %		15 %

Thus, lexical re-access again seems to be a costly procedure, despite of or maybe because it is depicting some selected information recall. Note also that the high rate of accommodation (spell-out) precludes an interpretation that will postpone lexical re-entry to later stages of processing. Therefore, monitoring is not the right way to describe lexical control, as we would simply not expect it to be that inaccurate. No one would need a monitoring or a control component that only took part of the information and produced results that possibly worsen normal production errors as is the case in category identity mistakes.

3. A higher degree of form relatedness for intermediate and erroneous word in lexical control when compared to similarities between target word and form substitution is predicted.
These findings come as no surprise, if one assumes that lexical control is a local, form-bound routine.

Table 3 Comparison of similarity in formal substitutions in German and English with similarity of intermediate and lexically controlled item

	formal substit.		interm./lex.control German (N = 39)
	German	English	
category identity	98 %	99 %	95 %
number of syllables	80 %	87 %	95 %
stress pattern	93 %	98 %	not counted
onset identity	67 %	87 %	74 %
peak			97 %
coda identity	70 %		28 %

4. There is a strong left to right similarity difference in lexical control errors between target and erroneous word and intermediary and erroneous word.

Table 4 Comparison of identity between target and lexically controlled item with identity between intermediate and lexically controlled item

	A. target/lex. control	B. interm./lex. control
(N = 39)		
Category	92 %	95 %
Syllables	87 %	95 %
stress	90 %	not counted
Onset	15 %	74 %
Peak	82 %	97 %
Coda	15 %	28 %

Recall that under our premiss the lexicon is accessed from left to right. The relevant aspects of tables 2 and 3, reassembled in table 4, thus support a linear lexical access mode.

The most striking difference to the pairs A. of table 4 which exhibit only minimal similarity is the onset congruity of the pairs in B. Note, that by onset we mean here: segments dominated by the onset constituent.[7]

The characteristics of lexical control seem to show that only limited information resources are available to this routine, namely of the phonological type. To illustrate this, we now give some examples:

(13b')	*spinn/stimm*	*spimm/spinn*
	different onset	common onset
	common peak	common peak
	different coda	different coda
(11d')	*kumm/fing*	*krumm/kumm*
	different onset	different onset
	different peak	common peak
	different coda	common coda

(13b') is the typical case, as table 4 clearly shows.

The high rate of identity between the peak of intended item and the resultant word and the still higher rate with respect to intermediary and resultant word might have consequences to depict the course of lexical access and for the internal structure of syllables. Absolute figures won't give all the cues, however, so we need to look at some relations that hold in lexical control. Then we will again address the fourth prediction.

5. The syllable we considered here consists of a flat structure of onset, peak, and coda, and is established through the melody bearing element. If lexical control 'reads' a flat syllable structure there should: (i) be no significant difference in agreement of either

Table 5 Co-occurrence relations between syllable constituents in lexically controlled item and target

lexically controlled item & target (N = 39)				
(NOT C) (BUT O)	8	(21 %)	AND P	6 (75 %)
(NOT O) (BUT C)	4	(10 %)	AND P	4 (100 %)
(NOT O, NOT C)	27	(69 %)	BUT P	22 (81 %)
(O AND C)	0		AND P	0
ONLY P	22	(56 %)		

Table 6 Co-occurrence relations between syllable constituents in intermediate and lexically controlled item

intermediate & lexically controlled item (N = 39)				
(NOT C) (BUT O)	28	(72 %)	AND P	27 (96 %)
(NOT O) (BUT C)	10	(26 %)	AND P	10 (100 %)
(NOT O, NOT C)	0		BUT P	0
(O AND C)	1	(3 %)	AND P	1 (100 %)

onset-peak or peak-coda sequences (table 5), (ii) exist a possibility to identify peaks (tables 5 and 6). If lexical access is from left to right, we expect to find (iii) a strong left to right similarity difference that shows up as an implicational relation between onset and peak (table 6). Finally, if lexical control is an access routine and not a separate processing level, we expect (iv) no further errors to be possible (table 6). Implication relations that bear on (i) and (ii) are given in tables 5 and 6.

Table 5 again shows the similarity of the lexically controlled item to the target item in terms of dependency relations between positions. The numbers seem to indicate that lexical control may access syllables by identifying peaks (ii), because in 56 % of the errors (i.e. three times more often than for onset and six times more often than for coda) there is only identity in the peak of target and controlled item, but in no other position.

There is some asymmetry, however, with respect to onset and coda identity with the peak (i). Onsets are identical in target and controlled item twice as often as codas, but this 'only' implies identity with peaks in 75 %, while if there is identity in coda there is also a 100 % identity with peaks. The same is true for peak-coda sequences in the relation of the intermediary non-word and lexically controlled item (table 6). Unfortunately, this leaves the question about the internal syllable structure still unanswered. Note finally that in 13 % of all errors there was no identity at all between target and controlled item.

As for the position-wise relations between intermediate and controlled item, table 6 strengthens the standard assumption of left to right lexical access (see prediction 4 above and (iii)). There is not a single case of a substitution in terms of non-shared positions; therefore, access is all that may happen, no three-step errors seem to be possible (iv). Therefore, lexical control does not have access to all information, i.e. it may not re-access the whole of the lexicon and may not re-compute all information, but only reads form entries. Given this, the high identity rate of the onset-peak sequences comes as no surprise and cannot on itself be an argument for a shallow syllable structure. By the way, this kind of selective information retrieval makes lexical control an unlikely candidate for current spreading activation processing models. This is not to say that one cannot arrange network layers in such a way. However, by doing so, everything hinges on that partition.

If there is anything that is unexpected, it is the 100 % implication of identical peak in case of coda identity (26 % of all cases). Again, we have to acknowledge that this may point to more structure. However, this question is independent of the status of lexical control.

Lexical control was shown to be an independent routine which uses purely formal information. It is a local process that computes segmental, syllable, and word-structure at most. As our analysis still rests on a rather slim data base, we naturally admit that the statistics may not be reliable yet. Still, to our belief, the qualitative aspects that render lexical control psychological reality will not be affected by a larger corpus.

4 Representation: Part two

We now want to address the question of what type of morphological structure a mental lexicon has to cope with in language processing, i.e. in production.

In neurolinguistic investigations, one very often refers to the logogen model, originally devised by Morton, which has the following properties:

- distinction of formal and semantico-lexical routes
- mapping graphemes to phonemes and vice-versa
- breakdown compatibility, that is, selective deficits can be predicted
- no internal structure of lexical items, therefore no finer analysis beyond phoneme-grapheme-correspondences can be based on it
- capability to distinguish processing of lexical items and non-words

Modifications of Morton's model all concern "boxes", that is, addition of further sub-components to the logogen.[8] We believe this model is not suitable for characterizing the internal structure of language processing units because it subsumes no interesting linguistic theory of the morphophonological construction principles natural languages make use of. Furthermore, as Pulvermüller (1992) argues, logogen models even seem to lack functional plausibility. Rather than simply adding further components one needs hypotheses concerning the domains these principles operate on during language processing.

In inquiries into the morphophonological make-up of Semitic languages, the expressive power of the grammatical lexicon was elaborated to a degree formerly not even thought of (McCarthy 1981; Keller & Leuninger 1993). Within this lexicon,

- the relation between morphological and phonological rules can now be expressed, e.g. word formation and syllabification;

- the rather vague distinction between diverse types of morpheme boundaries is motivated by level ordering;
- productive and non-productive word formations can be explained by this level ordering;
- various restrictions can be systematically described, e.g. the head condition.

With such a conception, phonological **and** morphological production errors receive a unified characterization, not only by assuming the lexicon to be the domain of operations, but also by exploiting the internal principles of the lexicon and its levels.
Up to now, we have tried to argue for the strong role of formal principles guiding language production. These can be simple and compound, as illustrated by the lexical control errors. We now want to have a closer look at the internal structure of lexical items, especially those items generated by morphological processes in lexical morphology. The above cited correction (27) is a first indicator to word level representations of considerable structural complexity.
This is the question of granularity. With respect to this question one illuminating example is found in Fromkin (1973). She notes a speech error – a rare one, but nevertheless one that has been processed and therefore needs explanation – which really is a challenge to all "surfacists":

(28) Rosa only date shranks ← Rosa only dated shrinks

This error has very interesting properties bearing directly upon our idea that the processor must compute "deep" representations and not only shallow ones, and that it must even do so on successive levels. The intended structure of (28) is something like (29):

(29) [$_{AGR\text{-}SP}$ [$_{NP}$ Rosa]$_i$ [$_{AGR\text{-}S'}$ [$_{TP}$ [$_{AGR\text{-}OP}$ [$_{AGR\text{-}O'}$ [$_{VP}$ only [$_{VP}$ t$_i$ [$_{V'}$ [$_V$ date] [$_{NP}$ shranks]]]]]]

The error results from an interaction of different components of the language capacity:
- perseveration of the I-Tense-feature;
- saturation of features;
- regular spell-out of features;
- categorial change.

To classify (28) as a perseveration is a direct consequence of the assumption that morphological spell-out is a rather late process, in analogy to accommodations such as (10), and that one doesn't find the phonetic form [*id*] in the resulting string.
Now, if syntactic features are saturated, the structure will satisfy all relevant well-formedness conditions of the syntax with respect to phonological form.[9] From the viewpoint of access to abstract lexical representations, this is a possible move, because *shrink* probably is noted with α-features, denoting N and V, or because [$_N$ *shrink*] is the outcome of a morphological derivation rule having [$_V$ *shrink*] as its base. The verbal form *date* inserted in AGR-S^0 leads to a syntactically correct result, as there are no non-saturated AGR- or TNS-features left.
Note that in such a structural approach the apparently missing accommodation of the verb *date* to the AGRS-/TNS-features is predicted, while in a shallow linear analysis

one would have to diagnose a strong grammatical violation, because no grammatic accommodation took place.
With the pending [+INFL]-feature the irregular past tense form of *shrink* can be "regularly" spelled out then as *shrank* on level I.
The stranding of the plural morpheme on *shrank* in the phonetic form of the error can only be regarded as evidence of a categorial change (V → N conversion) on level I/II.
An error, comparable in computational complexity to (28), is (2d) from our corpus, repeated here:

(30) (a) Die muß man mit rohen Handschuhen anfassen

The relevant structural parts of the alternatives underlying this blend are (30b) and (c):

(30) (b) wie ein **rohes** Ei behandeln
(c) mit **Samt**handschuhen anfassen

The fusion of the competing constructions presupposes a morphological reanalysis of *Samthandschuhen*, composed of an the head N (*Handschuhen*) and a modifying N (*Samt*), as a syntactic constituent N', [$_{N'}$[$_{A}$ *samtenen*][$_{N}$ *Handschuhen*]], consisting of A and N. This virtual structure must be temporarily generated internally so that the fusion (with subsequent grammatical control) is made possible (for a further grammatical analysis of blends containing affixes, cf. Gies 1993).
It seems evident, therefore, that representations may be very elaborated during language processing. Lexical information, including pairs of morphologically related forms, is available during the entire processing. This, then, is a variant of Kean's idea of lexical construal, a strategy even aphasic patients are able to use. The overall presence of the lexicon is perhaps comparable to the nowadays rather old-fashioned idea that the projection principle constrains all levels of syntactic derivation (cf. Chomsky 1981; but see Chomsky 1992). Note that neither the grammatical nor the functional projection principle is a global constraint increasing the expressive power up to non-learnability because this principle only checks strictly adjacent levels.

5 Morphologically complex words

Let us now extend the above sketched idea of fine granularity to morphologically derived words (cf. Bierwisch 1982). As we argued above, many speech errors do not require highly granular analyses, as e.g.:

(31) wieso wird sie nicht einfach *ausgemottet* ← ausgemustert/eingemottet

Nevertheless, the processing vocabulary at least needs such categories as "affix" and linear informations as "first" (prefix) or "last" (suffix), the latter obviously required for many stranding errors. Note that the break in a blend never falls into a prefix,

giving *aungemottet*, i.e. if the respective item is morphologically structured, this structure is in a sense retained (cf. Wiegand 1994, in prep.; Gies 1993).
Errors like (32) and (3) or (5a), repeated in (33), point to more structure because there must have been internal processes at work which cannot directly be read off the surface.

(32) (a) *saumsäumig* ← saumselig
(b) *lindernde* Umschläge ← mildernde Umstände
(c) *nerve die Nahrung, nähre die Nervung*, nähre den Nerv

(33) (a) da gibt's doch so einen *fliegenden Spruch* ← ein geflügeltes Wort
(b) wird das mit *Bindeschrift* geschrieben ← Bindestrich

(32a) is a perseveration with subsequent accommodation of the stem (Umlautung) to the suffix *ig*. (33a) requires a still more complex morphological analysis because a mere characterization as e.g. substitution wouldn't be sufficient. *Geflügeltes Wort* is an idiomatic N' which is formally broken up into constituents bearing specific semantic information. We leave the formulation of the precise relations between *geflügeltes* and *fliegender* and *Wort* and *Spruch* respectively to semantic theory. Anyway, both constituents have a common semantic core which can be spelled out in different ways by simultaneous loss of the specific semantic content. Errors of this type resemble the morphophonological algorithm proposed for Semitic languages where roots (semantic core) are the basis for all word formation processes (cf. McCarthy 1981).
Regularities of different lexical levels were used in the production of (33a), especially those of level I, where the non-productive nominalization *Spruch* is substituted by a non-derived noun. Another level I item is *geflügelt* which only apparently looks like a productive form. Contrary to that *fliegend* is a productively built item, which shows that the processor has accessed principles of level II. So, this error seems to be evidence for substituting non-productive forms by productive or non-derived forms. Note also that we find grammatical control, accommodating the gender feature of the adjectival modifier to its head in many errors here too.
One could analyze (32b) partially in analogy to (33a) because there is also a level II process deriving adjectives. But in this case, one is not compelled to do so. One could equally well analyze (32b) as a formal substitution of a collocational N'. In cases like this we adhere to a principle of structural adequacy the language production system seems to obey:

(34) Adapt granularity to structural needs

Following this principle, the processing device minimalizes its efforts to control (analyze, measure or otherwise correct) any of its outputs.[10] Going into depth is thus considered to be more costly than the processing of low granularity levels.
(33b) is caused by an anticipation of the stem underlying *schreiben* by reversing the inflectional process and deriving the non-productive nominalization *Schrift*, i.e. at least the relation between these two items must have been computed during language production. Formulated within the lexical framework assumed here, the speaker has simultaneous control of the lexical basis *schreib* and derived items, in our case, a nominaliza-

tion. As he now has to choose a form adequate for the intended noun position, he selects *Schrift* from level I.
Schematically this can be expressed as follows:
- schrieb-en → schreib-en (level I)
- anticipation in an N-position
- nominalization (level I) *Schrift*

Level-oriented speech errors are also found in the exchange (stranding) error (32c), this time the processor also makes use of the distinction between different productive and non-productive word formation structures, preferring the productive *ung* for nominalizing. Apart from this, (32c) is a combination of the processes involved in (32a) and (33b), schematically:

(32) (c) 1. nerve die Nahrung
2. nähre die Nervung
3. nähre den Nerv

1. - exchange of the stems *nahr* (reversing Umlautung, level I) and *nerv*;
   - spell-out of N-features for *nahr* by inserting *ung* (level II)

2. - exchange of the stems *nerv* and *nahr*
   - stranding *ung*

3. - spell-out of the irregular N- and V-forms of *nerv* and *nahr* with Umlautung (level I word formation)

All steps involve stranding of the inflection morpheme *e*.
Whatever position one may have with respect to the upper bounds of granularity, a morphological spell-out must have occurred in order to get the "right" item for a noun position in (32c). For this reason, a morphological analysis must have taken place during language production. Obviously, a mere surface oriented explanation is not sufficient here because *ung* is not present in the intended utterance. So, in contrast to Garrett's assumption, the processor must have access to a lexical entry for the clitic together with its subcategorization information (cf. Höhle 1982). In the same vein, Bierwisch (1970) notes that while processing

(35) Dem muß man ja seine eigene *Posterklärung ordnen* ← Postordnung erklären

the language production system must temporarily analyse [*erklärung*] and [*ordnung*] as being composed out of the respective verb-stems that are the basis for *-ung*-nominalization.

6 Conclusion: A unified model for representing language production data

A closer look at representational properties of language production data motivated our approach, namely, the overwhelming role played by lexical properties during language processing. This is only possible if it is assumed that the lexicon is modelled alongside lexical phonology and morphology. Such a model sharply contrasts with the usual functional models generally assumed in neuro- and psycholinguistic research, e.g. all variants of the logogen model.

In this article, we sketched an approach which allows for a unified description of all phonological and morphological, that is, form-based errors. We considered two components of a language production theory, representation and processes. The locus of all such errors is the lexicon.

The procedural component will incorporate the following planning types with the relevant psycholinguistic vocabulary:[11]

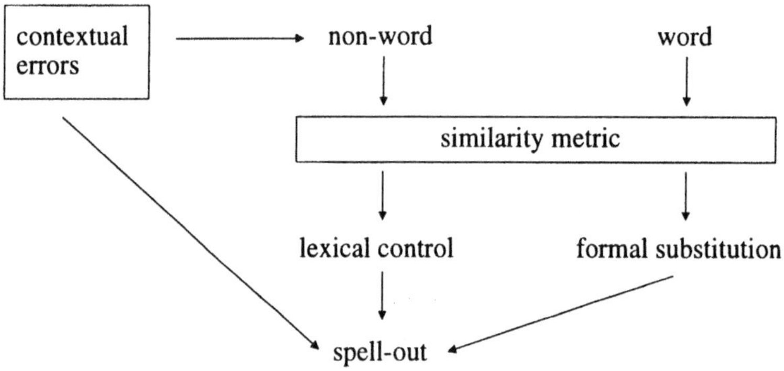

Such a unified treatment will contain a similarity metric which computes the lexical distance of error and intended item. This metric must be expressive enough to match the respective items against the following structural variables:

- category
- morphological constituency
- syllable structure (number, onset, peak, coda)
- metrical grid
- segmental structure (including features)

As formal word substitutions, lexical control errors are predicted to be strictly local, i.e. word-bound.

In general, form-based speech errors display maximal similarity, that is, minimal lexical distance. As Klein & Leuninger (1988, 1990) showed, the majority of speech errors do not differ in syllable structure and modify the intended item by at most two segmental changes. In other words, the lexical distance is minimal. In contrast, phonological paraphasias destroy the CV-structure which amounts to a maximal distortion of the structure of the intended item. This directly relates to the model of lexical phonology

and morphology with its strictly level-ordered representations. The earlier a distortion, the worse the resultant failure.
With respect to morphology, speech errors show the psychological plausibility of distinct levels of word formation. Even if a planning failure may land items in unintended syntactic positions, the processor has control of rich morphological vocabulary (affix, word, morpheme), so that by the means of morphological spell-out a moved item is accurately accommodated to its final position.

Notes

1 For connectionist processing models see e.g. Berg (1988); Blanken et al. (1988); Dell & Reich (1981); Dell (1986); Rumelhardt & McClelland (1986); Schade (1992); Stemberger (1985). Symbolic models are discussed in the following.

2 All examples of speech errors are from the *Frankfurter Versprecher Corpus*, unless indicated otherwise.

3 An investigation into the nature of this metric may possibly reveal decisive properties of representation formats, i.e. in parallel distributed processing a metric should be a cost-free adaption to the most likely, most salient (complex of) units, in (parallel) symbolic processing a metric is expected to use structural information.

4 This presumes syllabification on non-derived forms.

5 Again the mere possibility of multiple, distinct, and decomposable units asks for a representational system that is not a priori limited to specific content.

6 The expression "two-steps" is often used in another interpretation, meaning that lexical access first addresses the (semantics of a) lexical item and then its form (cf. Dell & Reich,1981). Contrary to that, we understand both steps as form-oriented processing; for aspects of statistical validity in error collections, cf. Ferber 1993.

7 The parallelism to the so-called "tip-of-the-tongue" phenomena is striking (Brown & McNeill 1966). The results show a dominance of first segments in lexical search procedures. Nevertheless, in most of the investigations considering the phonology of words no explicit assumptions with respect to syllable structure are made beyond mere linearity (for language production processes cf. Cutler 1982).

8 For applications to reading and writing cf. de Bleser 1991; Blanken 1992a; for aphasic processing of morphology and phonology cf. Nespoulous & Villiard 1992.

9 One could conceive of *shrank(s)* as being wrongly inserted in the INFL-position, but this would lead to a global destruction of sentence structure and begs the question of the plural morpheme.

10 One could well imagine that other aspects come into play here, e.g. processing time left in some situation, which might also have some impact on the depth of processing. This is in line with the following principle: Adapt granularity to time slice left for production. In the worst case, i.e. little time and necessarily deep analysis, the product will most likely remain a non-word; in the best case a close fit of an existing word will substitute the erroneous intermediary representation.

11 *Contextual* does of course not imply an unbounded error span, but in general means clause boundedness as in: *Und nun ein Blick auf den DAX. Der **LAX** liegt bei x Punkten* (cf. Garrett 1975).

References

Berg, T. (1988): Die Abbildung des Sprachproduktionsprozesses in einem Aktivationsflußmodell. Tübingen.

Bierwisch, M. (1970): "Fehler-Linguistik". Linguistic Inquiry 1, 397 – 414.

Bierwisch, M. (1982): "Linguistics and language error". In: A. Cutler, ed., Slips of the tongue and language production. Amsterdam.

Blanken, G. et al. (1988): Sprachproduktionsmodelle. Neuro- und psycholinguistische Theorien zur menschlichen Spracherzeugung. Freiburg.

Blanken, G. (1992a): "Die kognitive Neurolinguistik des Schreibens". In: G. Blanken, ed., 1992.

Blanken, G. (1992b): "Die Produktion geschriebener und gesprochener Wörter bei Aphasie. Eine Gruppenstudie". Working Papers of the Interdisciplinary Research Group on Neurolinguistics. Freiburg.

Blanken, G., ed., (1992): Einführung in die linguistische Aphasiologie. Theorie und Praxis. Freiburg.

Bower, G., ed., (1975): The psychology of learning and motivation. New York.

Browman, C.P. (1980): "Perceptual processing: Evidence from slips of the ear". In: V.A. Fromkin, ed., Errors in linguistic performance: Slips of the tongue, ear, pen, and hand. New York.

Brown, R. & D. McNeill (1966): "The 'tip of the tongue' phenomenon". Journal of Verbal Learning and Verbal Behavior 5, 325 – 337.

Caplan, D. u.a., eds., (1984): Biological perspectives on language. Cambridge/Mass.

Carlson, G. & K. Tanenhaus, eds., (1987): Linguistic structure in language processing. New York.

Chomsky, N. (1981): Lectures of government and binding. Dordrecht.

Chomsky, N. (1992): A minimalist program for linguistic theory. M.I.T. Occasional Papers in Linguistics 1. Cambrigde/Mass.

Clements, G.N. & S.J. Keyser (1983): CV-phonology. A generative theory of the syllable. Cambridge/Mass.

Cooper, W.E. & E.C.T. Walker, eds., (1979): Sentence processing: Psycholinguistic studies. Hillsdale.

Cutler, A. (1982): "The reliability of speech error data". In: A. Culter, ed., Slips of the tongue and language production. Amsterdam.

Cutler, A., ed., (1982): Slips of the tongue and language production. Amsterdam.

de Bleser, R. (1991): "Formen und Erklärungsmodelle erworbener Dyslexien". In: G. Blanken, ed., 1992.

Dell, G.S. & P.A. Reich (1981): "Stages in sentence production: An analysis of speech error data". Journal of Verbal Learning and Verbal Behavior 20, 611 – 629.

Dell, G.S. (1986): "A spreading-activation theory of retrieval in sentence production". Psychological Review 93, 283 – 321.

Dittmann, J. (1991): "Phonematische Störungen bei Aphasie". In: G. Blanken, ed., 1992.

Ellis, A.W. & A.W. Young (1988): Human cognitive neuropsychology. London u.a.

Ellis, A.W., ed., (1985): Progress in the psychology of language. Vol. 1. Hillsdale.

Fay, D. & A. Cutler (1977): "Malapropisms and the structure of the mental lexicon". Linguistic Inquiry 8, 505 – 520.

Ferber, R. (1993): Wie valide sind Versprechersammlungen? Bern.

Fodor, J.A. & Z.W. Pylyshyn (1988): "Connectionism and cognitive architecture: A critical analysis". Cognition 28, 3 – 71.

Fodor, J.A. (1975): The language of thought. New York.

Fodor, J.A. (1983): The modularity of mind. Cambridge/Mass.

Fodor, J.A. et al. (1980): "Against definitions". Cognition 8, 263 – 367.

Forster, K.I. (1979): "Levels of processing and the structure of the language processor". In: W.E. Cooper & E.C.T. Walker, eds.: Sentence processing: Psycholinguistic studies. Hillsdale.
Frith, U., ed., (1980): Cognitive processes in spelling. London.
Fromkin, V.A. (1973): "Introduction to Fromkin". In: V.A. Fromkin, ed., Speech errors as linguistic evidence. The Hague.
Fromkin, V.A., ed., (1973): Speech errors as linguistic evidence. The Hague.
Fromkin, V.A., ed., (1980): Errors in linguistic performance: Slips of the tongue, ear, pen, and hand. New York.
Garrett, M.F. (1975): "The analysis of sentence production". In: G. Bower, ed., The psychology of learning and motivation. New York.
Garrett, M.F. (1976): "Speech errors as linguistic evidence". In: R.J. Wales & E. Walker, eds.: New approaches to language mechanisms. Amsterdam.
Garrett, M.F. (1988): "Processes in language production". In: F.J. Newmeyer, ed., Linguistics: The Cambridge Survey. Vol. III: Psychological and biological aspects of language. Cambridge.
Garrett, M.F. (1992): "Lexical retrieval processes: Semantic field effects". In: A. Lehrer & E. Feder Kittay, eds., Frames, fields, and contrasts. Hove.
Gies, A. (1993): Was sich auch bei Kontaminationen passiert. Zum modularen Aufbau der Basiskomponente. Doctoral Diss., University of Frankfurt.
Grinberg Pla, V. (1994): "Zur hierarchischen Struktur der Silbe". Frankfurter Linguistische Forschungen 16.
Harley, T.A. (1984): "A critique of top-down independent levels of speech production: Evidence from non-plan-internal speech errors". Cognitive Science 8, 191 – 219.
Hillert, D. (1992): "Lexical semantics and aphasia: A state-of-the-art review". Journal of Neurolinguistics 7, 1 – 43.
Hillert, D. (1994a): The temporal course of semantic access in aphasia: Some explanations. Montréal TENNET V. Ms.
Hillert, D. (1994b): "Lexical selection in production: Reflections on spontaneous speech errors". Frankfurter Linguistische Forschungen 16.
Höhle, T. (1982): "Über Komposition und Derivation: Zur Konstituentenstruktur von Wortbildungsprodukten im Deutschen". Zeitschrift für Sprachwissenschaft 1, 76 – 112.
Hornstein, N. & D. Lightfoot, eds., (1981): Explanation in neurolinguistics. The logical problem of language acquisition. London.
Hotopf, W.H.N. (1980): "Semantic similarity as a factor in whole-word slips of the tongue". In: V.A. Fromkin, ed., Errors in linguistic performance: Slips of the tongue, ear, pen, and hand. New York.
Huber, W. (1981): "Semantic confusions in aphasia". In: B.B. Rieger, ed., Empirical semantics. Bochum.
Kean, M.-L. (1977): "The linguistic interpretation of aphasic syndromes. Agrammatism in Broca's aphasia: an example". Cognition 5, 9 – 46.
Kean, M.-L. (1981): "Explanation in neurolinguistics". In: N. Hornstein & D. Lightfoot, eds.: Explanation in neurolinguistics. The logical problem of language acquisition. London.
Keller, J. & H. Leuninger (1993): Grammatische Strukturen – kognitive Prozesse. Tübingen.
Klein, M. & H. Leuninger (1988): "Gestörtes und nicht-gestörtes Sprachverhalten: Zur Struktur lautlicher Fehlleistungen". Frankfurter Linguistische Forschungen 5, 1 – 19.
Klein, M. & H. Leuninger (1990): "Gestörtes und nicht-gestörtes Sprachverhalten: Zur Analyse lautlicher Fehlleistungen im Rahmen nicht-linearer phonologischer Theorien". Frankfurter Linguistische Forschungen 8, 1 – 17.
Laubstein, A. (1987): "Syllable structure: The speech error evidence". Canadian Journal of Linguistics 32, 339 – 363.
Leuninger, H. (1989): Neurolinguistik: Probleme, Paradigmen, Perspektiven. Opladen.
Levelt, W.J.M. (1983): "Monitoring and self-repair in speech". Cognition 14, 41 – 104.

Levelt, W.J.M. (1989): Speaking. From intention to articulation. Cambridge/Mass.
Marslen-Wilson, W.D. & L.K. Tyler (1980): "An interactive activation model of context effects in letter perception: Part 1. An account of basic finding". Psychological Review 88, 357 – 407.
McCarthy, J.J. (1981): "A prosodic of nonconcatenative morphology". Linguistic Inquiry 12, 373 – 418.
Meringer, R. & C. Mayer (1895): Versprechen und Verlesen. Eine psychologisch-linguistische Studie. Stuttgart. Reprinted 1978. Amsterdam.
Morton, J. (1980): "The logogen model and orthographic structure". In: U. Frith, ed., Cognitive processes in spelling. London.
Morton, J. (1984): "Brain based and non-brain based models of language". In: D. Caplan u.a., eds.: Biological perspectives on language. Cambridge/Mass.
Nespoulous, J.-L. & P. Villiard, eds., (1992): Morphology, phonology, and aphasia. New York.
Newkirk, D. et al. (1980): "Linguistic evidence from slips of the hand". In: A. Fromkin, ed., Errors in linguistic performance: Slips of the tongue, ear, pen, and hand. New York.
Newmeyer, F.J., ed., (1988): Linguistics: The Cambridge Survey. Vol. III: Psychological and biological aspects of language. Cambridge.
Pulvermüller, F. (1992): "Bausteine einer neurologisch-linguistischen Theorie". In: G. Rickheit et al., eds.: Linguistische Aspekte der Sprachtherapie. Forschung und Intervention bei Sprachstörungen. Opladen.
Rickheit, G. et al., eds., (1992): Linguistische Aspekte der Sprachtherapie. Forschung und Intervention bei Sprachstörungen. Opladen.
Rieger, B.B., ed., (1981): Empirical semantics. Bochum.
Rumelhardt, D.E. & J.L. McClelland, eds., (1986): Parallel distributed processing: Explorations in the microstructure of cognition. Cambridge/Mass.
Schade, U. (1992): Konnektionismus. Zur Modellierung der Sprachproduktion. Opladen.
Selkirk, E. (1982): "The syllable". In: H. van der Hulst & N. Smith, eds.: The structure of phonological representations. Vol. 2. Dordrecht.
Stachowiak, F.-J. (1979): Zur semantischen Struktur des subjektiven Lexikons. München.
Stachowiak, F.-J. (1982): "Haben Wortbedeutungen eine gesonderte mentale Repräsentation gegenüber dem Weltwissen? – Neurolinguistische Überlegungen". Linguistische Berichte 79, 12 – 29.
Stemberger, J.P. (1983): "Inflectional malapropisms: Form-based errors in English morphology". Linguistics 21, 573 – 602.
Stemberger, J.P. (1985): "An interactive activation model of language production". In: A.W. Ellis, ed., Progress in the psychology of language. Vol. 1. Hillsdale.
Treiman, R. (1989): "The internal structure of the syllable". In: G. Carlson & K. Tanenhaus, eds.: Linguistic structure in language processing. New York.
van der Hulst, H. & N. Smith, eds., (1982): The structure of phonological representations. Vol. 2. Dordrecht.
Wales, R.J. & E. Walker, eds., (1976): New approaches to language mechanisms. Amsterdam.
Wiegand, D. (1994): "Die Verfügbarkeit lexikalischer Informationen während des Sprachproduktionsprozesses". Frankfurter Linguistische Forschungen 15, 1 – 17.
Wiegand, D. (in prep.): Die Sprachproduktion als modular organisierter Prozeß: Zur Struktur und Berechnung von Kontaminationen. Doctoral Diss., University of Frankfurt.
Wiese, R. (1988): Silbische und lexikalische Phonologie. Studien zum Chinesischen und Deutschen. Tübingen.
Wiese, R. (1991): "Was ist extrasilbisch im Deutschen und warum?" Zeitschrift für Sprachwissenschaft 10, 112 – 133.

Spontaneous Language and Impairment of Communication in Alzheimer's Disease

Pierre Marcie, Michel Roudier, François Boller, Paris

Impaired communication is one of the main and most incapacitating symptoms of Alzheimer's disease and related dementias (referred to by the abbreviation AD). AD patients invariably loose in a progressive fashion their capacity to handle the various "instrumentalities" (Goldstein 1948) needed for verbal communication. These constitute a system which is the sum of knowledge shared by the members of the same community. This system could be represented as organized hierarchically and requires resources which vary according to the type of linguistic task. Studies of verbal communication in AD have documented most of the metalinguistic and basic linguistic functions, focusing mainly on tasks that imply the use of well known rules as is the case for naming and grammatical transformations. Since the rule is known, errors may be clearly described, thus leading to hypotheses concerning their generation.

The highest and most complex level of linguistic capacities is reached during the exchange of "spontaneous" language, where the speakers are concerned mainly with the content of the information rather than by its strict linguistic form. In spontaneous language, the speakers share a certain number of semantic values and linguistic rules. Spontaneous language can take many forms, depending on a variety of situations, a few examples being: "Job interviews, telephone calls, joke- and story-telling episodes, teacher-pupil exchanges, a range of recorded psychiatric, psychotherapeutic and psychological investigative abilities" (McGregor 1984). For each situation, the discourse needs to take its own form and follow its own rules. In a sense, spontaneous language is a misnomer since in most clinical situations the examiner must act as a "trigger" by initiating and maintaining the exchange. Nevertheless the term is deeply rooted in ordinary use and may be used simply to qualify "a 'semi-induced' verbal exchange" (Irigaray 1973).

In clinical situations involving the study of spontaneous language in cognitively impaired patients, one attempts to gather a corpus of speech under conditions which should be as free of constraints as possible. Linguistic analysis applied to such a corpus deals generally with the units or signs specific to each layer (Horejsi 1961), be it phonemic, morphologic, syntactic or at the discourse-level. These layers are organized hierarchically starting with a lower level (phonemic) and ending at the level of the utterance. The analysis is concerned mainly with the distributional properties of the units. At the level of the utterances, the problem is more complex because this component of discourse is realized through the integration of units originating from lower levels. Identical analyses may be used for the purpose of drawing inferences on the organization (or disorganization) of the informational content of the discourse. However, in analogy to what happens with the lower levels, utterances should be analyzed using units which in that case are based on informational content. This should provide an objective measure of the meaning implied during the verbal exchange. The distinction of normal from pathological speech relies on the measure of informational content of the verbal sequences.

Spontaneous language in dementia patients usually follows a pattern of turn-taking similar to that of normal subjects. As stated by Cutler (Cutler, Haxby, Duara, Grady, Kay & Kessler et al. 1985), various means are used in conversational exchanges, either in isolation or embedded, to perform this alternation. In the spontaneous language of AD patients, variations of prosodic contours represent the main index used to mark the end of the currently spoken sequence. In normals, a fall of FØ, a decrease of voice pitch and a lengthening of the last syllable (or of the last stressed syllable) constitute the main cues marking the end of an utterance. As in normal speakers, the end of an utterance can also be announced by stereotyped sentences usually devoid of meaning, such as "you know". These indices work equally well whether the sentence is grammatically complete or not. However, other more cognitively loaded indices seem to play a decreased role in AD patients as part of the impoverishment of available communicative tools. These include changes in gaze intensity, hand gestures, etc. However, even though these interactions are decreased, they reflect the preservation of a fundamental layer of generalized skills aimed at coordinating the behavior of two speakers. Quite obviously, there is more to social interaction than just language, but language occupies such an important position among the constituent "channels" of information exchange (gaze, gesture, posture, facial expression) that it has quite naturally come to provide a major focus for studies within the "Conversational Analysis tradition" (French & Local 1986). Therefore other ways must be sought to characterize the level of communicative disorders in the verbal expression of demented patients.

Prosody is a priori an equally poor way of differentiating normal from pathological speech. Despite the lack of systematic studies, it has been shown that in normal speakers, monosyllabic replies often have a prosodic contour characterized by a small range of pitch variation producing a standardized and monotonous result (Crystal 1969; Crystal & Davy 1969; Crystal & Quirk 1964). This probably applies to AD language. Prosodic falls which tend to occur frequently in normals may be more frequent in demented patients because their discourse is chopped and discontinuous. A tendency to generate short tonal units, also a constant feature of AD language, is frequently encountered in normals. The same applies to vocal hesitation like "hum". The pause system (Goldman-Eisler 1968) which is specific of each type of verbal expression and part of their identification is one of the few where changes have been documented. AD patients tend to show more frequent pauses which tend to occur at the point where content words are supposed to appear.

In view of the relative preservation of these conversational and melodic skills, differences must be sought elsewhere, i.e. information content.

In her landmark work on language in dementia, Luce Irigaray (1967, 1973) dealt more with the metalinguistic components of language than with spontaneous expression per se. She dealt particularly with verbal naming, reading aloud, writing on dictation, copying and with a set of metalinguistic tasks. All these tasks have in common that they imply the existence of a prototype of the performance model. Errors can be described, analyzed and possibly explained. The imbalance between her analysis of these tasks and that of spontaneous language is reflected by the disproportion between the 11 chapters dedicated to them and the single chapter (chapter 15), 17 pages long, dedicated to spontaneous language. In this chapter ("Etude du langage spontané et/ou semi-induit"), Irigaray points out that dementia patients often do not produce much "spontaneous" speech and that they have to be incited to engage into a verbal exchange. Hence the concept of "semi-induced language" which implies that the patient is encouraged by the examiner to talk on a topic familiar to him.
Linguistic performances were recorded in population recruited in two centers:

- 32 patients were examined in the research group directed by Dr. H. Hécaen at the Sainte-Anne Hospital in Paris;
- 20 patients had been examined following the same protocol at Bel-Air (the Psychiatry Department of the University of Geneva), directed then by J. de Ajuriaguerra. The diagnosis of AD had been established jointly by Drs. Ajuriaguerra, Tissot and Richard;
- a group of 20 normal control subjects received the same battery of linguistic tests.

Of course the diagnosis of "AD" is not mentioned in Irigaray's work because at that time, the disease was referred to with other names. The patients were diagnosed as having "senile dementia" on the basis of hospital admission due to a behavioral disorder, clear-cut mental deterioration (documented either by a WAIS or equivalent tests, or by Piaget's tests, the so-called "épreuves opératoires") and a neurological examination showing "diffuse cortical lesions" with the exclusion of focal signs.
The analysis of spontaneous language is limited to 7 subjects out of the 52, probably due to the methodological problem related to this type of data. The sample of speech consisted of about 150 "mots graphiques", i.e. graphemic strings enclosed between two graphic delimiters. Subjects had been chosen on the basis of a wide range of deterioration.
The bulk of her work dealt with the distribution of various types of words obtained from transcripts of spontaneous speech. The distribution of language elements in the demented discourse was thought to reflect systematic differences which could be considered characteristic features of the impact of dementia upon language generation.
Content words comprise 5 to 12 % of the output compared to about 45 % in controls. The reduction of the available lexical stock is correlated to the severity of dementia. The poverty of the demented language is felt to be due to a reduction in the "elements of the code" rather than their realization, since repetition is preserved.
Liaison words (inter- and intra-clause words, words used to indicate the various relationships associating speakers to each other in utterance course, or words used to link objects from outside into actual utterance) are more numerous and exceed the number of content words, a pattern opposite to that usually found in normals. These changes

Table 1 Distribution (percent) of parts of speech
(from L. Irigaray, Le Langage des Déments. Mouton: The Hague-Paris 1973: 278)

Subjects	Verbs			Substantives	Adjectives – Adverbs			Pronouns			Articles + adj. demo posses. indefinite etc.	Conjunctions	Prepositions	Interjections
	content	auxiliary & modal	auxiliary *be/have*		content	time place generic	negation	personal	relative	indefinite & others				
Font.	9.8	4.1	6.6	10.6	1.6	4.1	2.5	13.9	4.9	4.1	14.8	6.6	12.3	4.1
Mero.	10.0	4.0	7.0	6.0	8.0	12.0	7.0	13.0	4.0	7.0	10.0	9.0	2.0	1.0
Hard.	5.0	6.0	9.0	10.0	1.0	15.0	2.0	14.0	–	13.0	7.0	10.0	8.0	–
Blan.	6.7	5.0	5.8	10.0	3.3	5.8	4.2	20.0	3.3	5.8	10.0	9.2	4.2	6.7
Bour.	11.7	4.7	6.1	9.9	1.9	7.0	4.2	16.0	1.4	10.8	12.2	6.6	4.7	2.8
Chri.	6.1	10.7	5.6	8.2	1.5	8.2	4.1	18.4	2.0	8.7	11.7	9.7	3.1	2.0
Mach.	6.1	4.7	12.2	6.1	0.7	6.1	4.7	19.6	4.7	8.1	12.8	6.8	5.4	2.0

are linked to a deterioration of the sentence generating process and to the presence of numerous anacolutha. The number of verbs is greater in AD patients. The prevalence of purely function words over content words seems correlated to a decrease in semantic load and contributes to the impression of "semantic emptiness" provided by the patients' output.
When only the different lexical roots actually observed in the analyzed sample are taken into account, the ratio of root items versus content words appears even more unbalanced because of the high frequency of repetitions, stereotypes and perseverations.

Table 2 Occurrences of content words and lexical roots
(from L. Irigaray, Le Langage des Déments. Mouton: The Hague-Paris 1973: 280)

Subjects	Verbs		Substantives		Adjectives – Adverbs		Total	
	words	roots	words	roots	words	roots	words	roots
Font.	9,80	8,70	10,60	9,00	1,60	1,60	22,00	19,30
Mero.	10,00	10,00	6,00	5,00	8,00	5,00	24,00	20,00
Hard.	5,00	3,00	10,00	6,00	1,00	1,00	16,00	10,00
Blan.	6,70	4,20	10,00	8,30	3,30	1,70	20,00	14,20
Bour.	11,70	5,60	9,90	7,50	1,90	1,90	23,50	15,00
Chri.	6,10	5,10	8,20	7,70	1,50	1,50	15,80	14,00
Mach.	6,10	4,70	6,10	4,10	0,70	0,70	12,90	9,50

Another feature of pathological speech is the low specificity of semantic elements. One finds instead a high ratio of indefinite pronouns and adjectives, of auxiliary verbs, of modal auxiliary verbs (such as "to know", "to say", "to be able", "to do", etc.), of adverbs and adjectives (such as "very", "more", "also", etc.) which bear no precise information, contributing highly to that impression of a semantically empty discourse. Irigaray emphasizes that the range of lexemes present in the speech of demented belong to the 150-word-set the more frequently used in ordinary speech, as noted it in a previous work (Dubois, Marcie, Irigaray, Hécaen & Angelergues 1965).
Irigaray provides precise Tables summarizing the number and type of substantives present in the speech sample generated by one of her patients (Chri.). Out of 14 substantives, only 5 bear optimal level of lexical specificity ("frère", "père", "fille", "monsieur" as used to contextually indicate "docteur", "père Joseph") against 6 where the lexical specificity is rather shallow ("enfants", "gosses", "bonhommes", "bonnes femmes", "gens", "tout le monde") and 3 other ones ("choses" twice, "machins") which are "generic" lexical entities without any meaning at all.
Since they constitute linguistic utterances, theses fragments are syntactically structured. However, the syntax tends to be "simple and short", reflecting a reduction of the available syntactic schemes. Sentences are mainly of the kernel type, associating a

nominal phrase (subject) to a verbal more or less compounded phrase. Such a trend is still more effective as utterances are frequently incomplete. But, unlike what is found in normal speech, non verbal completion procedures are rarely observed. This may be related to the fact that utterances are often unfinished.

Irigaray notes the frequent usage of the first person pronominal form as sentence subject. The use of coordination particles to indicate the succession of the sentence components rather than the logical relations between ideas, contributes to a certain dissociation between the syntactic and logical articulation of the utterances. Words and particles of syntactic articulations are used in a way which tends to be automatic and independent of the actual logical relations implied in normal conditions.

On the basis on these distributional descriptions, Irigaray raises the question of what differentiates the discourse of the demented patients from the normal discourse. She concludes that the inadequacy of demented discourse is due to an inability of the speaker to insure a coherent transfer of information in the very context in which it can and must be understood. To what extent measures observed could allow to precisely define and characterize such an inadequacy of verbal expression? She describes two types of logico-verbal mechanisms eliciting verbal generation in demented patients. In terms then in use during this "generativist" period, she refers to "failure models". For each of them, she recognized the discourse sample of one her patients as the prototypical form of the given mechanism. The AD discourse is "incoherent" in either case, but the process responsible for it is different.

In the first case, (exemplified by the patient "Jall."), incoherence stems from a high rate of redundancy, as consecutive clauses follow each other with a minimal change from one clause to the next one. Generally the next clause is linked to the previous one in such a way that it is highly probable. This high probability contributes to lessen the distinctiveness which must be present in any new sentence to afford a new semantic meaning. Such a process can even reach a true tautological level, as shown in the following utterance: "Je ne boirai pas parce que je ne boirai" ("I shall not drink because I shall not drink"). Thus L. Irigaray schematized the actual process under the sequence of capitalized letters in which the closer the letters in the alphabet, the closer the semantic contents of one clause to the other. In the case just mentioned A = A. With many variations, this process can be found in many other instances of verbal expression.

Table 3 (from L. Irigaray, Le Langage des Déments. Mouton: The Hague-Paris 1973)

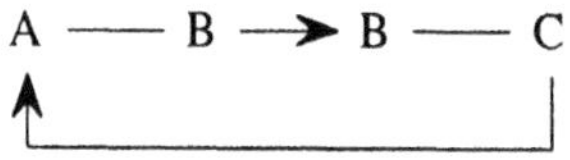

In the second case incoherence proceeds from a high level of improbability associating consecutive clauses, and lack of logico-syntactic relationships. Thus in Irigaray's words, the first utterance A is not followed by the highly probable A or B, but some very far L, or even X thematic element which prevents the receiver from understanding. The discourse could be schematized as follows:

Table 4 (from L. Irigaray, Le Langage des Déments. Mouton: The Hague-Paris 1973)

A —— B ⟶ B —— C ⟶ L —— X ⟶ P —— Z , etc.

Thus the two types of demented patients' discourse could be located on either side of the model of "normal" discourse, which can be understood as built up of an "optimal" degree of redundancy:

Table 5 (from L. Irigaray, Le Langage des Déments. Mouton: The Hague-Paris 1973)

A —— B ⟶ B —— C ⟶ C —— D ⟶ D —— E , etc.

As a conclusion to her analysis of spontaneous speech in demented patients, Irigaray proposes a theoretical model of discourse generation. It takes into account the semantic and informational content which cannot be extracted directly from the analysis of parts of a discourse or of syntagmatic levels. Her analysis of spontaneous speech has led her to propose a model essentially based on a semantic analysis based in turn on the coherence of the discourse in relation to the informational redundancy of the utterances. In normals, optimal redundancy allows transfer of new information while keeping a link with the previous informational element (or elements). Table 5 illustrates this process. The two forms of pathological discourse she recognizes are situated at both extremes of this coherence continuum. In the fist case, redundancy is excessive to the point of becoming reduced to tautological expressions where the conveyed information is too weak to bring new elements to the stream of discourse. In the second case, redundancy is insufficient. The extreme improbability of the elements or at least of some elements no longer allow one to identify a common thread linking the various elements of the discourse.

The problem with this approach is that it rests on data which do not measure directly the informational content of the discourse of AD patients. Semantic contents and meaning cannot be inferred directly from the analysis of segmental strings, even if one also analyses suprasegmental indices and paralinguistic events. Such an analysis requires integration of these elements within the contextual informations peculiar to the knowledge shared by the speakers.

This has led us to an attempt to define direct measure of the information included in AD discourse. The proposed measure is situated right at the level of expression of the deficit. First we have re-examined Irigaray's method on the basis of a corpus obtained from 2 AD patients and one normal hospitalized control matched for age and education level. Our goal was to verify the extent to which that method could produce similar results. Our linguistic corpus was larger than that of Irigaray consisting of 274 "graphic words" for the normal subject and 279 and 222 for the 2 AD patients. This represents a sample of about 5 minutes. We have counted words, types of words, pauses, and types of verbs. We have also evaluated the ratio between words and the number of different lexical roots.

Table 6 Number of pauses

	Pauses
control	3 (1,1 %)
AD patient (MMS 9)	12 (5,40 %)
AD patient (MMS 15)	22 (8,17 %)

The only measure which differentiates the two patients from the control is the number of pauses which is much greater in the output of the two AD patients (Table 6). Pauses do not play any special role and carry no insight either at the syntactic or at the stylistic level. They don't even provide information on the informational emptiness of the discourse, but they contribute to our perception of it. The pauses are a consequence of the difficulties that patients have to verbalize a given "idea" and to evoke the words necessary to express it.

Pauses were evaluated on the basis of a subjective assessment of the elapsed duration of silence. This index had not been systematically studied by Irigaray. It is true that it is not sufficiently pertinent to form the basis of a distinction between patients and normals. But Irigaray considered them as an index of semantic deficit which however is located out of the realm of semantic processing.

The same procedure used by Irigaray led us to different results. This difference may be due to the heterogeneity of the clinical expression of AD. These results, tentative as they are in view of the size of the sample, do not allow statements to be made concerning the semantic deficit or to provide an interpretation of it.

Table 7 Type of words

Subjects	Content	Fonctional	Empty	Paraphasic
control	109 (39,4 %)	161 (58,1 %)	3 (1,1 %)	4 (1,5 %)
AD patient (MMS 9)	88 (39,6 %)	128 (57,6 %)	2 (0,9 %)	4 (1,8 %)
AD patient (MMs 15)	99 (36,8 %)	160 (59,5 %)	8 (3,0 %)	2 (0,7 %)

Table 8 Lexical variety

Subjects	Total words	Total different lexemes
control	109	39 (35,8 %)
AD patient (MMS 9)	88	33 (37,5 %)
AD patient (MMS 15)	99	23 (23,2 %)

Table 9 Types of verbs

Subjects	Content	Modal	Auxiliary
control	17 (42,5 %)	6 (15,0 %)	17 (42,5 %)
AD patient (MMS 9)	9 (25,0 %)	7 (19,5 %)	20 (55,5 %)
AD patient (MMS 15)	18 (45,0 %)	10 (40,0 %)	12 (12,0 %)

Tables 7, 8 and 9 show the total number of words, verbs and the ratio between "total words" and the number of different words (which represents lexical diversity). They again diverge from the results obtained by Irigaray. None of these measures differentiate the patients from the control. These would therefore suggest a rigourously analogous discourse between the patients and the control.

Obviously this kind of measurement is not useful in specifying pathology. We therefore are forced to analyze the discourse at the level at which the information is expressed, seeking ways to measure the semantic deficit. In so doing, we have followed the approach of Tomoeda and Bayles (1993) who have recently sought ways to measure directly and objectively the information contained in elicited discourse such as the one produced during a three-minute observation of a painting.

They (Tomoeda & Bayles 1993) attempt to document the long-term effects of dementia evolution on the language production of AD patients. A set of three pairs of probable AD subjects and normal controls matched for sex, age and level of education, were followed over 5 years, one examination a year. Dementia was measured using the Global Deterioration Scale (Reisberg 1988). The task used to elicit speech production consisted in describing a picture, "Easter Morning", by N. Rockwell. The subject was asked to speak for 3 minutes. The examiner encourages him only if the subject finished speaking before the three minutes elapsed. Discourse performance was described along with 8 measures, of which the three main ones were (a) the total *number of words,* (b) the *number of "information units",* each of them defined as an information cue observed in the picture, and (c) *conciseness,* defined as a/b ratio. Other measures concerned marginal linguistic performances: circumlocutions, "frustrations", defined as complaints about his/her inability to speak, completion of phrases on a second attempt, uncompleted phrases, ideational repetitions in which the same idea is repeated back again, restated in identical or different words. Comparisons were conducted independently for each of the couples of matched subjects.

Results are closely parallel in the evolution of the couples of subjects. "The discourse samples revealed a common pattern of deterioration characterized by the diminution of total output and erosion of semantic substance". They emphasize that the measures used to analyze discourse are reliable and permit the disruption in semantic processing to be closely followed. In the authors' words, they are "sensitive to disease effects and not the result of differences in style and personality".

Total words decreased across examinations in patients. In normals no systematic variation was observed in wording. Nonetheless they found that using number of total words to differentiate mildly demented AD patients from normal elderly could be problematic.

Finally they point out that "verbosity and diminution of output are dependent on disease severity".
The pattern of deterioration in AD discourse was most effectively charted by measuring information units. The number of information units present in patients' discourse decreases dramatically with time. On the first examination the three patients identified a quantity of information units roughly similar to the three normal controls. They reached the level of no recognizable information units respectively on the 3rd, 3rd and 4th annual examination.

Table 10 Conciseness (information units/total words) of the discourse produced by the AD subjects and their respective NC subjects over the span of the 5-year study (from Tomoeda & Bayles (1993): Longitudinal Effects of Alzheimer Disease on Discourse Production. Alzheimer Disease and Associated Disorders 7(4), 223-236).

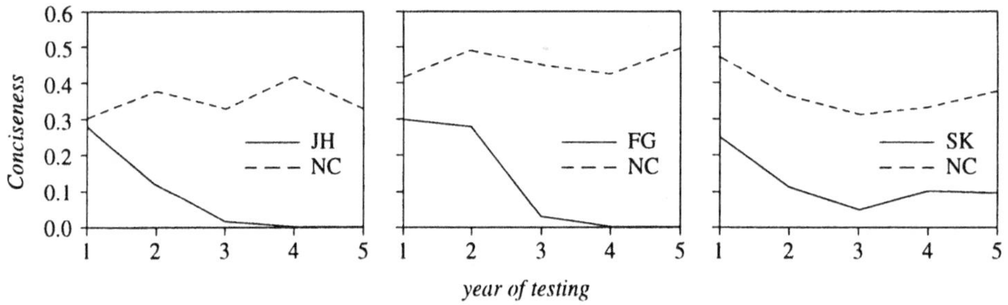

Conciseness of verbal expression, i.e. the ratio of the number of information units divided by total words, does provide reliable data only during the early phases of illness. At that time, that index allowed them to differentiate the discourses of patients from that of normal controls. On the first examination, the values of conciseness are quite similar in patients and normals. In normals a high variability appears from one examination to another, without any particular trend coming to light. On the other hand, in patients, that index worsened rapidly. That index probably represents the best measure of significant contents. Of course in later phases of illness, the ratio looses any meaning. The number of "true" information units tends to or even reaches zero. The number of words produced also decreases, even if it is not reduced in the same proportion. Furthermore, words no longer operate as components of information units "when subjects merely list items in the picture and provide no syntactic framework". Thus in demented patients, whose discourse typically lacks content, total words and information units tend to be unrelated.
The interest of Tomoeda and Bayles' (1993) approach is that information units provide the main source of difference between patients and controls. Furthermore, they are clearly and directly defined along the dimension where the main changes occur, i.e. the semantic processing of informations. Also the dissociation of the validity of information units from that of the conciseness index underscores the specificity of the

concept of information units as a unique and homogeneous level of linguistic performance.

Following this approach, we have attempted to define how these information units could be defined and characterized objectively in "spontaneous language". In our case, the patient's discourse was elicited by an open question such as "Tell me something about your past life". This situation differs from Tomoeda and Bayles' experimental setup. They were able to establish a correspondence between the verbal output and the content of the painting to be described (this is also the approach followed by Goodglass in the cookie theft test (Goodglass & Kaplan 1972)), thus allowing a precise definition of the information units as well as an objective basis for segmenting the discourse. This introduces an element of "authenticity" since only the units corresponding to a feature of the painting are counted. Our approach makes the verification process more difficult and perhaps less reproducible, but it comes closer to a situation of truly spontaneous speech.

In order to define semantically measurable units in minimally induced spontaneous speech (like in our setup), the only available possibility is to apply the same interpretation system used by all of us in everyday life during linguistic exchanges. This is a complex system which takes into account fragments of information, including paralinguistic indices, at different levels of the sequence of events that characterize verbal exchange. The linguistic processor uses these indices and integrates them into decisions used for interpretation and for the conduct of a conversation.

Within the corpus used for the present research, we have taken into account all the information units and have characterized three main types. Each type is defined in terms of its relationship with the main topic of the conversation.

- We first take into account *relevant* units. Each of them brings a significant element clearly associated with the actual theme of the verbal exchange. The information may be included in a phrase that has been produced directly or after self-correction which in turn may or may not include lexico-syntactic changes. We did not take into account the degree of redundancy of one unit compared to others.
- The second type is constituted by *irrelevant* units. These units do not carry any information linkable to the topic of the conversation. They cannot be considered as an introduction to a new topic. The units take different linguistic forms. They may be paraphasic or not. If present, the paraphasia(s) may involve one or more words. Irrelevant units may be incomplete after self-correction, whether the self correction is paraphasic or not. Finally they are called "empty" when the sentence (which may include a variable number of words) provides no usable information.
- The third type is made of a set of units *unrelated* to the present topic, generally uttered in a well-formed sentence, and often bearing a relevant information. They are often stereotyped phrases like "you know..." or "I can't say", inserted by the subject, knowingly or unknowingly within the conversation.

Table 11 summarizes the results.

As can be seen, the control subject only produced relevant information units. In a corpus of approximately similar length for the 3 subjects, the control produced significantly fewer units than the 2 patients, but the control had more relevant units and

Table 11 Distribution of information units

	Normal subject	AD patient (MMS 15)	AD patient (MMS 9)
relevant	32	26	24
relevant after self-correction			
without lexico-syntactic change	0	1	4
with lexico-syntactic change	4	0	0
sub-total	**36**	**27**	**28**
irrelevant	0	2	14
non-paraphasic	0	0	2
paraphasic incomplete	0	4	0
non-paraphasic self corrections	0	1	4
paraphasic self corrections	0	0	1
empty	0	3	0
sub-total	**0**	**10**	**21**
unrelated	0	7	6
total	**36**	**44**	**55**

relevant words. Also, as can be expected in such a relatively brief fragment, the control failed to produce unrelated units. At any rate their occurrence in a normal subject would probably only reflect a transient uncertainty concerning the conditions of the verbal exchanges.

Irrelevant sentences represent 27 % and 42 % of all units produced by the two patients. There are very few paraphasias. Self-corrections, by definition, do not produce relevant sentences. Self-correction tend to produce different results in patients and control. Patients go on with the same lexical-syntactic program while the control tend to perform transformations.

Self-corrections producing a relevant unit differ in the patients and in the control in that the patients simply follow the same syntactic or lexical program, without changing content, while the control can rearrange the sentence, implying an ability to shift at the content level.

Discussion

The analysis of spontaneous language presents problems which are not encountered with usual language tests such as naming or repetition which by definition include a comparison model and are therefore easier to quantify. However spontaneous language is the richest expression of language and the most important for interactions with others in everyday life.

Our purpose was to study language pathology in dementia at the level of spontaneous speech. Our proposed method which stresses information content as a key feature allows to clearly and objectively characterize discourse and separate pathology from normality in a manner which had not been undertaken before. We have identified a measurable entity expressed linguistically. The information units we propose identify the two possible entities (relevant and irrelevant) which contribute to the language.

In view of the small sample involved, this is clearly a pilot study. Further studies are necessary to better characterize irrelevant units. We have identified several linguistic forms for the irrelevant units. A future stage of the research will require an analysis of content as a first step for determining their "pathogenesis". The changes affecting spontaneous language seem to go out of the lexical and/or syntactic fields and to be closely linked to minute transformations bearing on the initial steps of thought processing ("Gesamtvorstellung" (Wundt 1904)). It seems therefore that the abnormal information units have to be defined according to the point where any semantic drift can be noticed. We feel however that despite the small sample, we have established the feasibility of the method. If its validity is confirmed, it could become part of the diagnostic work-up used by neuropsychologists as part of their effort to characterize and diagnose AD, especially in its early phases. A better understanding of the pathology of spontaneous language is important not only from a theoretical viewpoint but also for clinical reasons since it may affect functional prognosis and modify patients' care in everyday situations, whether at home or in institutions.

When trying to understand the mechanisms of pathological language in AD, we are confronted with the incapacity of these patients to express information on an evolving organized structure such as language. This has always been difficult to quantify, but preoccupation can be found in practically all previous studies of language in AD. Seglas (1892) was probably one of the first to study what was then called "aliénés" (insane), a disparate category of patients which certainly included what we now call AD. He distinguished *dyslogia,* "the results of intellectual deficits with preserved language functions" (this corresponds to what we call dementia), from *dysphasia* ("disorders of the language functions"), and *dyslalia* ("disorders of speech"). He clearly recognized the specificity of the semantic level, like us here.

Critchley (1964) quoted Sanford (1942) who had remarked on the ambivalence of language considered beyond its role of communication tool: "There are many indications that language is a vehicle of personality as well as of thought, for when a person speaks, he tells us not only about the world, but also, through both form and content, about himself". Critchley raised the problem of the interpretation of language when any deviation is introduced: "Deviations of the inner mental life consequently betray themselves in an unorthodox use of language. Any considerable aberration of thought or of personality will be mirrored in the various levels of articulated speech whether phonetic, phonemic, semantic, syntactic and pragmatic". When deviance occurs in language, its interpretation goes beyond the level of language itself.

After defining the relation between language and higher processes, Critchley goes back to linguistics to show that the poverty of demented subjects' language is due to "inaccessibility of those different vocabularies which ordinarily we can utilize and which we may term the speaking vocabulary, the writing vocabulary, and the reading vocabulary."

He refers for each of them "as the stock of terms which we are in the habit of employing". He considers that estimates or measures of word types may show the impoverishment of the semantic language of AD "The token-type ratio may prove revealing – and may demonstrate mathematically the poverty of the available vocabulary, and the great tendency towards verbal iterations, perseverations, and contamination". For Critchley, there are three types of language acts "requests for action (or commands); statements; descriptive-statements". In AD, "the stock reduction reflects the alteration of the semantic level. Analyzing the content of spontaneous speech in dementia, we can say that only the first of these classes (commands) survives".
Critchley therefore recognizes the specific nature of the AD deficit as being beyond language, but he attempts to demonstrate it with strictly linguistic measures. As for us, we have attempted to overcome this contradiction. We do not intend to deal with the philosophical issue of the relationship between thought and language, but have stayed at a strictly operational level. Our main question was how to account for the disorder observed in spontaneous language in AD.
One can propose a model in which language functions with its rules unaltered at the phonemic, syntactic, lexical, prosodic and even conversational. The actual "genesis of language" (Pick 1913) responsible for the elaboration of sentences is intact in AD (at least in its early stages). The deficit occurs, in the initial level of the microgenesis of language (Pick's "germ concept" or "thought content"), at the level of the interconnection between thought and its linguistic expression. The main characteristic of dementia is the destruction of some concepts or attributes of these concepts. This loss varies from one individual to another for a variety of reasons including the different location and progression of the lesions. The system of semantic values which forms the bulk of knowledge and competence acquired and maintained throughout an individual life, starts to be less tightly cohesive. Some pieces of this complex puzzle come to be altered and to induce a "cognitive instability" which contributes to disintegrate the cognitive relationships. This decreased cohesion of the system leads to decreased efficiency or even to a loss of the feedback controls, as noted by Seglas and Critchley. This loss has consequences at two levels. The patient no longer has the capacity to manage the totality of the semantic components of his discourse. In addition, he also loses his capacity for dynamic interactions within the development of his discourse. The result is that the spontaneous language of AD patients is characterized by meaningful sentences interweaved with fragments of uninterpretable discourse. The presence of these fragments wrecks the informational continuity of the whole sentence leading to "irrelevant information units".
There is therefore a dissociation between semantic and linguistic deterioration which appears most strikingly in the intermediate stages of the disease. Before that, it can be masked: "A patient with early dementia may preserve a façade of normality for quite a long time, by resort to a chatter of small talks" (Allison 1962). Then as the disease progresses language as a system is affected and disappears altogether.

References

Allison, R.S. (1962): The Senile Brain. London: Arnold.
Critchley, M. (1964): "The Neurology of Psychotic Speech". British Journal of Psychiatry 110, 353 - 364.
Crystal, D. (1969): Prosodic Systems and Intonation in English. Cambridge: Cambridge University Press.
Crystal, D. & D. Davy (1969): Investigating English Style. London: Longman.
Crystal, D. & R. Quirk (1964): Systems of Prosodic and Paralinguistic Features in English. The Hague: Mouton.
Cutler, N.R., J.V. Haxby, R. Duara, C.L. Grady, A.D. Kay, R.M. Kessler, M. Sundaram & S.I. Rapoport (1985): Clinical history, brain metabolism, and neuropsychological function in Alzheimer's disease 18, 298 - 309.
Dubois, J., P. Marcie, L. Irigaray, H. Hécaen & R. Angelergues (1965): "Analyse Distributionnelle en Neurolinguistique: le Comportement Verbal des Aphasiques et des Déments dans les preuves des Langage Répété". Langage et Comportement 1, 111 - 134.
French, P. & J. Local (1986): "Prosodic Features and the Management of Interruptions". In: C. Johns-Lewis, eds., Intonation in Discourse. San Diego, CA: College-Hill Press, 157 - 180.
Goldman-Eisler, F. (1968): Psycholinguistics: Experiments in Spontaneous Speech. London/New York: Academic Press.
Goldstein, K. (1948): Language and language disturbances. New York: Grune & Stratton.
Goodglass, H. & E. Kaplan (1972): The assessment of aphasia and related disorders. Philadelphia: Lea & Febiger.
Horejsi, V. (1961): "Les plans linguistiques et la structure de l'énoncé". Phologica 4, 193 - 203.
Irigaray, L. (1967): "Approche psycholinguistique du langage des déments". Neuropsychologia 5, 25 - 52.
Irigaray, L. (1973): Le langage des Déments. Paris: Mouton.
McGregor, G. (1984): Conversation and Communication. L 4, 71 - 83.
Pick, A. (1913): Die Agrammatischen Sprachstörungen. Berlin: Springer.
Reisberg, B. (1988): "Functional Assessment Staging (FAST)". Psychopharmacology Bulletin 24(1), 653 - 659.
Sanford, F.H. (1942): "Speech and Personality". Psychological Bulletin 39, 811 - 845.
Seglas, J. (1892): Les Troubles du Langage chez les Aliénés. Paris: Rueff.
Tomoeda, C.K. & K.A. Bayles (1993): "Longitudinal Effects of Alzheimer Disease on Discourse Production". Alzheimer Disease and Associated Disorders 7(4), 223 - 236.
Wundt, W. (1904): Völkerpsychologie. Eine Untersuchung der Entwicklungsgesetze von Sprache, Mythos und Sitte. Leipzig.

Speech corpus

Mr. Frém. Gustave (spontaneous language in a 91-year old normal subject)

(M.F., quelle est votre date de naissance?) **&** 19 mai 1899 **£** *(quel âge cela vous fait?)* **&** 91 ans passés **£** *(vous allez me raconter quelles études vous avez faites?)* **&** certificat d'études **£, &** après j'ai fait un an parce que ma mère voulait que j'apprenne un tas de choses **£, &** mais en fin de compte .. euh, euh, j'ai fait simplement un peu de chimie et un peu de physique **£ &** et j'ai même **£** + **&** il m'en est resté SO_4H_2 **£ &** et je ne sais pas ce que c'est, **£ &** je crois que c'est l'acide sulfurique **£, &** et [sypk] je ne sais

pas le restant **£, &** c'est tout ce que j'ai appris dans l'an **£ + &** avec tout ce qui me reste **£, &** après **£, &** eh bien, euh, après je me suis **£ + &** j'ai commencé à à travailler comme sertisseur en joaillerie **£, &** j'ai fait un an d'apprentissage **£, &** et c'était une maison qui débutait **£ &** et c'était deux excellents ouvriers qu'eux **£, &** mais comme on débutait il y avait des courses à faire toute la journée **£** .. **&** mes parents + mon + mon père, beau-père enfin, qui était [lsi] + joaillier **£, &** ma mère polisseuse en joaillerie **£, &** et moi, bien j'étais sertisseur **£, &** alors ils avaient beau chercher **£, &** ourtant les sertisseurs il y en a pas beaucoup **£, &** mais j'allais **£ + &** on trouvait pas à le .. d'autres maisons **£, &** en fin de compte on en a trouvé une **£, &** mais c'était chez le + un sertisseur qui était déjà plus jeune **£ &** et sa façon de travailler n'avait rien de moderne **£, &** il n'y avait que simplement que le chaton à griffes où là on pouvait faire du travail **£, &** parce que c'était comme pas de tèpe **£, &** malheureusement à peine commencé **£, &** c'était en face de la Banque de France **£, &** au 34 rue ..[akr] + Croix-des-Petits-Champs **£, &** et la maison a fermé parce que la guerre arrivait **£**

Ms. Lasc. Suzanne (spontaneous language in a 77-year old AD patient with an MMSE score of 15)

(qu'est-ce que vous avez fait aujourd'hui?) **&** qu'est-ce que j'ai fait seulement [zœr] **£** .. **&** j'ai fait un petit peu de bricolage dans ma cuisine **£** ... *(je vous écoute, allez)* **&** et puis j'ai **£** ... **&** je me suis fait euh **£** *(allez-y)* ... ... **&** combien **£ + &** comment que j'ai fait partie **£ &** alors, euh, j'ai voulu manger un peu **£ &** et puis j'étais ... déçue parce que ... le + le **£ + &** il y avait le voleur qui était passé encore pour, euh **£** ..., **&** pour prendre, euh, le **£ &** quelqu'un **£** ... **&** quelques affaires ... ... **&** je ne m'en rappelle plus **£** *(quelles affaires?)* **&** les vêtements .. le ... deux ... ... **£** *(est-ce que vous avez travaillé dans votre vie?)* **&** oh oui **£** *(qu'est-ce que vous avez fait comme métier?)* **&** comme métier? **£ &** ben j'ai fait un petit peu **£** ... **&** comment qu'on dit? **£ &** un peu tous les métiers **£** *(expliquez-moi ça?)* **&** oh oui **£** ... **&** ben, vous savez **£** ... **&** j'ai travaillé dans une sucrerie chez Sérieux **£** .. **&** après j'ai travaillé ailleurs dans le blanchiment, **£ &** oui j'ai travaillé .. à **£** .. **&** comment? **£** ... ... **&** on ne peut pas remettre ça à un petit peu plus tard, **£ &** je suis fatiguée **£** *(pourquoi vous portez deux alliances à la main?)* **&** parce que j'ai perdu mon mari, **£ &** il est mort d'un cancer **£** *(il y a longtemps?)* **&** il y a dix-sept ans **£** ... **&** j'ai toujours gardé son alliance, **£** alors comme elle était plus grande que la mienne, **£ &** alors euh .. je l'ai gardée **£** *(qu'est-ce qu'il faisait votre mari?)* **&** mon mari, il travaillait à la Ville de Paris **£** ... **&** il était **£** .. **&** il travaillait dans les Pompes Funèbres **£** *(et vous vous travailliez avec lui?)* **&** ah non pas du tout, **£ &** moi je travaillais dans la rue Denis-Papin **£**.. **&** euh euh c'était des transfo électriques, **£ &** des grands transfo électriques **£** .. **&** et puis il y a le licenciement chez quelqu'un, **£ &** mais mon mari il était content parce qu'il voulait plus que je travaille, **£ &** j'avais une petite fille [nwa] + très + très amie + très jeune, **&** alors euh, mon mari m'a dit tu resteras à la maison pour t'occuper des deux **£** ...**&** voilà.**£**

Ms. Mani. Virginie (spontaneous language in a 72-year old AD patient with an MMSE score of 9)

(quelle est votre date de naissance?) **&** 1919 **£** *(quel mois?)* & le ... le [zvoko], **£ &** pas le mois, **£ &** pas le [m m], **£ &** mais c'est un mardi **£**.. **&** 14 **£** .. **&** 14 le mardi **£** *(dans quel mois?)* **&** 14, **£ &** mais je ne sais pas **£** .. **&** ça doit être au mois de a **£ + &** de mars **£** .. **&** je ne sais tellement moi, **£ &** ça tombe le 14 **£**.. **&** ça tombe au mois de mars **£** .. **&** ou au mois d'avril, **£ &** je ne sais pas **£**.. *(on vérifiera)* **&** oui **£** *(ça vous fait quel âge?)* **&** 88 ans **£** *(et on est en quelle année aujourd'hui?)* **&** ah ... en quelle année **£ &** on est peut-être presque en quatre-vingt-neuf, hein **£** *(comment?)* **&** presque 89 **£** *(vous, vous avez presque 89 ans?)* **&** oui **£** *(et nous sommes en quelle année en ce moment?)* **&** oh ... c'est 1989 on doit être maintenant **£** *(mais vous êtes née en quelle année, vous?)* **&** en 1919, **£ &** vous me troublez, [ironic laughing] **£ &** hein, **£ &** oh oui, **£ &** vous me troublez, **£ &** vous ne m'avez pas eu **£** *(pas du tout)* **&** mais je suis contente de passer un moment avec vous **£** *(c'est bien)* **&** oui **£** *(vous allez me dire, vous avez été à l'école?)* **&** pas beaucoup **£** *(dites-moi)* **&** le temps du catéchisme **£** *(vous êtes née à quel endroit?)* **&** à Bruay-en-Artois **£** ... **&** on a eu vu des drôles hein, **£ &** je suis **£ + &** je suis l'ainée, **£ &** l'ainée de de [sat] **£ + &** de quatre enfants **£** ... *(que faisait votre papa?)* **&** ah, il était mineur **£**.. **&** il était pas normal **£** *(pourquoi?)* **&** d'abord elle a eu quatre enfants, **£ &** puis elle a été malheureuse comme les pierres **£** *(et pour quelles raisons?)* **&** hein **£** *(pour quelles raisons?)* **&** quoi, dans le Pas-de-Calais, Monsieur, **£ &** à Bruay-en-Artois **£** ... *(pourquoi a-t-elle été malheureuse?)* **&** parce qu'elle était seule avec les enfants, **£ &** elle était aidée par la Mairie, **£ &** mais elle était seule avec les enfants **£** *(et le papa il était où?)* **&** il fallait qu'elle aille faire des lessives le soir, **£ &** alors elle nous laissait seuls, **£ &** c'était moi qui fetais les vieux **£ + &** nettoyait mes frères et mes sœurs **£** .. **&** c'était pas une vie de château, **£ &** hein, je vous le dis.**£**

Transcription code

1 Within braces paraphasias are transcribed in phonetic notation.
2 Pauses are represented with a string of 2 or 3 colons depending of the subjective duration.
3 "+" symbol is used to mark any lexeme or phrase rewording.
4 Onset of an information unit is signalled with "&" symbol, end of an information unit with "£" symbol.
5 Within parentheses the examiner's words are written in italic.

The Time Course of Lexical Activation in Fluent and Nonfluent Aphasia

Penny A. Prather, Boston

1 Introduction

There is a remarkably consistent distinction between fluent and nonfluent aphasics in their performance on measures of semantic comprehension vs. lexical activation. Nonfluent aphasics perform "normally" – that is, similar to age-matched control subjects – on off-line semantic judgment tasks, e.g. grouping words based on semantic relatedness and matching pictures of individual objects to their category names (e.g. Goodglass & Baker 1976; Whitehouse, Caramazza & Zurif 1978; Zurif, Caramazza, Myerson & Galvin 1974). They do not perform normally, however, on measures of lexical priming that require rapid but ostensibly easier lexical ("word-non word") judgments. In direct contrast to nonfluent aphasics, fluent aphasics have significant difficulty making semantic judgments, but perform normally on measures of lexical priming.

On the face of it, these data seem to suggest some type of double dissociation between lexical and semantic processes, given the apparent preservation of semantic and disruption of lexical organization and/or access for nonfluent aphasics and the reverse profile for fluent aphasics. Such a dissociation clearly would have important implications in terms of theoretical models of the organization of language structures as well as for models of aphasia. The argument put forward here, however, is that the dissociation is not double and the distinction is not between "lexical" and "semantic". Rather, the dissociation is within the lexical domain, and reflects a distinction between slowed but direct access to lexical information (for nonfluent aphasics) vs. a fast but alternate route to lexical information (for fluent aphasics).

In the sections that follow, the argument for fundamental differences in lexical processing for fluent and nonfluent aphasics is made as follows: First, prior studies examining on-line lexical activation in aphasic populations are reviewed – data that generally have been interpreted as indicating that fluent aphasics are "normal" in automatic activation while nonfluent aphasics are different in some difficult-to-specify way. Second, studies examining the time course of lexical activation in normal populations of both college age and elderly subjects are reviewed, showing that automatic activation is rapid and short lived in those populations. Third, research is presented supporting an inference that lexical activation is rapid but not short-lived for fluent aphasics, and not rapid but short-lived for nonfluent aphasics. In the concluding section, these findings are discussed in terms of an hypothesis that lexical activation is abnormal for both fluent and nonfluent aphasics, but for quite different reasons. Nonfluent aphasics show a normal route of lexical activation but a protracted rise time relative to that seen in normal populations. Fluent aphasics, on the other hand, speculatively do not access the "normal" lexicon at all; rather, they access the "sense" but not the detailed semantic and syntactic knowledge of a word. In that sense, the surface differences in ability to make semantic judgments reflect underlying differences in both what and how quickly fluent and nonfluent aphasics access lexical information. The distinguishing characteristics for these groups are respectively in the *route* and *rate* of lexical access.

2 Lexical priming in fluent and nonfluent aphasics: A review

As noted above, a number of studies conducted in the late 1960's and early 1970's demonstrated that fluent aphasics, in contrast to nonfluent aphasics, had difficulty making semantic judgments. When asked, for example, to decide which two words in a triad went together "best", fluent aphasics had much more difficulty than either nonfluent aphasics or control subjects in applying semantic classification schemes (Zurif et al. 1974). These failures suggested some type of underlying disorganization or disturbance in semantic organization that distinguished fluent from other aphasics. Based on those findings, Milberg, Blumstein and their colleagues undertook a number of pioneering studies examining semantic organization in aphasics populations. Their findings were not at all what was expected, and have been a major influence in re-directing conceptualizations of disturbances in lexical processing among aphasics.

To examine the hypothesis that fluent aphasics were somehow deviant in their semantic organization based on their performance on off-line judgment tasks, Milberg & Blumstein (1981) used lexical priming methodology to examine semantic organization and access in real time. Essentially, "priming" refers to the fact that words are processed more quickly when they are preceded by a related word or "prime" than when they are preceded by an unrelated word or "control". Most often, priming, that is, "speeding up" of lexical activation has been measured in terms of relative lexical decision times (although other types of judgments have also been used), that is, deciding whether a string of letters (e.g. "slumpf"; "edit"; "blfk"; "doctor"; "nurse") is or is not a real English word. Lexical decision times for target words are faster in "related prime-target" pairs (e.g. "doctor-*nurse*") than in "control prime-target" pairs (e.g. "table-*nurse*"). With respect to semantic organization, the premise in using priming is that it reflects strength of connections among words, and thereby reveals something about the underlying organization of lexical and semantic knowledge by reflecting what nodes are "close to" and what nodes are"distant from" each other. The general claim based on a large body of priming studies is that the underlying organization of semantic space is essentially a network in which related words are "closer" than unrelated words, with semantic "clusters" defined in part by hierarchical relations (Collins & Loftus 1975; Smith, Shoben & Rips 1974).

Relevant to examination of semantic organization in aphasic subjects, Milberg & Blumstein (1981) were primarily interested in examining the hypothesis that fluent aphasics failed semantic judgment tasks because of an underlying impairment or deviance in lexical/semantic organization. To examine that hypothesis, subjects were presented with experimental word pairs in which a target word was preceded by a related prime or by an unrelated prime, as well as pairs that included non-words. Stimuli were presented visually, with the following temporal relations:

prime . . . . target . . . . prime . . . . target
├ 2000 msec ┤ ├── 4000 msec ──┤ ├ 2000 msec ┤

Using that paradigm, Milberg & Blumstein hypothesized that fluent aphasics would show deviant lexical priming (relative to control subjects), if in fact they had an underlying deviance in lexical/semantic organization. Nonfluent aphasics were expected to show normal priming effects, consistent with an inference of normal semantic organization. The results, however, were just the opposite of those predicted. Fluent aphasics showed "normal" lexical priming, that is, their performance was no different from that of elderly controls; nonfluent aphasics, on the other hand, failed to show lexical priming.

Based on their normal performance in making semantic judgments, it is assumed that nonfluent aphasics access lexical information. Milberg et al. speculatively inferred from their failure to prime that nonfluent aphasics may have a deficit in *automatic* activation of lexical information. Instead, they may access lexical information "intentionally", in some effortful way. Subsequent priming studies did not, however, clearly support that hypothesis – nor did they clearly contradict it. Rather, they found that sometimes but not always, nonfluent aphasics showed priming. In a follow-up study using auditory rather than visual stimuli, and with a shorter delay between words in a pair (500 msec between words in a pair, 8000 msec between pairs), Blumstein, Milberg & Shrier (1982) found that nonfluent as well as fluent aphasics showed lexical priming. In a third study again using an auditory presentation and a 500 msec delay between words but presenting words in triplets (e.g. "money-bank-teller") rather than pairs, Milberg, Blumstein & Dworetzky (1987) found that nonfluent aphasics failed to show priming, while normal control and fluent aphasics showed priming under some, although not all, conditions. The one general finding across these initial priming studies was that under all conditions where normal elderly subjects showed priming, fluent aphasics also showed priming. Changes in inter-stimulus interval (ISI), using pair vs. triplet contexts, using auditory vs. visual presentation of stimuli – none of those changes affected priming for fluent aphasics any more or less than it did for normal controls. Something about those changes did, however, differentially affect performance of nonfluent aphasics.

Subsequent studies examining lexical priming effects in fluent and nonfluent aphasics have continued to support the initial generalization from Milberg and Blumstein's studies: (1) In all cases where elderly control subjects prime, fluent aphasics prime. Whether words are presented in pair, triplet or sentence contexts, and whether the delay between prime and target words is short or long, fluent aphasics prime reliably. (2) In some studies, nonfluent aphasics showed the same priming effects as normal controls; in others they did not (see Table 1 for summary of studies). Priming in that sense has not been absent but rather has been less "stable" for nonfluent aphasics than for other aphasics and for normal controls (Hagoort 1993).

While Milberg and Blumstein's priming studies began as an attempt to understand why fluent aphasics fail semantic judgment tasks, they raised a very different set of questions: Why are nonfluent aphasics unstable in their priming? And why are fluent aphasics so stable in their priming when there is little evidence that semantic knowledge is reliably available to them?

One potential explanation for the findings of nonfluent aphasic's unstable priming is methodological: The instability is not with nonfluent aphasics, but rather with the variability in the procedures used to examine lexical activation in that population. No two studies have used the same methodology (see Table 1). Studies have varied in modality of presentation (auditory vs. visual), in contextual framework (one word vs. two word vs. sentence contexts preceding the target word), in interstimulus delays (from 100 to 2000 msec), in delays between pairs or triplets (from 4000 to 8000 msec) – and these variations have been completely unsystematic. Clearly none of these changes affected performance of fluent aphasics relative to performance of age-matched control subjects, while some or all of them did affect performance of nonfluent aphasics. The difficulty, given the lack of systematic variation, is in inferring which are the relevant factors in understanding nonfluent aphasics' deviant performance.

There are some potentially interesting almost-generalizations noted in reviewing these lexical priming studies. Considering just those studies that used a pair priming methodology, that is, where target words were preceded by a single prime word ("doctor-nurse"), nonfluent aphasics showed priming when words were presented *auditorally*, but not when they were presented *visually* (see Table 1). That was true despite variations in the ISI between words. Studies presenting words visually seemed more sensitive, on the other hand, to temporal factors. There is as yet no data to interpret modality differences, but they are an intriguing and potentially important difference, one about which we will speculate later in the paper.

Another potentially relevant factor, and one for which there are at least some relevant data, is temporal effects. The potential relevance of this factor was proposed speculatively by Swinney, Zurif & Nicol (1989), following yet another serendipitous priming result. They conducted a study designed to test Milberg and Blumstein's hypothesis that nonfluent aphasics may be impaired in automatic activation of lexical information. Consistent with the general inconsistency of nonfluent aphasics' priming, Swinney et al. found that nonfluent subjects both did and did not show automatic priming – and concluded that disrupted automatic processing may be a *result* rather than the fundamental *explanation* for nonfluent aphasics' lexical deficits. They proposed that a more fundamental process, rate of access, may instead be at the heart of those deficits.

To examine automatic lexical activation in aphasics, Swinney and his colleagues adapted a paradigm that had reliably demonstrated automatic effects in young normals (college age subjects). In their research, Swinney and his colleagues had shown that when young subjects hear an ambiguous word, all meanings of that word are automatically activated, regardless of prior knowledge or expectations. Even when an ambiguous word is presented in a strongly biasing context, all of its meanings are activated briefly. This

Table 1 Summary of priming results across studies using different priming paradigms, temporal factors, and modality of input

Authors	Year	Subjects	Method (context; time factor)	Modality	Results (FL = Fluent NF = Nonfluent NC = Controls)
Milberg & Blumstein	1981	FL NF, conduction Controls	PPP 2000 ISI 4000 betw pairs	visual	FL: primed NF: did not NC: primed
Blumstein et al.	1982	7 FL 3 NF 4 TM 4 glbl 5 conduction	PPP 500 ISI 8000 betw pairs	auditory	All primed
Milberg, Blumstein Dworetzky	1987	6 FL 7 NF	triplets 500 msec ISI 8000 msec betw triplets	auditory	FL: yes NF: no
Katz	1988	7 NF 19 undergrads	ambig pairs, PPP 500 ISI 6000 between pairs	auditory	NF: yes NC: yes
Swinney, Zurif, Nicol	1989	FL NF NC	ambig words sent context	visual	FL: both meanings NF: hi freq only NC: both meanings
Hagoort	1993	7 NF 4 FL 12 NC	ambig triplets 100, 500, 1250 ISI 6000 msec between	auditory	FL: yes at 100, 500 NF: yes at 100, 500 (priming for concordant and neutral only)
Kramer Ostrin, Tyler	1993	4 NF NC, young (24 to 40) NC, old (60 to 80, all F)	PPP 250 msec ISI 6000 msec between pairs	auditory	NF: primed (semantic & assoc) NC: primed (also both types)

was demonstrated using a cross-modal priming technique (Swinney 1979). Subjects listen to sentences a subset of which contain target ambiguous words; for those sentences, immediately after hearing the ambiguous word, the subjects see a word related either to the a priori most frequent (primary) interpretation of the ambiguity or towards the least frequent (secondary) meaning of the ambiguity, or they see a control word matched in length and frequency to the related words but unrelated to the target ambiguity. For example,

The gardener was responsible for watering every **plant*** on the enormous estate.
*tree vs. page
factory vs. funeral

(See Swinney 1979, for details on this methodology.) Using this technique, Swinney has found that regardless of the direction or strength of the prior sentence context, subjects reliably show faster lexical decisions for words related to both meanings of the ambiguity (here, "tree" and "factory") than for their matched control words (here, "page" and "funeral"). These data were interpreted as strong evidence that, once a lexical item is activated, all of its relevant meanings are activated; activation is in that sense "full", not selective or directed. These data have been cited as convincing evidence that lexical activation is a modular process, that is, a process that is rapid, obligatory and informationally encapsulated (Fodor 1983). Relevant to investigations of lexical activation in aphasic subjects is the *automaticity* of this process. One cannot *choose* not to activate both meanings, nor can prior context serve to inhibit activation of both meanings either actively or passively; activation of both meanings is, at least normally, automatic and obligatory. If, then, both meanings are *not* activated in nonfluent aphasics, that would be strong evidence in favor of an argument that that population is impaired in automatic activation.

Briefly, what Swinney, Zurif and Nicol found was, first, consistent with all prior studies, fluent aphasics performed "normally", showing rapid activation of both meanings of ambiguous words, regardless of direction of sentence bias. Second, nonfluent aphasics did not prime "normally". Rather, they showed priming for the primary but not secondary meaning of ambiguous words, regardless of context. Context did not direct access – they did not access the secondary meaning even when the context cued them to that meaning, nor did they inhibit the primary meaning when the context cued them away from that meaning. In that sense, their lexical activation was automatic and informationally encapsulated. But neither did they show activation for both meanings. Why not?

Here, Swinney et al. invoked a temporal explanation. While young subjects do show obligatory activation of both meanings of ambiguous words, Simpson (1984) provides evidence that that activation is temporally ordered; for non-equibias ambiguities of the sort that Swinney used, where one meaning is stronger than the other, the primary meaning is accessed slightly more quickly than the secondary meaning. It may be, Swinney et al. reasoned, that nonfluent aphasics show selectively slowed activation. If there is a generally protracted rise time in activating words in the lexicon, then nonfluent aphasics might have time to get to the first but not second meaning of ambiguous words under the constraints of the cross-modal priming task.

This temporal explanation is elegant in its simplicity. It offers a parsimonious way to account for the instability rather than absence of lexical priming in nonfluent aphasics; they would show automatic priming only under conditions that allowed sufficient time for them to activate words, which varies across studies and paradigms.

There have now been several studies examining time course of lexical activation in aphasic populations – again with variable findings, and claims both for and against slowed activation. In order to consider those findings critically, however, it is necessary first to consider investigations of the time course of lexical activation in "normal" young and elderly populations, and the methodological concerns addressed in that research.

3 Time course of lexical activation in non-aphasic, "normal control" populations

In the preceding section, "automatic" lexical activation was defined as a rapid, obligatory, informationally encapsulated process. Automatic activation is driven by sensory input; hearing or seeing a particular phonemic code like "plant", the related lexical node is automatically activated, which in turn automatically activates an ordered spread of activation to its near associates (e.g., Collins & Loftus 1975). Automatic activation is not, however, the only route by which lexical information can be accessed. It is also possible to intentionally search the lexicon, and by that route, to initiate spread of activation from specific nodes to their associates. It is the availability of this alternate "intentional search" route that Milberg and Blumstein invoked, for example, as a possible explanation for nonfluent aphasics' lack of rapid automatic priming but preserved ability to access lexical information in order to make semantic judgments.

In addition to differences in source of initial access, and relevant to considerations of the time course of lexical activation, automatic and intentional lexical access differ in the rates at which they are initiated. In a now classic study, Neely (1977) devised a paradigm that allowed separation of the relative contributions of automatic vs. intentional access to lexical priming effects. Neely used a traditional pair priming paradigm in which subjects saw a prime and target word presented sequentially; the new twist in his application of this paradigm was the opposition of associative vs. anticipatory priming. Subjects were specifically instructed that when the prime word in a pair was from a particular category (e.g. "vehicles"), then the target word would be an exemplar from an unrelated but specified category (e.g. "anatomy"). That is, subjects were specifically instructed that seeing a prime word from the category "vehicles" signaled that the target word would be from the category "anatomy". That instructed connection potentially allowed initiation of an intentional search and activation of words in the targeted semantic category. While subjects were not informed of this, in some instances, words from the prime category "vehicles" were followed by semantic associates (e.g. "car – windshield") that is, by "unexpected but related" words. These semantic associates are the relations, of course, that normally prime automatically. Varying the stimulus onset asynchrony (SOA) across word pairs, ranging from 250 to 2000 msec, Neely found that priming was accounted for by automatic or associative priming alone at 250 msec; anticipatory activation did not contribute to priming effects until SOAs of at least 500 msec. By a 2000 msec SOA, however, *only* anticipatory activation was observed; associative primes actually *inhibited*, that is, effected *longer* lexical decision times for target words at that delay. Inhibition is, of course, assumed to reflect the result of an inaccurate expectation, and therefore is interpreted as a reflection of intentional processes.

Several investigators since, using Neely's paradigm, have supported Neely's basic finding with respect to the relative time course of automatic vs. intentional priming (e.g., den Heyer, Briand & Smith 1985; Favreau & Segalowitz 1983). Generally, using a pair priming paradigm and lexical decision task, automatic priming seems to operate by 200 msec; priming by intent initiates later, at about 500 msec or so; and inhibition of automatic by intentional priming occurs somewhere between 1100 and 2000 msec.

The apparent establishment of the relative time course of automatic vs. intentional priming has had important implications for research in this area. Most relevant to the work in aphasia, it is frequently cited as support for claims that pair priming paradigms in which short SOAs or ISIs (inter-stimulus intervals) are used (250 msec or less) *necessarily* reflect automatic lexical processes, since those delays are too short to allow intentional processing.

There are two cautionary notes to be made about that claim. First, studies investigating the time course of automatic vs. intentional priming using Neely's paradigm include a critical condition: opposition of intentional and associative priming effects. Subjects are instructed to anticipate a particular relation that conflicts with or distracts from associative priming. Using this paradigm, it is clear that intentional priming does not occur at short SOAs or ISIs and that automatic or associative priming does. Importantly, however, when subjects are told to anticipate a relation, presumably they put all of their "intentional effort" into the instructed task. As they have more time – either between word pairs or after seeing a word pair – presumably any strategic attempts to find relations will focus on the instructed relation. What, however, about studies using associative primes and short SOAs (< 300 msec)? When the only systematic relation across a set of word pairs is associative, what is to prevent subjects from "intentionally" noticing and looking for that relation, whether or not they are instructed to do so? If the delay between words in a pair is short enough, arguably subjects would not have time to look intentionally for associative relations, even if they noticed them. If, however, the delay between word pairs were long enough (and there are as yet no empirical data to indicate what "long enough" might be), then arguably subjects could intentionally look for relations – as they must, for example, in studies demonstrating that priming effects increase as the proportion of associated words increases (den Heyer, Briand & Dannenbring 1983; Tweedy, Lapinski & Schvaneveldt 1977). As de Groot (1984) demonstrated, using a pair priming paradigm even with very short SOAs (240 msec), proportion effects are observed, which arguably indicates application of intentional strategies.

It is also of importance that the basic studies examining the time course of lexical activation have used visually presented materials. While certainly one would hope that the *relative* temporal relations between automatic and intentional priming would hold, it is not at all clear that *specific* temporal values could be applied directly to other modalities, notably to auditory presentation of materials – the modality used most commonly with aphasic populations.

An alternative paradigm developed to examine the time course of *automatic* lexical activation is the single or List Priming Paradigm (LPP) (McNamara & Altarriba 1988; Prather & Swinney 1988; Shelton & Martin 1992). Rather than distract subjects from intentionally looking for associative relations as Neely's does, this paradigm operates by reducing the amount of time available to look for relations. Using this paradigm, subjects are presented letter strings (words and nonwords) serially, and instructed to make lexical decisions on each letter string as quickly as possible. As soon as the subject responds, a specified ISI is initiated, and then the next letter string presented. Shelton & Martin conducted several experiments in which the ISI was held constant at 500 msec and the nature of the materials varied to include associative vs. semantic relations (e.g. "bread-butter" vs. "bread-cake") and forward vs. backward associations (e.g. "fly-paper" vs. "paper-fly"). They consistently found associative and only associative priming using the LPP, while associative, semantic, forward, and backward relations all yielded priming effects when words were presented in a pair priming paradigm (PPP). In addition, when a neutral prime condition was included, inhibition effects were found when using the PPP but not the LPP. These data were taken as strong evidence that the LPP yields priming only for automatic associations, at least at a 500 msec ISI, and prevents either anticipatory or backward priming effects.

Prather introduced one other manipulation to the LPP: a word (e.g. the word "WORD") repeated at random intervals throughout the list (on average every 15th item). Prather and her colleagues were most interested in using the LPP to examine the time course, that is, the rise and fall time of automatic lexical activation. At short ISIs, the LPP restricted priming to automatic effects by not allowing time to invoke intentional strategies. At longer ISIs, however, potentially there would be sufficient time to allow anticipation or other automatic effects. The intention in including the repeated word was to provide a kind of "decoy" that was easily noticed so that, if subjects were going to develop intentional strategies, they would be most likely to develop them around the repeated word. Using that paradigm with both college age and elderly subjects, Stern, Prather, Swinney & Zurif (1991) found that for both subject groups, priming obtained at 500 msec, but not at earlier (300 msec) or later (800, 1100 and 1500 msec) ISIs. The loss of priming at the longer ISIs supports the claim that the LPP, unlike the PPP, taps primarily automatic priming effects, which diminish unless they are sustained in some intentional way (Prather & Swinney 1988; Simpson & Burgess 1985).

Note, importantly, that the specific times at which priming obtained differed from the times report in studies using PPP, including Neely's "conflict" PPP. Subjects prime "earlier" when words are presented as isolated pairs rather than in a continuous list. That finding underscores the point made earlier: one cannot assume that there is a fixed time at which priming obtains; rather, the time course must reflect at least the effects of the input modality, lexical rise and fall time, and specific task demands. While lexical rise and fall times are assumed to be fixed, input modality and specific task demands vary – and those variations need to be taken into account in comparing temporal data on "automatic" priming across studies.

4 Examination of time course in aphasic subjects

We now return to the question raised earlier: do nonfluent aphasics show a protracted rise time in automatic lexical activation? And does that distinguish them from fluent aphasic as well as non-aphasic control subjects?

As noted above, claims about non-aphasics' rapid automatic lexical activation have been equivocal. Most recently, Kramer Ostrin & Tyler (1993) cite their own findings as well as those of Hagoort (1993) and Blumstein et al. (1982) as strong evidence in favor of the preservation of rapid automatic activation for this group; these are all studies in which nonfluent aphasics showed priming at short SOAs. In truth, there are at this point more studies claiming that nonfluent aphasics *do* show automatic activation than studies claiming they do *not* (see Table 1.). The difficulty in accepting these claims, however, is that none of the paradigms used in these studies offers convincing evidence that they rule out the possible influence of strategic priming effects. Also, the issue is not simply whether nonfluent aphasics show "automatic" activation, but whether they do so within a "normal" time frame.

Consider the four studies in which short SOAs were used and in which nonfluent aphasics showed priming. The first, Blumstein et al. (1982), presented stimuli auditorally in a PPP with an SOA of 500 msec and inter-pair interval of 8000 msec; the second, Katz (1988), also used a PPP with an SOA of 500 msec and an inter-pair interval of 6000 msec; the third, Hagoort (1993), presented words auditorally in a triplet paradigm with SOAs ranging from 100 to 1250 msec and an inter-triplet delay of 6000 msec; and the most recent, Kramer Ostrin & Tyler (1993), used a PPP with an ISI of 250 msec and inter-pair delay of 6000 msec. While all of these studies obtained priming for nonfluent aphasics at short SOAs (500 msec or less), they all also allowed long inter-pair or inter-triplet delays (4000 msec or longer).

In short, while priming has been demonstrated with nonfluent aphasics at very short delays using pair and triplet priming paradigms that arguably interfere with "anticipation priming", no consideration has been given to checks on"post-lexical priming". Studies using long inter-pair and inter-triplet delays may reflect automatic priming, but they also may not. Kramer Ostrin & Tyler consider this issue explicitly, and cite prior studies (particularly Neely's work) using short SOAs and low proportion of related pairs as support for claims that their findings reflect automatic priming. Without including, as Neely did, explicit conditions that allow a check on the presence of strategic effects when using a PPP, however, the question of strategic effects remains. And, overall, the most parsimonious explanation for otherwise "unstable" findings with nonfluent aphasics to date is that those studies showing priming at short SOAs with nonfluent populations have not ruled out, and probably allow, some type of strategic priming.

One difficulty in assuring that one is getting automatic priming when using pair and triplet paradigms is that the empirically demonstrated "check" on post-lexical priming

Figur 1 Difference scores as a function of interstimulus interval (ISI). Comparison of data for nonfluent aphasic (from Prather et al. 1992) with neurologically intact elderly and college-age subjects (from Stern et al. 1991)

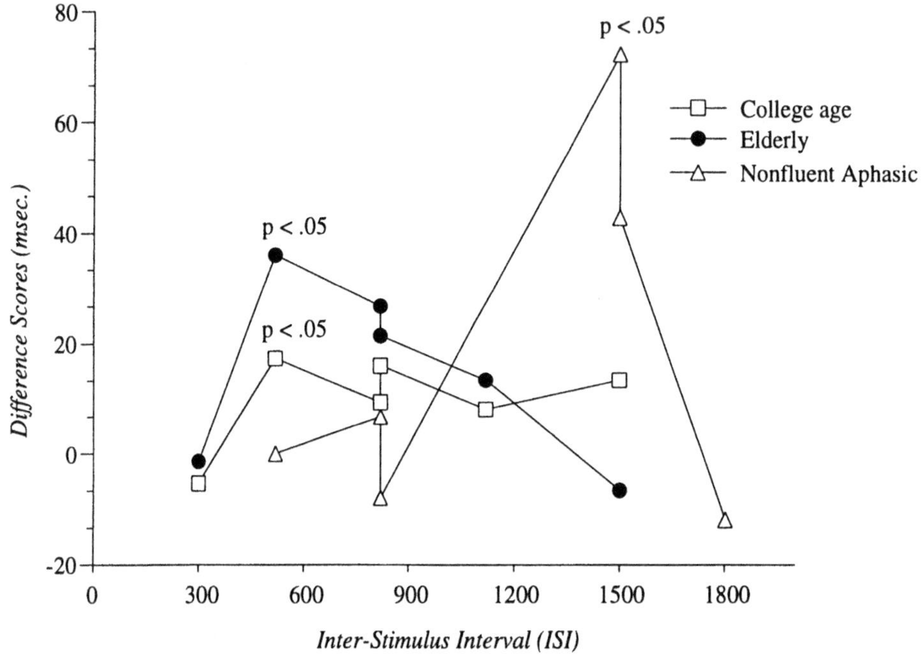

is to introduce a condition that conflicts with looking for associative relations, as Neely did. That is not a viable condition to introduce with aphasic populations. The alternative approach, and the one that we have adopted in our lab, is to use an LPP. This paradigm does allow explicit checks on strategic priming that are applicable with both aphasic and control populations. As described above, using the LPP with both young and elderly subjects, priming effects obtained at 500 msec ISIs, and not at either earlier or longer delays, with a rise-and-fall pattern characteristic of both young and elderly subjects (see Figure 1). Critical here is the *loss* of priming at long ISIs. If strategic priming effects were a factor, priming would be expected to *increase,* not *decrease,* over time (Neely 1977, 1991; Prather & Swinney 1988; Shelton & Martin 1992). To test the hypothesis that nonfluent aphasics have a protracted rise time for automatic lexical activation using the LPP, the specific prediction was that nonfluent aphasics would be slower in accessing information in the lexicon, and consequently that automatic priming would obtain later in time than is normally found, but that they would show a similar rise-and-fall pattern. The "fall" in priming is critical in making claims that automatic activation is being examined. If, using an LPP, aphasics showed a later rise time than controls but also continued to show priming as ISIs increased, clearly the possibility would remain open that strategic, not automatic, effects were being tapped.

To date in our lab, we have used an LPP and case study methodology to examine the time course of lexical activation in aphasic populations. The assumption in beginning with case studies was that, while we were predicting slowed activation as a general characteristic of nonfluent aphasics, there was no reason to assume equivalent slowing for all nonfluent aphasics. Individuals with different lesion sites and/or severities and with different premorbid skills might well have different degrees of slowing as a function of their injury, effects that would be missed and, if present, would diminish rather than enhance effects based on averaging across subjects in a group.

Using the LPP and case study approach, Prather, Zurif, Stern and Rosen (1992) obtained support for the hypothesis of slowed but preserved automatic lexical activation for a nonfluent aphasic. This study essentially replicated the Stern et al. (1991) study in which young and elderly subjects were presented with associatively related word pairs embedded in the context of a list of words and nonwords. Letter strings were presented visually on a computer monitor; subjects were instructed to make a word/nonword decision as quickly as possible. As soon as they made their response, that letter string was removed, a fixed ISI was initiated, the next letter string was presented, and so on, with occasional breaks for feedback. In Stern et al., 12 elderly and 12 young subjects each saw target words once in one of 12 possible conditions (6 ISIs (range 300 to 1100 msec) x 2 Relatedness (related vs. control) conditions). Both young and elderly subjects showed significant priming at, and only at, an ISI of 500 msec. Prather et al. used the same materials and the same basic procedure (although different specific ISIs), but tested a single subject (L.D., a 61 year old male nonfluent aphasic) who saw each target word in each of its 12 conditions across 12 visits. Using that paradigm, L.D. showed priming at an ISI of 1500 msec, but not at either shorter (500 and 800 msec) or longer (1800 msec) ISIs.

Critical in claims of *selectively* slowed activation for nonfluent aphasics, of course, is demonstrating that activation is *not* slowed for other aphasics. More recently, Prather, Zurif & Love (1992) replicated the first case study with a second nonfluent aphasic, and also extended this research to include a fluent aphasic. Findings with a second nonfluent aphasic again supported the prediction of slowed activation. The surprising finding in this second study was the lack of a normal priming curve for our fluent aphasic subject.

Briefly, the same materials and basic procedure were used as in our earlier work (Prather, Zurif & Love 1992). Subjects included FC, a 58 year old right-handed male with nonfluent aphasia, and JM, a 54 year old right-handed male with a fluent aphasia. Both subjects were presented initially with word lists that included ISIs of 500, 1100 and 1500 msec ISIs; as in Prather, Zurif, Stern & Rosen (1992), across six sessions (separated by a minimum of two weeks), each subject saw each target word preceded once by a related and once by a control prime at each of the three ISIs. Similar to findings with LD, FC was just beginning to show priming at 1500 msec (although those effects were not significant); JM, on the other hand, showed priming at both 500 and 1100 msec and did not show a decline until 1500 msec. In a second study, priming was examined at ISIs of 1500 to 2100 with FC, who did not show reliable priming until an ISI of 2100 msec. For JM, priming was obtained at 300 and 500 msec, and again did not diminish until 1500 msec. To summarize, FC, a nonfluent aphasic showed a reliable priming effect at an ISI of 2100 msec but not at shorter ISIs; JM, a fluent aphasic, showed reliable priming at ISIs ranging from 300 to 1100 msec, but not at longer ISIs. Clearly neither of these findings is "normal". Both case studies with nonfluent subjects to data have, as predicted, shown a protracted rise time in lexical activation[1] relative to findings with both young and elderly subjects. Unexpectedly, our case study with a fluent aphasic showed a rise time that was too rapid, and also that extended for too long. Normally, using the LPP to examine the time course of lexical activation, priming did not obtain until an ISI of 500 msec (see also Shelton & Martin 1992), and quickly diminished.

Again, a serendipitous finding with an aphasic population. We now come full circle. Milberg & Blumstein set out to understand why fluent aphasics were "deviant" in semantic judgments, expecting to find deviant priming and instead finding "normal" priming with that population and "deviant" findings for nonfluent aphasics. We set out to understand why nonfluent aphasics were unstable in their priming effects, expecting to find a "normal" time course with fluent aphasics, and instead obtaining at least preliminary indications that they are somehow deviant in their time course. In effect, our findings could represent support for what Milberg & Blumstein originally hypothesized: there is something unusual about fluent aphasics' access to lexical/semantic information.

5 Concluding Remarks

The introductory remarks prefaced the following conclusion: that the distinctive deviations for nonfluent and fluent aphasics, at least with respect to lexical processing, were respectively in *rate* and *route* of lexical access. Let me elaborate on those points in light of the data presented above.

Based on findings to date, the most parsimonious account for the variable lexical priming effects obtained with nonfluent aphasics remains that proposed by Swinney, Zurif and Nicol: a delayed rise time in lexical activation, or at least in obtaining detectable activation. At present, there is insufficient data to make strong claims, but initial findings are strongly suggestive that while they are slower to activate lexical information, nonfluent aphasics are like normal controls in showing a rapid decline in activation once peak activation is achieved. In that sense, they show a slower rise time but normal dampening or inhibition of automatic lexical activation over time.

This hypothesis of delayed rise time in no way contradicts published findings showing priming for nonfluent aphasics, and indeed offers the strongest support for a claim that nonfluent aphasics demonstrate automatic lexical activation. The constraint placed by our findings is on time: nonfluent aphasics show automatic activation *given sufficient time*. That is critical in considering the implications of delayed lexical activation on real-time sentence comprehension. As Lenneberg pointed out, the time course of real-time sentence processing is tightly constrained; phonological, lexical, syntactic and semantic information all need to be available at the right time, as well as in the right form, in order to support normally rapid sentence comprehension. If that timing is disrupted, then sentence comprehension should be disrupted – as it is known to be for nonfluent aphasics. While their comprehension can be quite good on off-line tasks where there are no time constraints and where information can be repeated and pondered, there are clear failures in comprehension of particular syntactic forms under time constraints. Recently, for example, on-line investigations of gap-filling have supported the expectation that, arguably because of their slowed activation, nonfluent aphasics fail to activate information that is critical to on-line sentence comprehension at the time that it is needed. Briefly to describe the premise of this research, according to government and binding theory (Chomsky 1981), movement of a constituent leaves a trace (an abstract, phonetically empty marker) in the position it vacated, e.g. in the sentence:

The priest enjoyed the drink$_i$ that the caterer was serving (t)$_i$ to the guests.

there is a "trace" following "serving" that refers back to the object of "serving", which is "drink". The presence of that trace, and its association to "drink", is actually detectable through priming techniques (see Swinney & Fodor 1989; Swinney & Osterhout 1990, for reviews of this work). Normally, immediately following (but not preceding) the verb "serving", associates to the object of "serving", i.e. "drink", are primed, consistent with the hypothesis that there is an active trace in the gap following "serve" that references the object of "serve", i.e. "drink". On the assumption that nonfluent aphasics are slowed in their activation, one could expect that they would be slowed in filling the trace, that is, in activating "drink" – a prediction currently being investigated by Swinney, Zurif and their colleagues. To date, they find that, in contrast to fluent aphasics and elderly controls, nonfluent aphasics do not show priming at gaps that should be filled by traces (Swinney, Zurif, Prather & Love 1993; Zurif 1994), consistent with predicted findings. Importantly, the prediction that the trace would not be active immediately for nonfluent aphasics based on the hypothesis of slowed activation fits well with linguistic analyses suggesting that an underlying feature of nonfluent aphasics' syntactic deficits is failure to represent traces (Grodzinsky 1990). What remains to be determined is whether the trace is not represented at all, or rather (consistent with the hypothesis of temporal delay) is activated "later" than normally is the case – and later than is necessary for rapid sentence comprehension.

Much work clearly remains to be done, but we would argue that the hypothesis of slowed activation of lexical information is unique to nonfluent aphasics, and that it accounts for many of their failures in production as well as comprehension. The apparent discrepancies between their "on-line" and "off-line" performance capabilities and the variability in their performance across tasks that vary in processing rate and load certainly lends itself to an explanation based on processing rate rather than on a deficit in underlying lexical/semantic organization or availability.

Fluent aphasics, on the other hand, present a priming pattern that may be best understood as a failure to access lexical information normally, or failure to access normal lexical information. All studies examining priming in nonfluent aphasics report that they prime routinely; our recent findings with one case study showed that, at least for that subject, priming obtained sooner and longer than for either nonfluent aphasics or age matched controls. Consistent with that finding, we are currently conducting studies examining cross-modal priming at various delays following presentation of ambiguous words in sentence contexts; our findings to date indicate that priming for the contextually inappropriate meaning of an ambiguous word dampens relatively quickly for normal controls (as Swinney, Onifer, Prather & Hirshkowitz 1979 found), but not for fluent aphasics.

Failure to show a decline in automatic priming over time might be accounted for in terms of failure in some inhibitory control mechanisms. Inhibitory controls could not easily explain early as well as late priming, however. Indications to date are that fluent aphasics prime much more – sooner as well as longer – than control subjects. One possible account of their overall priming profile is that fluent aphasics access lexical information in a completely different manner from nonfluent aphasics and controls. Relevant to that speculation, studies examining lateral differences in priming have suggested that the right hemisphere may do a different kind of analysis of lexical information, a kind of "coarse coding" (Beeman 1994), analogous to getting a global impression rather than detailed knowledge of individual words. Speculatively, the priming effects obtained with fluent aphasics may reflect access to "right hemisphere" rather than "left hemisphere" knowledge. That is, fluent aphasics may be operating on a different data base – in effect, the "different lexical organization" initially proposed by Milberg and Blumstein, although a somewhat based on a different account than they may have had in mind. It is an intriguing notion, one that is clearly underspecified theoretically as well as empirically at present, but that bears consideration. Of course, consideration of that hypothesis in turn requires consideration of the relation between syntactic form and lexical activation. Fluent aphasics show preserved appreciation of syntactic relations, including rapid activation of traces; if "coarse coding" is an accurate description of their lexical information, then either that coarse code includes relevant syntactic information, or syntactic relations – at least some syntactic relations, like traces – are specified independently of lexical information.

What is not speculative is that much of the empirical discrepancy across studies examining lexical processes in aphasic populations reflects inconsistencies in methodology across studies. It is simply not possible to compare studies that use different priming techniques, different temporal parameters, different modalities of presentation, and different subject populations. A report of priming in one study using a PPP but visual presentation of materials cannot be compared directly to a "similar" study using an auditory presentation; it is quite possible that auditory processing is much faster, or that reading is much slower, and consequently that a "simple" shift in modalities completely changes the temporal parameters involved. Similarly, studies using pair vs. triplet vs. sentence contexts cannot be compared directly, particularly in terms of temporal parameters. Much of the "controversy" surrounding the issue of automatic lexical activation in fluent and nonfluent aphasic populations seems grounded in making comparisons across studies that are fundamentally different and consequently not comparable – and most of which, in addition, failed to control for the possibility of strategic factors. Understanding lexical processes in aphasic populations promises important insights into lexical processing generally as well as into neurological underpinnings of those processes, but advances are not likely without more systematic procedural considerations.

Note

1 In making claims about "automatic" activation using the LPP, it is important to show a decline as well as rise in priming effects. We are for that reason cautious in making claims of automatic activation for FC, who showed priming at an ISI of 2100 msec only, which was the longest ISI examined with that subject. Based on all other findings with the LPP, we feel justified in assuming that this does reflect automatic priming, but clearly must remain cautious until extending this finding through several additional case studies where we are able to show a fall in rise time after peak priming.

References

Beeman, M., R. Friedman, J. Grafman, E. Perez, S. Diamond & M. Lindsay (1994): "Summation priming and coarse semantic coding in the right hemisphere". Journal of Cognitive Neuroscience 6.

Blumstein, S., W. Milberg & R. Shrier (1982): "Semantic processing in aphasia: Evidence from an auditory lexical decision task". Brain and Language 17, 301 – 315.

Chomsky, N. (1981): Lectures on government and binding. Dordrecht: Foris.

Collins, A. & E. Loftus (1975): "A spreading-activation theory of semantic processing". Psychological Review 82, 407 – 428.

de Groot, A. (1984): "Primed lexical decision: Combined effects of the proportion of related prime-target pairs and the stimulus-onset asynchrony of prime and target". The Quarterly Journal of Experimental Psychology 36A, 253 – 280.

den Heyer, K., K. Briand & G. Dannenbring (1983): "Strategic factors in a lexical-decision task: Evidence for automatic and attention-driven processes". Memory & Cognition 11, 374 – 381.

den Heyer, K., K. Briand & L. Smith (1985): "Automatic and strategic effects in semantic priming: An examination of Becker's verification model". Memory & Cognition 13(3), 228 – 232.

Favreau, M. & N. Segalowitz (1983): "Automatic and controlled processes in the first- and second-language reading of fluent bilinguals". Memory & Cognition 11(6), 565 – 574.

Fodor, J.A. (1983): The Modularity of Mind. Cambridge, Mass.: The MIT Press.

Goodglass, H. & E. Baker (1976): "Semantic field, naming, and auditory comprehension in aphasia". Brain and Language 3, 359 – 374.

Grodzinsky, Y. (1990): Theoretical perspectives on language deficits. Cambridge, Mass: MIT Press.

Hagoort, P. (1993): "Impairments of lexical-semantic processing in aphasia: Evidence from the processing of lexical ambiguities". Brain and Language 45, 198 – 232.

Katz, W. (1988): "An investigation of lexical ambiguity in Broca's aphasics using an auditory lexical priming technique". Neuropsychologia 26(5), 747 – 752.

Kramer Ostrin, R. & L. Komisarjevsky Tyler (1993): "Automatic access to lexical semantics in aphasia: Evidence from semantic and associative priming". Brain and Language 45, 147 – 159.

Milberg, W. & S. Blumstein (1981): "Lexical decision and aphasia: Evidence for semantic processing". Brain and Language 14, 371 – 385.

Milberg, W., S. Blumstein & B. Dworetzky (1987): "Processing of lexical ambiguities in aphasia". Brain and Language.

McNamara, T. & J. Altarriba (1988): "Depth of spreading activation revisited: Semantic mediated priming occurs in lexical decisions". Journal of Memory and Language 27, 545 – 559.

Neely, J. (1991): "Semantic priming effects in visual word recognition: A selective review of current findings and theories". In: D. Besner & G. Humphreys, eds., Basic processes in reading visual word recognition, Hillsdale: Erlbaum, 264 – 336.

Neely, J.H. (1977): "Semantic priming and retrieval from lexical memory: Roles of inhibitionless spreading activation and limited capacity attention". Journal of Experimental Psychology: General 106, 226 - 254.

Prather, P. & D. Swinney (1988): "Lexical processing and ambiguity resolution: An autonomous process in an interactive box". In: S.L. Small, G.W. Cottrell & M.K. Tanenhaus, eds., Lexical Ambiguity Resolution California: Morgan Kaufman.

Prather, P.A., E. Zurif, C. Stern & T.J. Rosen (1992): "Slowed lexical access in nonfluent aphasia: A case study". Brain and Language 43, 336 - 348.

Prather, P., E. Zurif & T. Love (1992): "Time course of lexical access in fluent and nonfluent aphasia". Academy of Aphasia.

Shelton, J. & R. Martin (1992): "How semantic is automatic semantic priming?" Journal of Experimental Psychology: Learning, memory, and cognition 18(6), 1191 - 1210.

Simpson, G. (1984): "Lexical ambiguity and its role in models of word recognition". Psychological Bulletin 96, 316 - 340.

Simpson, G. & C. Burgess (1985): "Activation and selection processes in the recognition of ambiguous words". Journal of Experimental Psychology: Human Perception and Performance 11, 38 - 39.

Smith, E.E., E. Shoben & L. Rips (1974): "Structure and process in semantic memory: A featural model for semantic decisions". Psychological Review 81, 214 - 241.

Stern, C., P. Prather, D. Swinney & E. Zurif (1991): "The time coures of automatic lexical access and aging". Brain and Language 40, 359 - 372.

Swinney, D., E. Zurif & J. Nicol (1989): "The effects of focal brain damage on sentence processing: An examination of the neurological organization of a mental module". Journal of Cognitive Neuroscience 1, 25 - 37.

Swinney, D. & J.D. Fodor (1989): Journal of Psycholinguistic Research (Special Issue on Sentence Processing), 18(1).

Swinney, D., W. Onifer, P. Prather & M. Hirshkowitz (1979): "Semantic facilitation across sensory modalities in the processing of individual words and sentences". Memory & Cognition 7, 159 - 165.

Swinney, D. & L. Osterhout (1990): "Inference generation during auditory language comprehension". In: A. Graesser & G.H. Bower, eds., The Psychology of Learning and Motivation. New York: Academic Press.

Swinney, D., E. Zurif, P. Prather & T. Love (1993): The neurological distribution of processing operations underlying language comprehension. Manuscript, Dept. of Psychology, University of Cal., San Diego.

Swinney, D.A. (1979): "Lexical access during sentence comprehension: (Re)consideration of context effects". Journal of Verbal Learning and Verbal Behavior 18, 645 - 659.

Tweedy, J., R. Lapinski & R. Schvaneveldt (1977): "Semantic-context effects on word recognition: Influence of varying the proportion of items presented in an appropriate context". Memory & Cognition 5(1), 84 - 89.

Whitehouse, P., A. Caramazza & E. Zurif (1978): "Naming in aphasia: Interactivity effects of form and function". Brain and Language 6, 63 - 74.

Zurif, E. (1994): Brain regions of relevance to syntactic processing. In: Invitation to Cognitive Science, 2nd Edition.

Zurif, E., A. Caramazza, R. Myerson & J. Galvin (1974): "Semantic feature representations for normal and aphasic language". Brain and Language 1, 167 - 187.

Interactive/Activation in Normal and Brain-damaged Individuals: Can Context Penetrate the Lexical 'Module'?

Arturo Hernandez, Elizabeth Bates, San Diego

Anomia is defined as a pathological deficit in finding and producing words. It is the one symptom that appears in every form of aphasia. It is also an early and ubiquitous symptom in dementia of the Alzheimer's type, and milder forms of anomia are among the most common complaints in normal aging. Classically, anomia has been explained as a disconnection or deterioration in the links between semantic and lexical representations (i.e. between meaning and phonological/orthographic forms – (Farah & Wallace 1992; Gainotti, Silveri, Villa & Miceli 1986; Hadar, Jones & Mate-Kole 1987; le Dorze & Nespoulous 1989; Lucchelli & de Renzi 1992). In fact, some studies have found that training can greatly improve the performance of anomic aphasics, (Colby, Chrisinaz, Parkinson, Graham & Karpf 1981) a clear indication that semantic representations themselves have not been damaged in anomia. Since the residual language deficit in anomic patients seems to revolve around lexical access (i.e. naming), it would be useful to know whether these patients show normal forms of facilitation and/or inhibition in real-time lexical processing. The same is true for the milder word-finding deficits that are often found in normal aging. Is this deficit restricted entirely to word production, or can we find correlates and (perhaps) a possible cause in other aspects of lexical access? And if so, what is the nature of the disturbance in lexical access that underlies this common disorder?

In the present study, we will examine the interaction between discourse and word-level priming in a cross-modal naming paradigm (i.e. pronunciation of visually presented words in an auditory context), in young normal controls, in healthy older adults, and in eight aphasic patients with documented deficits in word finding. We will show that lexical access in context involves a complex, dynamic interplay of facilitative and inhibitory processes. Aphasic patients and older adults display the same qualitative pattern observed in college students, but there is also evidence for increased reliance on context and a reduced ability to overcome or inhibit forms of priming that interfere with the task of word pronunciation – a tendency that is evident in normal aging, and even more prominent in patients with focal brain injury. Before presenting results of this experiment, we will provide a brief overview of the theoretical issues that are at stake in the study of lexical access in normal populations, followed by an even briefer review of the relevant research on lexical access in aging and aphasia.

1 On Lexical Access in Normal Adults

The nature of lexical-semantic processing is a hotly debated issue in the psycholinguistic literature. On one side stand those who believe that lexical processing is highly modular (Fodor 1983; Forster 1981). In this view, the steps leading from the perception of letters or sounds to the code of the word and the subsequent activation of all core meanings must occur before lexical items can be integrated into a larger sentential or discourse context. In other words, context cannot pre-select lexical items This "autonomy" of lexical processing has received support from a series of studies showing that all meanings of an ambiguous word are immediately accessed regardless of contextual bias (Onifer & Swinney 1981; Seidenberg, Tanenhaus, Leiman & Bienkowski 1982). It is only after a short delay (about 500 ms between prime and target) that the contextually appropriate meaning is accessed. The inference drawn is that associative links along a semantic pathway are activated immediately and that any context effect is post-lexical. The result of these studies have firmly placed the autonomy of lexical processing as a necessary consideration for any theory of on-line lexical-semantic processing.

Despite the strong evidence in favor of the modularity hypothesis, many have opposed this interpretation of reaction time studies with ambigous words. Van Petten and Kutas (Van Petten & Kutas 1987), for example, used event-related potentials (ERP's) to look at the processing of homophones. The authors found that priming (as measured by component of the ERP called the N400) of the semantically inappropriate word began later and was smaller than that of the semantically appropriate word at a short stimulus onset asynchrony (SOA). At long SOAs, only the contextually appropriate meaning was primed. Since all of this occurred before the average time required to register a button press, it is clear why reaction times would not serve to clarify this point. This is not to denigrate reaction time tasks. The present study involves reaction times. The important point to be taken from the Van Petten and Kutas study is that language processing may involve multiple processes that occur well before the collection of reaction times.

The modularity hypothesis also carries a number of additional assumptions regarding the nature of priming effects, with particular emphasis on the contrast between facilitation and inhibition – yet another controversial issue in psycholinguistics. Some authors have proposed that insights into real-time language use must come from the study of language processes that are fast, automatic, and unconscious; methods that elicit slower, controlled and conscious processes are subject to experiment-specific strategies and hence may not generalize to language use outside of the laboratory. For example, some investigators have found that semantic priming effects can be influenced by the subject's expectations about the stimuli, induced by varying the proportion of related/unrelated items and/or the proportion of words to non-words (Neely 1976; Tweedy, Lapinski & Schvaneveldt 1977). Hence, although there is a certain amount of automatic, facilitative priming that occurs regardless of expectations, some contribution to semantic priming may be due to conscious processes. These conscious processes can cause both inhibition and facilitation. These arguments rest, in turn, on two additional assumptions (following Posner's suggestions for attentional processes outside the verbal domain – Posner & Snyder 1975): all automatic processes are based on facilitation, and the presence of inhibition always implies some form of controlled, strategic processing. Because claims about modularity pertain only to automatic processes, it follows that studies investigating the autonomy hypothesis should avoid methods that induce inhibitory processing.

However, other theorists have argued against the traditional automatic/controlled processing distinction. In an interactive/activation framework, for example, both inhibition and facilitation are thought to occur early in processing (Colombo 1986; Grainger 1990; McClelland & Rumelhart 1981). In fact, evidence for very rapid and automatic forms of inhibition have been reported in non-verbal priming studies (Marangolo, Dipace, & Pizzamiglio 1993). In the same vein, it could be argued that well-known phenomena like the Stroop effect provide evidence for fast, automatic forms of inhibition in the language domain. Thus there is good reason to believe that both facilitation and inhibition can occur early in language processing. If this view is correct, then we need not assume that expectations always lead to slow, strategic and experiment-specific forms of processing; rather, expectations could be used to set up rapid and relatively unconscious patterns of inhibition and facilitation that do generalize to language performance outside of the laboratory.

Investigators have studied facilitation and inhibition (and automatic and controlled processes) by manipulating subject expectancies or SOA's with normal controls, and/or by looking at populations in which there is some reason to believe that these processes are differentially impaired. The relevant populations have included individuals with diffuse or focal brain damage (i.e. Alzheimer's patients or aphasics) as well as normal geriatric populations. In the following section, we will review some of the literature on the effects of aging and neurological insult on 'real-time' language processing, with a particular focus on the relative contribution of facilitation and inhibition.

2 Language Processing in Older Adults and Brain-Damaged Individuals

Recent studies have revealed a number of differences between older adults and younger college controls. These include impairments in short-term and long-term memory (Mitrushina & Satz 1991; Salthouse 1991) which can affect both the ability to remember detailed information of previous discourse or interpret sentences correctly (Hasher & Zacks 1988; Light & Burke 1988; Salthouse 1991). Age-related changes have been attributed to efficiency of processing brought about by a general cognitive slowing (Nebes & Brady 1992; Salthouse 1991), a decline in processing capacity or attentional resources (Hasher & Zacks 1988), or the inability to inhibit irrelevant information, a special case of the reduced capacity theory (Hasher, Stoltzfus, Zacks & Rypma 1991; Hasher & Zacks 1988). These theories imply that a more general processing change (i.e. limited short-term memory) is responsible for impairment in more specific domains of cognitive processing (Salthouse 1991).

Within this framework, the older adult population can provide an important test case for the theories of lexical processing described above. Presumably, changes in general processing should have no effect on automatic semantic priming, since automatic processes (like reflexes – Fodor 1983) are not affected by general processing demands. Therefore a change in general processing capacity should only influence post-lexical processes. Studies with older adults have revealed that automatic semantic priming remains unchanged in older adults (Chiarello, Church & Hoyer 1985) and adults with Alzheimer's disease (Ober, Shenaut, Jagust & Stillman 1991). In addition, syntactic processes which are thought to be even less subject to strategies (i.e. more automatic) have shown little or no decrement with aging when memory load is controlled (Zurif, Swinney, Prather, Wingfield & Brownell 1993). Within this view, effects of aging should only be observed on syntactic processes that involve long-distance relationships (i.e. processes that require the listener to hold several elements in memory). Taken together, these studies support a view in which automatic processes are not affected by changes due to aging or diffuse neurological damage.

In aphasia, a much more localized and focal type of brain damage, differential impairment of automatic and controlled processing has been proposed. Specifically, it has been argued that Broca's aphasics fail to show automatic semantic priming, but can use a set of heuristic (i.e. conscious) processes. By contrast, Wernicke's aphasics show no decline in automatic priming but fail to employ heuristic strategies (Milberg, Blumstein, Katz & Gershberg 1993). This is an interesting proposal that could account, in principle, for many of the double dissociations that are observed between Broca's and Wernicke's aphasia (Bates, Wulfeck & MacWhinney 1991). However, other studies have shown that Broca's aphasics do show evidence for forms of semantic and syntactic priming that are usually assumed to reflect automatic processing (Hagoort 1993; Ostrin & Tyler 1993). As an alternative to the automatic/controlled dichotomy, it has been argued that Broca's aphasia represents a general slowing of activation for linguistic information, with serious and rather specific consequences for the coordination of parsing operations and/or for efficient integration of lexical items into contextual frames (Friederici & Frazier 1992; Friederici & Kilborn 1989; Kolk & Van Grunsven 1985; Ostrin & Tyler 1993).

In contrast with the growing literature on lexical processing in Broca's and Wernicke's aphasics, there are surprisingly few 'on-line' studies of lexical access in patients who suffer from milder forms of language impairment due to a focal lesion. In many cases, these patients have evolved from a more severe fluent or non-fluent aphasia in the first few months after their injury, to a milder form of aphasia restricted primarily to word finding deficits (i.e. anomia). Because these patients themselves often represent a developmental continuum from more serious forms of aphasia, it is reasonable to ask whether their word-finding deficits reflect a milder variant of the deficits in "on-line" lexical access reported for Broca's and/or Wernicke's aphasia. And the continuum may extend in the other direction to include healthy older adults.

In the present study, a cross-modal naming paradigm was used to study lexical access in college-aged adults, older adults, and a group of higher-level aphasic patients (i.e.

anomic aphasics). We have departed from other real-time studies of lexical processing, in two respects. First, most studies with impaired and normal populations have used lexical decision, which may be susceptible to post-lexical search strategies (Balota & Lorch 1986) and is less naturalistic than other tasks such as naming. In order to avoid some of these problems, the current study used cross-modal naming (i.e. time required to pronounce a visual word in an auditory context). Naming is thought to provide a deeper and less strategic measure of lexical access; whether or not this is the case, it is certainly true that cross-modal naming produces faster latencies than lexical decision. Second, most studies have used minimal semantic contexts, i.e. word pairs or a brief sentence. Instead, we will assess priming in a discourse context. The use of discourse-level priming should help to provide subjects with robust semantic expectations, while insuring a more naturalistic mode of language processing (Foss 1982).

In the procedure adopted here, visual word pairs (a prime followed by a target) are embedded in an auditory context that is several sentences long. The word pairs may be semantically related to each other or not (W+ vs. W–). The target may or may not be a good completion of the discourse context up to that point (C+ vs. C–). Finally, a neutral control condition will be used in which subjects will see an unrelated pair in which neither word is a good completion of the context. We will assume that reaction times which are significantly faster than this neutral control reflect some form of facilitation (from the context and/or the prime word), while reaction times that are significantly slower than this neutral control reflect some form of inhibition. An example of these items can be seen in Table 1.

In essence, we are placing discourse-level priming in competition with word-level priming. To ensure this competition, the word pairs will be presented at a 200 ms stimulus onset asynchrony (SOA), an interval at which there should be little or no contextual penetration according to a purely modular lexical-semantic account. If the modular account is correct, we may find a main effect of word-level priming (an automatic form of activation) and a main effect of contextual priming (a post-lexical effect), but no interaction. Above all, contextual effects should not eliminate or reduce word-level effects in the rapid stimulus-response windows adopted in the present study.

The second point of this study is to investigate how contextual integration and lexical-access are affected by aging. Previous results have offered a number of possibilities with regard to the effects of aging on language processing. Some theories imply large changes in language processing with age (Hasher & Zacks 1988) while others find little or no change in language processing with age (Ober et al. 1991; Zurif, Swinney, Prather,

Table 1 Sample conditons from the experiment

"The boy was driving the car down the"	
ROAD-STREET (W+/C+)	APPLE-STREET (W–/C+)
APPLE-ORANGE (W+/C–)	STREET-APPLE (W–/C–)
Neutral Control = APPLE-KNOB	

Wingfield & Brownell 1992). The present experiment should help to disambiguate these positions by observing the way in which two robust phenomena (local word-level semantic priming and global discourse-level priming) when placed into competition are affected by aging. If the failure-of-inhibition account of cognitive impairments in aging is correct, then it should be particularly difficult for older adults to suppress discourse-level or word-level effects that slow word naming in the young; at the same time, we may expect a sparing and (indeed) an augmentation of the facilitative context effects that are observed in younger subjects.

Finally, we hope to shed some light on the nature of the underlying processes that characterize the naming deficit shared by anomic patients. If anomic patients display quantitative or qualitative changes in the normal patterns of lexical facilitation, inhibition and competition observed within this paradigm, then we may infer that these processes play some role in naming disorders. On the other hand, if these patients show the same patterns of word- and discourse-level priming displayed by age-matched normal controls, we must conclude that the locus of their naming deficit lies elsewhere.

3 Method

Subjects

Sixty-two subjects were tested using the cross-modal word pair paradigm. The young controls were twenty undergraduates at the University of California, San Diego, recruited through the subject pool of the Department of Psychology. The older adult group was made up of fifteen right handed individuals between the ages of 63 and 85 (mean = 68.6429, sd = 10.2553).

The aphasics comprised of eight subjects with slight to moderate word-finding difficulties. These were mainly recruited from the San Diego Veterans Administration Hospital but also from surrounding hospitals. The patients all were between the ages of 39 and 79 (mean = 65.54, sd = 10.48) and all had suffered a single stroke to the left hemisphere. All Eight patients were classified as anomic aphasics. Classification of aphasia type was based on subjects' performance on the Western Aphasia Battery (WAB). Patients were all at least six months post stroke onset (mean = 5, sd = 3.66), had no history of alcohol or drug abuse, no history of psychiatric illness, no other significant brain disorder or dysfunction, normal visual acuity, normal hearing acuity, minimal limb apraxia, minimal motor speech involvement. A summary of patient information can be seen in Table 2.

Table 2 Aphasic Patient information

ID #	Age	Sex	Handed-ness	Etiology	WAB Classification	WAB AQ (naming)	Lesion
JS084	68	M	R	CVA	A-mild	97.5 r (8.8)	Frontal Parietal
HP139	75	M	R	CVA	A	94.4 r (9.3)	Left Frontal-Parietal
TB247	65	M	R	CVA	C/A	73.0 r (8.9)	N/A
BU252	79	M	R	CVA	A	84.3 r (8.3)	N/A
PB405	67	M	R	CVA	Trace A	98.0 r (10)	Anterior
ES406	71	M	R	CVA	A	85.6 r (7.5)	N/A
JW410	65	M	R	CVA	A	85.5 r (8.6)	N/A
MC421	66	M	R	CVA	A	83.2 r (8.1)	N/A

A = Anomic, W = Wernicke, B = Broca, C = Conduction

Apparatus

Subjects were run on a Macintosh IIsi computer connected to a Carnegie-Mellon button box. The experimental trials were administered using the *PsyScope* experimental shell developed at Carnegie-Mellon University by Brian MacWhinney and Jonathan Cohen (Cohen, MacWhinney, Flatt & Provost 1993). All of the experimental materials were placed on a Syquest removable cartridge drive.

Test Materials and Design

The materials in this task consisted of fifteen texts chosen from third-grade-level textbooks. All texts were 7-8 sentences long. The passages were chosen to address a number of culturally neutral topics (i.e. animals, space, firefighters, etc.). Between six and eight words were extracted from every text (approximately one per sentence). The words that were extracted from the texts (all common nouns) were replaced with a word pair (also common nouns). The word pairs were placed in one of five conditions and coded according to the relationship of the target to the text (context+ or context–) and to itself (word+ or word–). In the first condition, both prime and target were good completions of the discourse up to that point (W+/C+). In the second condition, the prime was a bad completion but the target was a good completion (W–/C+). In the third condition, the prime and target were both bad completions but were related to each other (W+/C–). In the fourth condition, the prime and target were unrelated semantically to each other, but the prime was a good completion (W–/C–). Finally, the neutral control consisted of word pairs that were neither related to themselves nor to the context (neu). There were 20 items per condition. Congruent words were all the original words in the text. Incongruent words were chosen so as to not match the text. When a second congruent word was needed, a synonym of the completion which was close in frequency was chosen. The incongruent word pairs were chosen to be strongly associated. Conditions were randomly assigned across the experiment. Every subject received the same random order.

The word targets were all balanced for frequency of occurrence using the Kucera and Francis norms (1982). In addition, they were balanced for length. Although the stimuli where not randomized across subjects (one cannot randomize sentences in a discourse paradigm), the conditions that appeared were randomized so that subjects could not predict which of the five conditions would appear next.

The baseline condition consisted of 30 word pairs (fifteen related and fifteen unrelated). These were presented in the same order to each subject, but like the experiment these conditions were randomized. The baseline was used primarily as a way to provide subjects practice with perceiving and reading word pairs in isolation before the more difficult task of seeing similar items in context. Therefore, we will not present analyses of priming data for these out-of-context pairs.

Procedure

All of the undergraduate students were tested in Experimental rooms located at the Center for Research in Language at the University of California, San Diego campus. Both older adults and Aphasic patients were tested at the VA San Diego.

Each session consisted of two parts. In the baseline section, subjects were instructed that two words would appear one after the other and that they should pronounce the second word into the microphone as quickly as possible. The word pair was presented at a 200 msec SOA. After the baseline section, the participants were told that they would be hearing a set of texts in which they had to answer a multiple-choice question. Thus they should pay attention to the content of the passage. In addition, they were also advised that during the text the recording would stop and two words would appear on the screen. Subjects were told that they should pronounce words as quickly and accurately as possible. They were informed that the words might or might not fit with the text. The texts were presented auditorally. At a predetermined point during the text the sound would stop and a visual word was immediately presented on a computer screen for 200 ms followed by a target word. College normals were given a response window of 1 second while older adults and aphasics were given two seconds to respond. If he/she responded before the elapsed time had passed, then the text continued. If the subject did not respond within the response window, a no response was recorded, the word would come off the screen and the auditory text would resume. At the end of the text a question would appear on the screen. These questions asked about the text that had just been presented, and served as a rough measure of the level of comprehension. Once the question was answered the next passage would begin.

Table 3 Mean Reaction Times in ms and percentage of errors for each group

	Context +	Neutral	Context–	Facilitation	Inhibition
Young Adults					
Word+	530 (0.29 %)	537 (0.29 %)	536 (1.17 %)	6.95	–1
Word–	509 (0.58 %)	537 (0.29 %)	549 (0.58 %)	27**	12*
Older Adults					
Word+	668 (0 %)	669 (1.33 %)	661 (3 %)	1	–8
Word–	620 (0.33 %)	669 (1.33 %)	697 (0.33 %)	48**	27*
Aphasics					
Word+	922 (1.33 %)	989 (1.17 %)	963 (1.17 %)	67*	–26
Word–	868 (0.83 %)	989 (1.6 %)	1005 (1.5 %)	121**	16

* $p < 0.05$, ** $p < 0.01$

4 Results and Discussion

College Controls

Experimental reaction times: The raw data for normal controls can be seen in Table 1. The raw reaction times were placed into a 2 (word relationship) x 2 (context relationship) within-subjects ANOVA. There were main effects of word relationship, $F(1,19) = 4.949$, $p < 0.038$, contextual relationship of the target word, $F(1,19) = 35.49$, $p < 0.000$, and a word relationship by contextual relationship interaction, $F(1,19) = 25.83$, $p < 0.000$. The contextual relationship was significant over items, $F(1,76) = 7.04$, $p < 0.01$, and the word relationship by contextual relationship interaction was marginally significant over items, $F(1,76) = 3.19$, $p < 0.078$. The results showed that W+ words were read in 533 ms while W– words were read in 529 ms. Furthermore, C+ words were read in 519 ms while C– words were read in 542 ms The word relationship by contextual relationship interaction revealed that for W+ words contextual relevance was unimportant (530 vs. 536 ms). For W– words contextual relevance was very important (509 ms vs. 549 ms). In addition, notice that W–/C+ words are read faster than W+/C+ words (509 vs. 530 ms).

A set of t-tests was run in order to compare across conditions and to compare each condition to the neutral control. These confirmed the findings in the general ANOVA. First of all, for W– words the C+ condition was faster than the C– condition, $t(19) = 7.978$, $p < 0.000$. In addition, it was found that W+/C+ condition was significantly slower than the W–/C+ condition, $t(19) = 5.32$, $p < 0.000$. In addition, comparisons with the neutral control revealed that the W–/C+ condition was significantly faster than baseline, $t(19) = 5.96$, $p < 0.000$, and that the W–/C– condition was significantly slower than baseline $t(19) = 2.39$, $p < 0.02$.

Figure 1 Word relationship by contextual relationship interaction for college controls

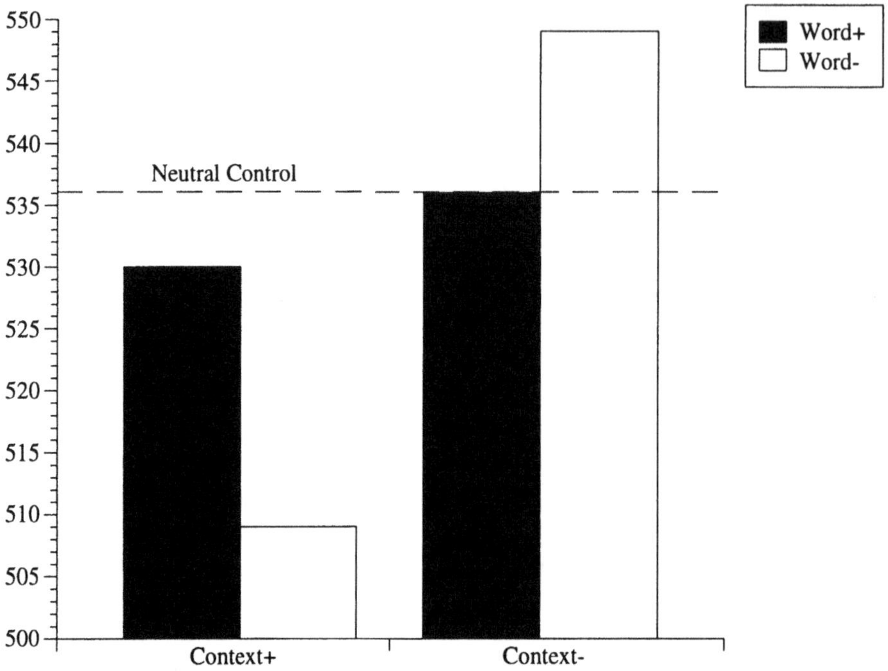

To simplify analyses across groups, the mean RT for neutral control items for each subject was subtracted from each reaction time for that subject in the four experimental conditions. These adjusted reaction times for the college controls were placed into a 2 (word relationship) x 2 (context relationship) within-subjects anova. This yielded a significant main effect of word relationship, $F(1,19) = 4.949$, $p < 0.038$, contextual relationship of the target word, $F(1,19) = 35.49$, $p < 0.000$, and a word relationship by contextual relationship interaction, $F(1,19) = 25.83$, $p < 0.000$. The contextual relationship was significant over items $F(1,76) = 7.14$, $p < 0.009$, and the word relationship by contextual relationship interaction was marginally significant over items, $F(1,76) = 3.32$, $p < 0.072$. These results revealed that the W+ words were read only 3 ms faster than baseline while W– words were read only 7 ms faster than baseline When the target was a good completion (C+) it was read 17 ms faster than neutral, and 5 ms slower than neutral when it was not (C–). In addition, the WxC interaction revealed that the difference between C+ and C– words was larger for W– words (–27 ms vs. +12 ms) than for W+ words (–6 ms vs. 0 ms). It also was clear that the W–/C+ words were read about 21 ms faster than W+/C+ words.

The results from the college controls seem very clear. The data do not support a purely modular model in which word-level and discourse-level priming cannot interact, and they also show that discourse effects can operate very early. However, it is clear that there are constraints on the nature of the interaction between context and word primes. First, there is a significant amount of facilitation (i.e. RTs faster than baseline) when

Figure 2 Word relationship by contextual relationship interaction for older adult controls

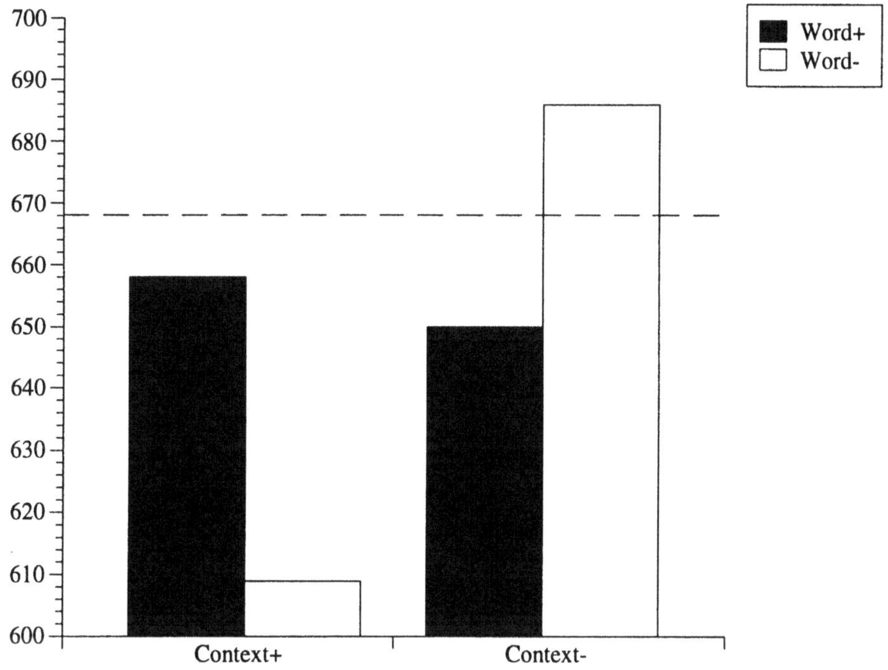

the target is contextually relevant and the prime is not (W–/C+), and a significant amount of inhibition (i.e. RTs slower than baseline) when the prime is contextually relevant and the target is not (W–/C–). Hence there do appear to be early and rapid forms of contextual facilitation and inhibition. However, W+ words are neither facilitated nor inhibited relative to the neutral control. Thus, at least for normal controls, words which are locally semantically related (W+) are apparently unaffected by context. The apparent "encapsulation" of local semantic priming from context appears to provide evidence in favor of a modular view. However, this view is hard to maintain when the W+ and W– conditions are compared within and across discourse conditions. If local semantic priming were truly modular, then W+ items should be faster than W– items regardless of contextual constraints. This was clearly not the case. In fact, W+/C+ words were actually significantly *slower* than W–/C+ words. In other words, the usual "automatic" effect of priming at the local level has been thwarted and even reversed by context; or, conversely, the usual facilitative effect of context has been thwarted or suppressed by a local relationship.

Further evidence in favor of an interactive account comes from the various C– conditions. First, there was no difference in reaction times between neutral control items (unrelated words that are both unrelated to the context) and the W+/C– condition (related words that are both unrelated to the context). Hence it does look as though the expected "local" effects of word-word priming have been blunted when neither of these words fit the discourse context, suggesting that context can exert some kind of inhibitory effect on "automatic" local priming. Second, the slowest reaction times across all experimental and control conditions were observed for unrelated word pairs in which the prime fits the context but the target does not (W–/C–). The significant difference between W–/C– items and the neutral control also suggests that context has some kind of competitive or inhibitory effect.

We propose that the interactions between discourse-level and word-level priming observed in this study reflect a competition between the two items in a word pair for the role of "best completion" at the discourse level, as follows.

In the W–/C+ condition, the first word (i.e. the word prime) is a bad completion of the context. In a model that permits contextual pre-selection, we could argue that the first word has not been facilitated by context, and may indeed have been actively suppressed. In a model that has "bottom-up priority" with no pre-selection, we would have to argue (at best) that the first word receives no post-access boost (i.e. there is no effort to integrate it into the context). Indeed, there may be active efforts to inhibit incongruent primes as soon as they are recognized. In either case, these incongruent primes are so weak that they cannot provide much activation *or* inhibition for the target word that follows. Thus subjects quickly pronounce the second word, which is a good completion that can be integrated easily into the context.

By contrast, in the W+/C+ condition, the first word (the prime) is an excellent completion of the context. In a model that permits contextual pre-selection, we could argue that the first word is recognized early because its threshold was lowered by spreading activation. In a model that precludes contextual pre-selection, we would have to argue that these congruent primes receive a very rapid post-access boost, with rapid integration into the context. When the second word (the target) appears, it is at a considerable disadvantage, for two reasons. First, there is a slight delay because the first word is still being integrated into the context (where it fits so well). (This delay would presumably hold whether the target word fits the context or not.) Second, because the target and the prime are both good completions of the sentence, they are strong competitors – and this competition takes some time to resolve. In a sense, the second (target) word is like a rightful heir that has been (temporarily) supplanted by an impostor.

A similar logic can be used to explain why W–/C– items are significantly slower than neutral controls. In both these conditions, there is no "local" semantic relationship between prime and target, and in both cases the target is not a good completion at the discourse level. However, in the W–/C– condition (but not in neutral controls), the prime word *is* a good completion. In a model that permits pre-selection, we could argue that the prime was already activated by the context before it could be recognized. In a model that precludes pre-selection, we would have to argue that the first word in the pair received a post-access boost, and that efforts began to integrate it into the context. However, in the task that we have imposed upon our subjects, they are required to read the second word. That word has little chance in a competition for "best completion", because it is semantically incongruent and because the congruent prime has already made it in the door. Therefore the target word receives inhibition from the context, and from its competitor. This is the worst possible circumstance for word recognition, a fact that shows up in the exceptionally slow reaction times for W–/C– items.

Finally, consider the finding that word-level priming fails to occur when neither word fits the context (i.e. W+/C–/is not faster than the neutral control). Why has this supposedly automatic local priming failed? We suggest that this phenomenon can be explained if we assume that discourse context exerts an early and powerful inhibitory influence on words that are bad completions. Because the prime is a bad completion in both these cases, it is quickly suppressed (whether this occurs before or after lexical access is irrelevant to this point). As a result, the prime is so weak that it cannot exert a facilitative effect on the target word that follows, and hence no local priming occurs. As we have pointed out, these effects can be explained with or without invoking preselection. However, at the very least, it is clear that discourse effects are very strong, very fast, and inhibitory in nature (Marslen-Wilson & Tyler 1987). It would be easier to explain how such powerful effects get off the ground within a 200-ms window if we were able to assume some form of pre-selection. Such pre-selection may come from the discourse level, or it may represent a build-up of lexical activation from the related words that invariably occur in a long discourse passage. If the latter is true, then we might expect rapid facilitative and inhibitory effects of this kind following scrambled prose or random word lists. Other studies using lists of lexically related but syntactically unrelated words have failed to find such strong priming effects (Kilborn 1987), but to our knowledge, none of these have used the cross-modal naming paradigm. Hence the nature of the context effects observed in the present study is still open to debate. For present purposes, we can conclude that discourse does have inhibitory and facilitative effects on lexical access, and these effects fall within the time window that is usually reserved for automatic processes. This brings us to the next part of our study, where the paradigm is extended to elderly controls and aphasic patients.

Older Adult Controls

Experimental reaction times: The raw reaction times for the older adult controls were placed into a 2 (word relationship) x 2 (context relationship) within-subjects anova This yielded a significant main effect of contextual relationship of the target word, $F(1,14) = 10.38$, $p < 0.006$, and a word relationship by contextual relationship interaction, $F(1,14) = 24.62$, $p < 0.000$, but (in contrast to our findings for young normals) no main effect of word relationship. The main effect of contextual relationship, $F(1,76) = 7.26$, $p < 0.009$, and contextual relationship by word relationship interaction, $F(1,76) = 5.16$, $p < 0.026$ were also significant across items The target was read in 683 ms when it was a good completion (C+), and 736 ms when it was not (C–). In addition, the WxC interaction revealed that for W– words, the difference between C+ and C– condition was large, (658 ms vs. 759 ms). For W+ words, both the C+ words and C– condition elicited equal reaction times (706 ms vs. 714 ms). In short, subjects showed contextual priming for unrelated words but not for related words. In addition, like normal young controls, older adult controls read W–/C+ words faster than W+/C+ words (658 ms vs. 706 ms).

A set of t-tests were conducted on the raw reaction times in order to compare across conditions, and to compare each condition to the neutral control. Comparisons with the neutral control revealed that the W–/C+ condition was significantly faster than baseline, $t(14) = 4.09$, $p < 0.001$, and that the W–/C– condition was marginally slower than baseline $t(14) = 2.07$, $p < 0.057$. Further analyses revealed that the W+/C+ condition was significantly slower than the W–/C+ condition, $t(19) = 4.58$ $p < 0.000$.

Adjusted reaction times: Once again a set of analyses was conducted on reaction times with the neutral control subtracted out. The adjusted reaction times for the older adult controls were placed into a 2 (word relationship) x 2 (context relationship) between-subjects anova. This yielded a significant main effect of contextual relationship of the target word, $F(1,14) = 10.58$, $p < 0.006$, and a word relationship by contextual relationship interaction, $F(1,19) = 24.73$, $p < 0.000$. Furthermore, both effects were also significant across items, $F(1,76) = 8.65$, $p < 0.004$, and $F(1,76) = 6.26$, $p < 0.014$. These analyses mirrored the raw reaction time analyses. The target was read 25 ms faster than baseline when it was a good completion (C+), and 9 ms slower than baseline, when it was not (C–). In addition, the WxC interaction revealed that for W– words, the C+ condition was 48 ms faster than baseline and the C– condition was 27 ms slower than baseline. For W+ words, both the C+ words and C– condition were slightly faster than baseline (1 ms and 8 ms respectively). In short, subjects showed contextual priming for unrelated words but not for related words. In addition, like normal young controls, older adult controls read W–/C+ words faster than W+/C+ words.
The results from elderly controls reveal essentially the same qualitative pattern of data that was present in the young controls. To investigate any quantitative differences that may exist between groups, an ANOVA was run with both groups included.

Comparisons between younger and older adult controls: The adjusted rt data was placed into a 2 (group) x 2 (word relationship) x 2 (context relationship) mixed design ANOVA with group as the only between subjects factor. The ANOVA yielded a main effect of context relationship, $F(1,33) = 30.63$, $p < 0.000$, a word relationship by contextual relationship interaction, $F(1,32) = 45.75$, $p < 0.000$, and a group by word relationship by contextual relationship interaction, $F(1,32) = 9.73$, $p < 0.004$. The word relationship by context relationship interaction revealed the same pattern that was seen in each separate group analysis. Namely, subjects were faster than baseline when the target word was contextually related than when it was not. Furthermore, subjects showed contextual priming effects only when there was no local word relationship. The three-way interaction revealed that older adults showed a considerable amount of increased facilitation in the W–/C+ condition (48 vs. 27 ms), increased inhibition in the W–/C– condition (27 vs. 12 ms). In addition, there was a slight reversal in the W+ conditions. W+/C+ were equally facilitated for both groups but W+/C– words were more facilitated for older adult controls than for younger controls. The three-way interaction therefore arises from a considerable increase in the size of effects for W– words, and a slight reversal in the W+ conditions for elderly controls relative to young controls.
To summarize, so far. Normal aging does seem to have small effects on the nature of both local and global facilitation and inhibition in the present experiment. First of all, aging seems to increase both facilitation and inhibition when there is no local word relationship. Second, the rapid form of inhibition between both words seems to increase slightly (21 ms vs 48 ms). Once again it is difficult to understand how elderly subjects

Figure 3 Word relationship by contextual relationship by group interaction for old and young controls

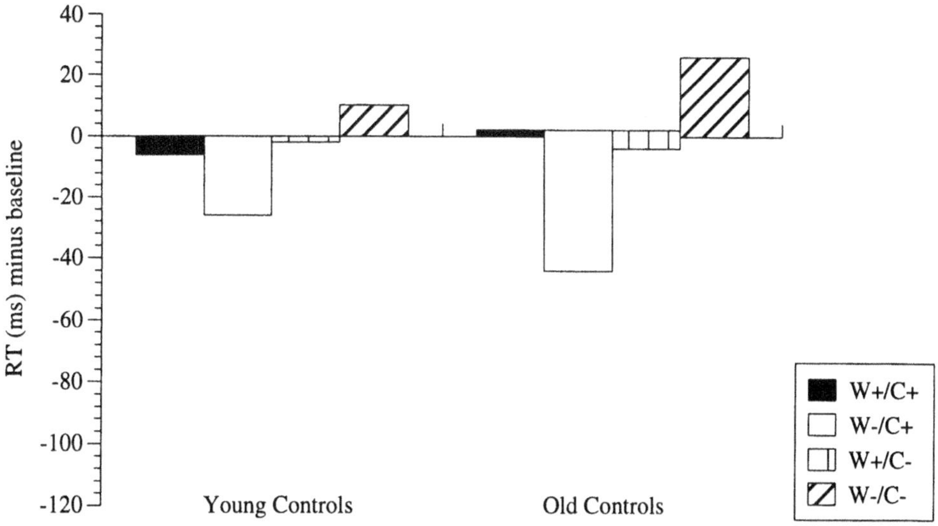

could be more facilitated for two words that are unrelated. Thus it appears that elderly controls are attempting to integrate the first word and that there is an inability to 'let go' or inhibit the activation of the second word as quickly. Thus the second word is pronounced even slower. This raises an interesting possibility. Is the increased inhibition between good sentence completions caused by a breakdown in the ability to inhibit the first word? This does seem to be confirmed by the fact that elderly controls show more inhibition in the W–/C– condition. That is, older adult controls are less able to suppress the integration of a good completion when it is followed by a bad completion. Thus it becomes even clearer that inhibition and facilitation relative to baseline may be a product of many overlapping effects which are occurring before reaction times are collected.

To better understand the nature of these multiple effects, a group of high-level aphasics were run on the same task. In using a more impaired group of subjects, it may become clearer which forms of suppression and excitation are affected by a decrease in language processing capability.

Aphasic Individuals

Eleven subjects were run on the experiment. Three were dropped because of high error rates and a high number of no responses. For these reasons all analyses involved only eight subjects.

Experimental reaction times: The raw RT's were placed into a 2 (word relatedness) x 2 (context relatedness) within-subjects anova. The results yielded a significant effect of context relatedness, $F(1,7) = 6.36$, $p < 0.040$ and a significant word relationship by context relationship interaction, $F(1,7) = 7.13$, $p < 0.032$. The main effect of context relationship was significant over items, $F(1,76) = 10.63$, $p < 0.002$ while the context relationship by word relationship interaction was marginally significant, $F(1,76) = 3.775$, $p < 0.056$. In addition, a set of t-tests was conducted in the same fashion as had been done with both control groups. The t-tests showed that the W–/C+ condition, $t(8) = 5.87$, $p < 0.0002$ and the W+/C+ condition were faster than baseline. In addition, it was found that the W–/C+ condition was marginally faster than the W+/C+ condition, $t(10) = 1.86$, $p < 0.09$. Although the data are considerably noisier (and reaction times are very large, mean = 964) aphasics show the same general pattern presented by both control groups. Namely,

W–/C+ < W+/C+ < W+/C– < W–/C–

Adjusted reaction times in context: The adjusted RT's were placed into a 2 (word relatedness) x 2 (context relatedness) within-subjects anova. The results yielded a significant effect of context relatedness, $F(1,7) = 6.37$, $p < 0.04$ and a significant word relationship by context relationship interaction, $F(1,7) = 7.13$, $p < 0.032$. Both the main effect of context relationship, $F(1,76) = 14.52$, $p < 0.000$, and the word relationship by context relationship interaction, $F(1,76) = 5.37$, $p < 0.023$. This showed the same general pattern which was seen in the raw reaction time data and of both control groups. Despite the fact that the ordering of the results are essentially the same, it is important to note that Aphasics as a group appear to be showing more facilitation. This is especially true for words which are contextually related. Note, however, that W+/C– words are showing the beginnings of facilitation. The results suggest that while the ordering of conditions relative to themselves is maintained, there is a change in the magnitude of effects when compared to Older adults and young adults. To further evaluate this a set of analyses was run with group as a variable.

Comparisons between older adults and aphasics: The adjusted reaction times for both groups were put into a 2 (group) x 2 (context relationship) x 2 (word relationship) ANOVA with group as the only between subjects factor. The analyses yielded a main effect of group, $F(1,21) = 6.32$, $p < 0.02$, contextual relationship, $F(1,39) = 14.79$, $p < 0.001$, an interaction of word relationship by contextual relationship, $F(1,39) = 34.31$, $p < 0.000$, and a marginally significant group by contextual relationship interaction, $F(1,39) = 3.73$, $p < 0.033$. The results reveal that aphasic patients show a larger amount of facilitation relative to baseline, especially for target words which are contextually relevant. In fact, Aphasic patients show a 94-msec facilitation for C+ words whereas older adults show a 24-msec facilitation effect for those same words. Finally, it appears that W+/C– words are slightly facilitated for Aphasic patients but only at baseline for the other two groups. Clearly, the Aphasic patients, while preserving the same general pattern, are being facilitated by any condition in which there is either a local word relationship or a global contextual relationship. Thus the locus of their deficit appears to lie not in the absence of local or global forms of priming, but in the ability to coordinate and integrate these sources of information in an efficient manner.

Figure 4 Word relationship by contextual relationship interaction for aphasics

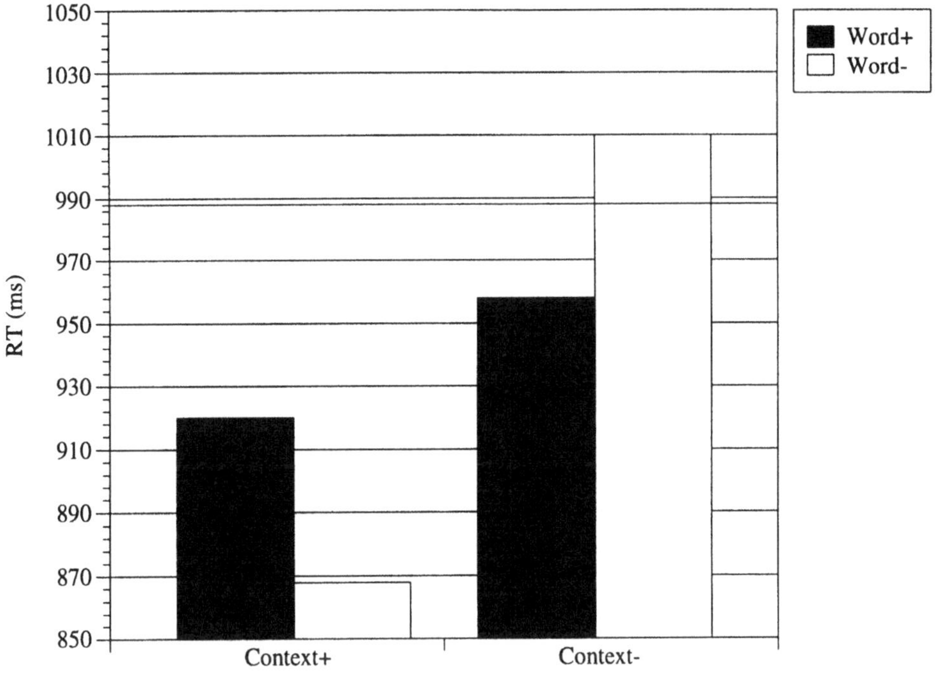

Figure 5 Contextual relationship by group interaction for old controls and aphasics

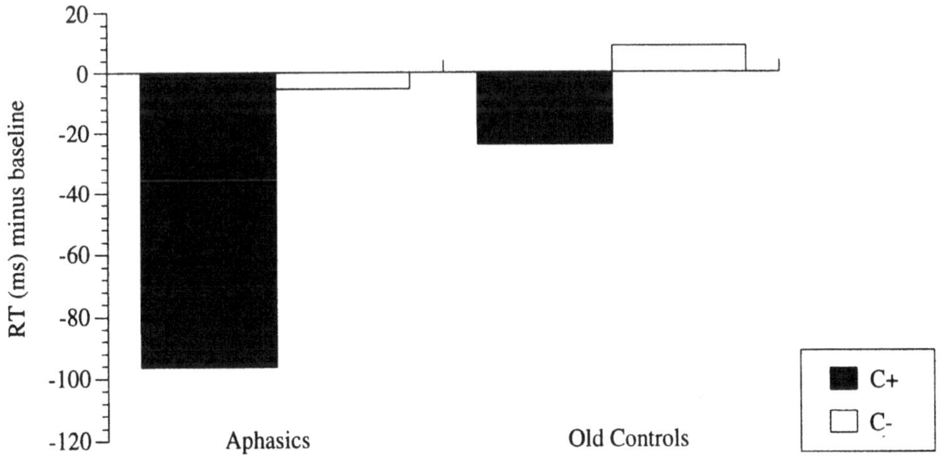

Indeed, it is fair to say that these aphasic patients experience too much priming, so that they are affected by competitive effects that normals weed out quickly in the comprehension process. Under this interpretation, we might argue that the locus of anomia (at least in these patients) has to do with the unchecked spread of activation. Target words are indeed active, but so are their competitors. The resulting traffic control problem may result in word substitutions, and/or in a failure to come up with the target word quickly.

General Discussion

The present study attempted to shed light on the issue of lexical autonomy and lexical access in normals and anomic patients, by placing word-level priming in competition with discourse-level priming. This design yielded a number of interesting interactions between word-level and sentence-level factors, as follows.

First, there was a reversal of the expected relationship between W+/C+ items and W–/C+ items In contrast to the predictions of an additive model, reaction times were significantly slower when prime and target were related to each other *and* to the discourse context (W+/C+), compared with a condition in which the target fits the context but the prime does not (W–/C+). We explained this counterintuitive finding by postulating a competition between the prime and target for the role of "best completion" at the discourse level. In the W+/C+ condition, both are good completions and therefore the competition between related words is fierce. In the W–/C+ condition, the prime is unrelated to the context and therefore provides no competitive inhibition of the target.

Second, we failed to find "automatic", local priming effects between related words when neither of the words fit the context (i.e. W+/C– items were no faster than neutral controls, where the two words are unrelated to each other and the context). We suggest that this occurs because the discourse context can suppress incongruent word primes, which in turn prevents those primes from exerting a facilitative effect on their single-word targets.

Third, the slowest reaction times of all were observed in the W–/C– condition, where the target is unrelated to the context and to the prime word, but the prime serves as a good completion. We argued that this condition is slower than neutral control items (where nothing is related to anything else) because the prime does indeed serve as a good completion, boosting its activation and suppressing pronunciation of the target word.

It is not clear whether these effects are lexical or post-lexical, a point which is further discussed below. But it is clear that context can have powerful effects on lexical access, in the time window that is usually described in studies that lay claim to automaticity. Furthermore, it is clear that these early context effects involve inhibitory processes, in contrast with previous claims that inhibition always reflects slow, controlled, strategic forms of processing.

The second objective of this study was to observe the changes in language processing that occur with aging and aphasia. Normal aging had a slight but significant impact on the ability of subjects to perform the cross-modal word pair task. First of all, older adults showed an increase in the size of the competitive inhibition between congruent prime and target (W+/C+ vs. W–/C+). The size of this effect was 48 ms, vs. 21 ms in young adults. Yet this seemingly contradicts results in the literature which indicate that aging should provide a breakdown in inhibition. This can be explained in two ways. The first regards the speed at which words are integrated. Presumably, young college controls are faster at integrating the first word and are less slowed in the pronunciation of the second word. If this were the case then it would be expected that older adults should be approximately twice as slow as young controls. This was not the case. The second possibility is that older adults were unable to adequately inhibit the first word. In this case, a breakdown in inhibition of the prime leads to an increase in inhibition between prime and target. In other words, it is the older adults' inability to suppress the prime that led to the larger competition between prime and target. This is further confirmed by the older adults' increased inhibition in the W–/C– condition. In this case, younger adults are better able to suppress the congruent prime to name the incongruent target.

Results for aphasic patients were somewhat more complex. In terms of competitive inhibition, these subjects are about 300 ms slower than older adults but only show a slight increase in the size of competitive inhibition. This is further evidence against a general slowing-of-processing account. However, these subjects seem to show a huge increase in facilitation. In fact, it is clear that contextually related targets significantly facilitated response (–96 ms in Aphasics vs. ~ –24 ms in older controls). This is reminiscent of a finding reported by Nebes, Boller & Holland (1986) for another population with naming deficits, i.e. patients with Alzheimer's disease. Furthermore, Nebes, Boller, & Holland found that subjects had more difficulty in producing a response for sentences with low and medium cloze probability. The present results further confirm that neurologically impaired patients may benefit from highly supportive contexts. If aphasics are more context-dependent (like the AD patients) than normals, then it may be particularly difficult for them to process items in the neutral control condition, in which (in essence) nothing is related to anything else. If this is the case, then the use of this condition as a neutral control may be misleading, inflating our estimates of facilitation and reducing our estimates of inhibition. Thus (for example), the 16 msec. inhibition effect for W–/C– words in the aphasic patients may be an underestimate.

Is there a better candidate to serve as the neutral control in studies of priming at the discourse level, in aphasic patients or any subject population? In fact, there may be no good solution to this problem (West & Stanovich 1988), since there is no such thing as a "neutral paragraph". This opens an even deeper issue, which was alluded to earlier. How much does the neutral control tell us about the interplay of facilitation and inhibition? In the current experiment, the W+/C+ condition was slower than the W–/C+ condition. At first glance, one would have to conclude that the W–/C+ condition is more facilitated (i.e. incongruent primes facilitate the pronunciation of an unrelated word). This implausible situation led us to propose a competitive inhibition between two words which were attempting to fill the same location in a sentence. This seems to confirm an interactive/activation model of language processing in which selection of a candidate involves inhibition of semantically related neighbors. The results, however, could be placed within a purely facilitatory model in which activation of one candidate leads to a slower activation of a second candidate. Thus a congruent or incongruent target is slower to pronounce because the system must 'reset' before pronouncing the second word. That is 'inhibition' can arise from the a system which is over-'activated' and must wait for resting state to be reached before activation of a subsequent word. In either case, the present results suggest that language processing may be made up of multiple forms of facilitation and inhibition which sum in ways that appear to be purely inhibitory or purely facilitatory. In this view, facilitation and inhibition observed may be a much more complex and dynamic phenomenon than that which is proposed in traditional automatic/controlled models (Posner & Snyder 1975). In fact, facilitation and inhibition may be two sides of the same coin.

Another more controversial issue surrounding modular systems involves the notion of automaticity. For a process, to be automatic it must occur within a fast timeframe and be absent of strategic processes. Furthermore, facilitation is considered to be a central property of modular automatic systems Thus it is unclear if the effects we have captured are lexical or post-lexical. As was mentioned earlier, the majority of studies have used single-word presentation with a sentence or a single word as a prime. In these studies, it was clear that the locus of the study was the access of the target. In this study, however, we used both of these methodologies together. This presents a problem because the results indicate that both the prime and the target may be affected by the sentence context. For example, the results from the experiments presented show that processing of a contextually relevant word (200 SOA) can slow the naming of the subsequent word. Presumably we could accept that a contextually relevant word is accessed within 200 ms but that this has post-lexical effects on the naming of the target. In other words, does access of the first word slow the integration or access of the second word? Further studies which manipulate SOA, ISI and perhaps even the number of related trials might better disambiguate whether these effects are lexical or post-lexical. What the present study does suggest is that the processes involved in sentence integration are rapid and robust.

The locus of the effects are somewhat disambiguated by the data from anomic aphasics. These subjects showed about the same competitive inhibition effect (54 vs. 47 ms) but where markedly faster for semantically congruent words in general. Thus an impairment in naming which seems to slow processing speed does not have an effect on the competition between two 'good' completions. Thus it seems that natural aging and not mild focal brain damage may be responsible for an impairment in the ability to inhibit good completions. An impairment in access, however, does seem to slow the naming of semantically incongruent words more than semantically congruent words. Thus anomics have more problems with access of incongruous targets. Hence, it is clear that the effects we have captured involve to some extent problems with lexical access (i.e. naming) and not with contextual integration. What the current study seems to suggest is that anomia to some extent is alleviated by the presence of good contextual support. The use of a larger discourse context can provide anomics the type of contextual support necessary for relatively unimpaired language processing.

The present study has provided a number of insights into the language processing of normal, aging and brain-damaged adults. First of all, it has shown that local priming takes on a very different form when placed in a full sentence context. Specifically, it appears that word-level priming can be overwhelmed by higher forms of priming. Second, these context effects appear to involve rapid forms of inhibition. This form of inhibition may be the product of residual activation of the prime or inhibition of competitors. Third, the word-finding deficits experienced by aphasic patients (and, to a lesser degree, by some older adults) may involve an over-reliance on context, coupled with an inability to suppress inappropriate competitors. Perhaps, the most interesting part of this over-reliance on context is that it led to an apparent increase in facilitation which may actually be caused by the inability of aphasics to inhibit incongruent stimuli (which includes the baseline).

We suggest that current models of on-line psycholinguistic processing should consider more carefully the role of inhibition and facilitation. More specifically, these models should consider the possibility of multiple forms of facilitation and inhibition which can sum across the time window generally employed in psycholinguistic processing. The long-standing debate regarding autonomy vs. interaction may be an oversimplification of the complex and dynamical processes involved in language processing, a finding which was further confirmed by the increase in 'facilitation' in anomics. Finally, it is clear that discourse-level contexts can serve as a vehicle for understanding the nature of processing at the word-level. The future use of these contexts should help to clarify existing questions and propose new possibilities. The current study is only the first step in what will hopefully be a rich new source of information for understanding real-time language processing.

References

Balota, D.A. & R.F. Lorch (1986): "Depth of automatic spreading activation: Mediated priming effects in pronunciation but not in lexical decision". Journal of Experimental Psychology: Learning, Memory & Cognition 12, 336 – 345.

Bates, E., B. Wulfeck & B. MacWhinney B. (1991): "Cross-linguistic studies in aphasia: An overview. Special Issue: Crosslinguistic studies of aphasia". Brain & Language 41, 123 – 148.

Chiarello, C., K.L. Church & W.J. Hoyer (1985): "Automatic and controlled semantic priming: Accuracy, response bias, and aging". Journal of Gerontology 40, 593 – 600.

Cohen, J., B. MacWhinney, M. Flatt & J. Provost (1993): "PsyScope: An interactive graphic system for designing and controlling experiments in the psychology laboratory using Macintosh computers". Behavioral Research Methods 25, 257 – 271.

Colby, K.M., D. Chrisinaz, R.C. Parkinson, S. Graham & C. Karpf (1981): "A word-finding computer program with a dynamic lexical-semantic memory for patients with anomia using an intelligent speech prosthesis". Brain & Language 14, 272 – 281.

Colombo, L. (1986): "Activation and inhibition with orthographically similar words". Journal of Experimental Psychology: Human Perception & Performance 12, 226 – 234.

Farah, M.J. & M.A. Wallace (1992): "Semantically-bounded anomia: Implications for the neural implementation of naming". Neuropsychologia 30, 609 – 621.

Fodor, J. (1983): The modularity of mind: An essay on faculty psychology. Cambridge, Mass.: MIT Press.

Forster, K.I. (1981): "Priming and the effects of sentence and lexical contexts on naming time: Evidence for autonomous lexical processing". Quarterly Journal of Experimental Psychology: Human Experimental Psychology 33A, 465 – 495.

Foss, D.J. (1982): "A discourse on semantic priming". Cognitive Psychology 14, 590 – 607.

Friederici, A.D. & L. Frazier (1992): "Thematic analysis in agrammatic comprehension: Syntactic structures and task demands". Brain & Language 42, 1 – 29.

Friederici, A.D. & K. Kilborn (1989): "Temporal constraints on language processing: Syntactic priming in Broca's aphasia". Journal of Cognitive Neuroscience 1, 262 – 272.

Gainotti, G., M.C. Silveri, G. Villa & G. Miceli (1986): "Anomia with and without lexical comprehension disorders. First European Workshop on Cognitive Neuropsychology" (1983, Bressanone, Italy). Brain & Language 29, 18 – 33.

Grainger, J. (1990): "Word frequency and neighborhood frequency effects in lexical decision and naming". Journal of Memory & Language 29, 228 – 244.

Hadar, U., C. Jones & C. Mate-Kole (1987): "The disconnection in anomic aphasia between semantic and phonological lexicons". Cortex 23, 505 – 517.

Hagoort, P. (1993): "Impairments of lexical-semantic processing in aphasia: Evidence from the processing of lexical ambiguities". Brain & Language 45, 189 – 232.

Hasher, L., E.R. Stoltzfus, R.T. Zacks & B. Rypma (1991): "Age and inhibition". Journal of Experimental Psychology: Learning, Memory & Cognition 17, 163 – 169.

Hasher, L. & R. Zacks (1988): "Working memory, comprehension, and aging: A review and a new view". In: G.H. Bower, eds., The psychology of learning and motivation. (Vol. 22). San Diego: Academic Press, 193 – 225.

Kolk, H.H. & M.M. Van Grunsven (1985): "Agrammatism as a variable phenomenon". Cognitive Neuropsychology 2, 347 – 384.

le Dorze, G. & J.-L. Nespoulous (1989): "Anomia in moderate aphasia: Problems in accessing the lexical representation". Brain & Language 37, 381 – 400.

Light, L.L. & D.M. Burke (1988): "Patterns of language and memory in old age". In: L.L. Light & D.M. Burke, eds., Language, memory and aging. New York: Cambridge University Press.

Lucchelli, F. & E. de Renzi (1992): "Proper name anomia". Cortex 28, 221 – 230.

Marangolo, P., E. Dipace & L. Pizzamiglio (1993): "Priming Effect In A Color Discrimination Task". Perceptual And Motor Skills 77, 259 – 269.

Marslen-Wilson, W.D. & L.T. Tyler (1987): "Against Modularity". In: J.L. Garfield, eds., Modularity in Knowledge Representation and Natural-Language Understanding. Cambridge, Massachusetts: The MIT Press.

McClelland, J.L. & D.E. Rumelhart (1981): "An interactive activation model of context effects in letter perception: I. An account of basic findings". Psychological Review 88, 375 – 407.

Millberg, W., S.E. Blumstein, D. Katz & F. Gershberg (1992): Semantic facilitation in aphasia: Effects of time and expectancy. Unpublished Manuscript, Boston University School of Medicine, Aphasia Research Center, Boston.

Mitrushina, M. & P. Satz (1991): "Effect of repeated administration of a neuropsychological battery in the elderly". Journal of Clinical Psychology 47, 790 – 801.

Nebes, R.D., F. Boller & A. Holland (1986): "Use of Semantic Context by Patients with Alzheimer's Disease". Psychology and Aging 1, 261 – 269.

Nebes, R.D. & C.B. Brady (1992): "Generalized cognitive slowing and severity of dementia in Alzheimer's disease: Implications for the interpretation of response-time data". Journal of Clinical & Experimental Neuropsychology 14, 317 – 326.

Neely, J.H. (1976): "Semantic priming and retrieval from lexical memory: Evidence for facilitatory and inhibitory processes". Memory & Cognition 4, 648 – 654.

Ober, B.A., G.K. Shenaut, W.J. Jagust & R.C. Stillman (1991): "Automatic semantic priming with various category relations in Alzheimer's disease and normal aging". Psychology & Aging 6, 647 – 660.

Onifer, W. & D.A. Swinney (1981): "Accessing lexical ambiguities during sentence comprehension: Effects of frequency of meaning and contextual bias". Memory & Cognition 9, 225 – 236.
Ostrin, R.K. & L.K. Tyler (1993): "Automatic access to lexical semantics in aphasia: Evidence from semantic and associative priming". Brain & Language 45, 147 – 159.
Posner, M.C. & C. Snyder (1975): "Facilitation and inhibition in the processing of signals". In: P. Rabbitt & S. Dornic, eds., Attention and Performance. (Vol. V). New York: Academic Press, 669 – 683.
Salthouse, T.A. (1991): "Mediation of adult age differences in cognition by reductions in working memory and speed of processing". Psychological Science 2, 179 – 183.
Seidenberg, M.S., M.K. Tanenhaus, J.M. Leiman & M. Bienkowski (1982): "Automatic access of the meanings of ambiguous words in context: Some limitations of knowledge-based processing". Cognitive Psychology 14, 489 – 537.
Tweedy, J.R., R.H. Lapinski & R.W. Schvaneveldt (1977): "Semantic-context effects on word recognition: Influence of varying the proportion of items presented in an appropriate context". Memory & Cognition 5, 84 – 89.
Van Petten, C. & M. Kutas (1987): "Ambiguous words in context: An event-related potential analysis of the time course of meaning activation". Journal of Memory & Language 26, 188 – 208.
Zurif, E., D. Swinney, P. Prather, A. Wingfield & H. Brownell (1992): An on-line analysis of syntactic processing in the elderly. Unpublished manuscript, Brandeis Univesity, Department of Psychology and Center for Complex Systems, Waltham, Massachusetts.

On Lexical Properties, Syntax, and Brain Damage*

Lewis P. Shapiro, Florida; Cynthia K. Thompson, Illinois

This manuscript describes how lexical and syntactic properties contribute to the process of producing and understanding sentences. The logic to our approach takes the following line: We assume that language processing exploits a mind/brain data base consisting of representations, rules, and principles specific to the language domain. Our best bet on the proper characterization of this data base is given by linguistic theory. We thus use aspects of a linguistic theory as a set of deductions about how sentence processing might operate. We also use the information gleaned from investigations of normal language representation and processing to help investigate what goes awry in the language system subsequent to brain damage, and to develop targets for treatment. In principle we can also use the evidence gathered from our neurolinguistic studies to further develop normal models of sentence production and comprehension. We begin with some representational issues; we follow with a discussion of sentence comprehension in both normal and disordered populations and end with a discussion of our work in sentence production.

1 Representational Issues

Our purpose in this section is to characterize the mentally represented linguistic information that our subsequent sentence comprehension and production work has exploited. We begin, then, with an overview of one current linguistic theory – the principles and parameters approach of Government and Binding (GB) theory (e.g., Chomsky 1981,1986; van Riemsdijk & Williams 1986; Haegeman 1992). GB distinguishes four major levels of representation with the sentence as the unit of analysis: D-structure (an underlying form), S-structure (something like a surface realization of a sentence, though more abstract), LF (logical form), and PF (phonology-syntax interface). Lexical items, along with their associated predicate-argument structure, are inserted at D-structure. A transformational rule (Move-alpha) applies freely to convert D-structure representations to S-structure representations. At D-structure, thematic relations are specified; at S-structure binding relations (referent-argument position links) are

* The work reported in this paper was supported by NIH grants DC00494 and DC01809.

specified. LF characterizes the logical form or structural meaning of a sentence. And PF specifies the sound component of the sound-meaning relation.
A few principles and theories apply to each representational level. For example, X-bar theory (the phrase structure component) and theta-theory (assignment of thematic roles) apply at D-structure. Case, Binding, and Control theories apply at S-structure. The output of move-alpha affects S-structure. The Theta-Criterion and the Projection Principle apply to all levels of representation. In this section we will only describe those aspects of the theory that are (directly) relevant to the present work.

1.1 X-bar theory

Phrase structure (PS) rules characterize the possible phrasal geometry of sentences allowable in a language. Each PS rule must contain a *head* that is related to its phrasal counterpart. The head is a lexical category that forms part of a larger unit (a phrasal category or clause) and passes on its properties to that larger unit. A verb (V) is the head of a verb phrase (VP), a noun (N) is the head of a noun phrase (NP), a preposition/postposition (P) is the head of a prepositional or postpositional phrase (PP), and so on. A *complement* – part of the larger unit of which the head is a part – is idiosyncratically selected by (or "subcategorized" by) the head. For example, a verb – the head of a VP – may subcategorize for an NP complement (and other phrases and combinations of phrases, as well):

(1) $[_{V''}$ $[_{V'}$ $[_{V}$ fixed] $[_{NP}$ the car]]]

In (1), the V' – *fixed the car* – is headed by the V – *fixed*; the NP embedded within the V' – *the car* – is the complement of the head.
PS's are hierarchically organized with a maximal projection, intermediate projections, and the head. The generalized schema is shown in (2) (substitute any lexical category type for X, such as V, N, or P; substitute any phrasal category XP, such as NP, VP, etc., for an X'):

(2) X" (maximal projection) → Spec (specifier; e.g., articles), X' (intermediate projection) X' → X (head), complement

Since every PS must abide by the X-bar schema in (2), the range of possible PS rules – and therefore sentences – in any language is limited. Ordering of the head and specifier are parameters that allow variation among languages: The head can either fall to the left (e.g., head-initial English) or to the right (e.g., head-final Japanese) of the complement. The specifier can either come before or after the X" it modifies. Languages 'chose' one or the other for their entire set of PS rules. It turns out that recent versions of GB (Chomsky 1986) have done away with PS rules altogether, and X-bar theory and other principles determine well-formedness in a language. For present purposes we will continue to use PS rules in their more standard form (as is common in psycholinguistics).

There is one serious limitation to PS rules, however: If left as is, PS rules will freely overgenerate the allowable structures in a language; that is, they will generate not only the grammatical sentences of a language but some ungrammatical ones as well. Consider the PS in (3):

(3) $[_{S}$ $[_{NP}$ the boy] $[_{VP}$? $[_{NP}$ the ball]]]

Given the PS configuration in (3), any verb may fill the verb slot via *lexical selection*. But our intuitions about what structures are grammatical and what are not tell us that this cannot be so:

(4) The boy $[_{VP}$ $[_{V}$ hit] $[_{NP}$ the ball]]

(5) *The boy $[_{VP}$ $[_{V}$ [put] $[_{NP}$ the ball]]

There must be some way to limit the output of the PS component to conform to only the well-formed instances of a language; there must be some way to disallow, for example, (5) – lexically inserting the verb *put* in a PS rule of the form: VP → V NP – while allowing (4). One important filter that limits the output of the PS component is the lexicon.

1.2 The Lexicon and Theta-theory

In this section we consider the lexical properties of verbs (and prepositions) and how such information interacts with the syntax of sentences. That is, we ask: What information is represented with a lexical item and how does this information interact with the structure of a sentence? In this vein we consider three types of representation: subcategorization, argument structure, and thematic roles. It may turn out that one or another of these lexical properties are predictable from other information and thus are not really representational *primitives*. For example, Jackendoff (1987, 1990) makes a strong case that thematic roles are derived from lexical-conceptual structure and thus thematic roles are to be considered as "mnemonic devices" that stand for a more richly specified, and primitive, set of conceptual representations (e.g., CAUSE, PATH, etc.). For the time being, however, we consider each level of representation separately.

1.2.1 Subcategorization

Consider again the verbs *hit* and *put*. Our grammatical intuitions tell us that *hit* allows an NP, shown in (4), and that *put* must take an NP PP as in (6):

(6) The boy $[_{VP}$ $[_{V}$ put] $[_{NP}$ the ball] $[_{PP}$ on the shelf]]

Such information is represented as part of the verb's entry in the lexicon, or our mental dictionary. Partial entries, then, for *hit* and *put* are shown in (7) and (8):

(7) hit_V [__ NP]

(8) put_V [__ NP PP]

Hit is said to *subcategorize* for an NP, and *put* for an NP PP. If we assume that the subcategorization frame for each verb must be satisfied in the sentence in which the verb is contained (that is, if a verb is represented with an [__NP] subcategorization in the lexicon, then the NP must also be represented in the sentence), then we ensure that the correct verb will be inserted in its proper structural configuration. We thus limit the output of the PS component to form only grammatical sentences of the language. Since (8) shows that *put* must subcategorize for an NP PP, and since (5) has *put* embedded in a sentence with only a direct object NP, the theory rules out (5) as grammatical.
Indeed, there is a formal principle – the *Projection Principle* – that states that the lexical properties of a verb (at this point in our discussion, the subcategorization frame) must be satisfied in the syntax:

(9) The Projection Principle: Lexical representations (e.g., subcategorizations) are projected to each syntactic level (e.g., s- and d-structure).

Given the lexical representation in (8), (5) is ruled out by the Projection Principle. This principle is quite powerful and rationalizes syntactic structure in the following sense: When we acquire a lexical item, we acquire facts about the lexical item's syntactic privileges of occurrence (perhaps from the real-world contingencies of use; see below).

1.2.2 Predicate-argument structure

From a logical standpoint, most sentences can be considered representations of relations between a predicate and its arguments, hence the term *argument structure*. An NP (or S) in a sentence can be an argument of the verb if it occupies an *argument position* (i.e., subject and complement positions) in the sentence. While strict subcategorization supplies information about the syntactic form (and ordering) of arguments, argument structure characterizes how many arguments a verb selects. In effect, argument structure specifies how many participants occur in the 'action' described by the verb. Consider again the verbs *hit* and *put*. The transitive verb *hit* needs two participants, a "hitter" and a "hittee", thus it selects for two arguments and hence a two-place argument structure. The verb *put* selects for a three-place argument structure. Arguments can either be *external* or *internal*. External arguments (i.e., the subject) fall outside the domain of the VP while internal arguments fall within the domain of the VP, that is, are often sisters to the head.
Arguments and argument structures are often represented as variables:

(10) [The boy $_x$] [$_{VP}$ hit [the ball y]]

(11) [The boy $_x$] [$_{VP}$ put [the ball y] [on the shelf $_z$]]

(10) shows that *hit* selects for an (x y) argument structure where the NP *the boy* is the x-argument (external) and the NP *the ball* is the y-argument (internal); (11) shows that *put* selects for an (x y z) argument structure where the NP *the boy* is the x-argument, the NP *the ball* is the y-argument, and the PP *on the shelf* contains the z-argument. Verbs that allow sentential clauses can also be described using argument structure. For example:

(12) [Dillon $_x$] knew [$_{NP}$ the answer $_y$]

(13) [Dillon $_x$] knew [$_S$ the answer was wrong $_y$]

The verb *know* allows a two-place argument structure of the form (x y) in either (12) or (13). In (12) the y-argument is served by an NP in the syntax; in (13) it is served by a sentential clause (S). Each argument can also have a different "semantic" status as well, as is shown in the next section.

1.2.3 Thematic and semantic roles

Each argument takes on a certain *thematic* or semantic type (e.g., Agent, Theme, Patient, Goal, Experiencer). Each verb selects sets of thematic roles assigned to its arguments; each set of roles is called a *thematic grid*. Like subcategorization and argument structure, thematic properties are written into the lexical representation of the head. The verb *kiss*, for example, allows a two-place (x y) argument structure; assigned to these arguments from one thematic grid is both an Agent and a Patient:

(14) (a) [Dillon $_{Agent}$] kissed [$_{NP}$ Joelle *Patient*]
(b) kiss $_V$ [__ NP] – subcategorization
(x y) – argument structure
(Agent Patient) – Thematic grid

(14a) shows that the verb *kiss* allows a two-place argument structure with Agent and Patient assigned to the arguments; the representation in (14b) reflects the lexical properties of the verb.
Consider now sentences (15)-(18):

(15) Dillon kissed Joelle (active)

(16) Joelle was kissed by Dillon (passive)

(17) It was Dillon who kissed Joelle (subject cleft)

(18) It was Joelle who Dillon kissed (object cleft)

Despite appearing in different grammatical positions, *Dillon* is the Agent and *Joelle* is the Patient in each of these sentences (such similarities among the roles played by arguments placed within different syntactic structures, in effect, rationalizes the need for theta-roles). *Theta Theory* states that the predicate assigns its associated thematic roles to particular grammatical positions at D-structure. A transitive verb like *kiss*, for example, will have two thematic roles to assign, one associated with the subject position and one associated with the object position (in GB, subject and object are defined configurationally; object position is always VP internal, while subject position is located outside the VP. Currently under debate is whether or not both the subject and object NP are base-generated internal to the VP). Two important principles constrain assignment of thematic roles in the syntax: the Projection Principle (9) and the *Theta Criterion:*

(19) Theta Criterion: Every argument (i.e., NP) in a sentence must receive one and only one thematic role. Each thematic role associated with a predicate must be assigned to one and only one argument.

(19), much like the Projection Principle, ensures that a verb's thematic properties – specified in it's lexical entry – will be assigned one-to-one to the arguments represented in the syntax.

Consider again (15)-(18). In each of the sentences the thematic role of Agent is assigned to *Dillon*. In (16), for example, the direct object NP – *Joelle* – is displaced from the canonical post-verb position to sentence initial position. But the Projection Principle (9) and the lexical entry for *kiss* (14b) require that *kiss* have a direct object argument position to which the Patient role can be assigned. And the Theta Criterion (19) requires that each argument position be assigned a thematic role represented in the verb's thematic grid. It appears, then, that (16) and, indeed, (18) are ruled out by both of these principles. But our intuitions tell us that this cannot be so since (16) and (18) are well-formed, grammatical sentences. So, there must be some mechanism allowing the assignment of thematic roles to NP's that have been moved out of their canonical argument positions. This mechanism in GB theory is the *trace*.

1.3 Trace theory and thematic role assignment

The Projection Principle ensures proper thematic role assignment by requiring insertion of an empty category or trace into the position from which a category has moved. The trace is then linked or *coindexed* with the originally moved category. The thematic role is assigned to the trace in the original position. Coindexation then allows the moved constituent to inherit the thematic role assigned to the trace. The trace of movement and the NP that moved (the *antecedent*) form a *theta-chain*, and the theta-criterion is revised to include theta-chains:

(20) All thematic roles are assigned to theta-chains, and each theta-chain receives one and only one thematic role.

Consider the following:

(21) Who did Dillon kiss?

Skipping the details, the D-structure representation for (21) captures the lexical properties of *kiss*. *Who* is in the direct object argument position and assigned the Patient role by *kiss*:

(22) $[_{S'}$ [Dillon kissed who]]

To derive its S-structure, *who* is moved into complementizer (COMP) position (actually, the Specifier position of COMP), leaving behind a trace in the direct object argument position:

(23) $[_{S'}$ $[_{COMP}$ Who$]_i$ did $[_S$ Dillon kiss t_i]]

Who is coindexed (represented by *i*) with the trace (*t*), forming a theta-chain. The Wh-element receives its thematic role *indirectly* via the trace-antecedent chain. Sentences (15)-(18) receive a similar analysis, shown by the S-structures in (24)-(26):

(24) [Joelle$]_i$ $[_{VP}$ was kissed t_i] by Dillon]

(25) [It was Joelle$_i$ $[_{S'}$ $[_{COMP}$ who$]_i$ $[_S$ Dillon kissed t_i]]

(26) [It was Dillon $[_{S'}$ $[_{COMP}$ who$]_i$ $[_S$ t_i kissed Joelle]]

Skipping the details, in (24) the Patient is assigned by the verb to the chain represented by the coindexed direct object argument position (*t*) and the displaced argument *Joelle*. In (25) the NP is moved to a position (COMP) not directly assigned a thematic role (a *non-argument* position) and is linked with a trace in a canonical position (an argument position) that has been assigned its proper thematic role. In (26) there is no trace in object position (though there is one in subject position), thus Patient is assigned directly. There are two major types of movement (subsumed under Move-alpha): NP-movement and *Wh*-movement. NP-movement occurs in the derivation of the passive (24) and so-called NP-raising structures (e.g., *Dillon seems to Joelle to be crying*). NP-movement moves an NP from an argument position to another argument position, leaving behind an NP-trace. *Wh*-movement derives *Wh*-questions, relative clauses, and relative clefts. Unlike NP-movement, *Wh*-movement involves displacement of *Wh*-phrases from argument positions to non-argument positions (Specifier position in COMP), leaving behind a *Wh*-trace (e.g., (25)). The *landing site* of the moved constituent (i.e., argument or non-argument position) is a potentially important variable to consider in the thematic assignment process since direct assignment of thematic roles is possible *only when constituents are in argument positions.*

1.4 Sentences as arguments and their semantic status

Sentential clauses can also serve as arguments of a verb. On some accounts (Grimshaw 1979; Pesetsky 1983) these arguments take on specific semantic realizations. Consider the verb *know*:

(27) (a) Joelle knows [$_{S'}$ that Dillon broke the glass]
(b) Joelle knows [$_{S'}$ why Dillon broke the glass]
(c) Joelle knows [$_{S'}$ what a destructive kid Dillon is]!

The versions of *know* in (27) (arguably, each has the same 'sense') are not differentiated by either subcategorization or argument structure since in each case *know* subcategorizes for a sentential clause that is associated with an internal y-argument. In each case, however, the sentential argument has a distinct semantic status. In (27a) the argument is realized as a Proposition (headed by a *that*-clause); in (27b) it is realized as an Interrogative (headed by a *wh*-clause); and in (27c) the argument is realized as an Exclamation. Since it appears that verbs select among a small corpus of such semantic types (e.g., *know* allows three of these types; *ask* allows one – an Interrogative) much like they do for thematic roles, for the time being we suggest that these 'complex semantic types' form a part of the thematic-semantic representation of the verb.

1.5 Arguments and adjuncts

It is necessary to make one more distinction before we move on to a description of the relevance of this work to normal and disordered language processing. Implicit in this organization of lexical entries is the distinction between *arguments* and *adjuncts*. This distinction is not an easy one to make, but it has been found to have processing implications. An argument is idiosyncratically selected by the verb; it forms part of the verb's entry in the lexicon. An argument is thus assigned its thematic role by the verb. An adjunct is not selected by particular verbs; any verb can appear in a sentence with an adjunct and thus the adjunct does not need to be specified as part of the verb's entry. Consider:

(28) Mitzi sent the car *to the garage*

(29) Mitzi fixed the car *in the garage*

In (28) the three-place predicate (ditransitive or "dative" verb *send*) assigns three thematic roles to its arguments – an Agent to the NP *Mitzi*, a Theme to the NP *the car*, and a Goal to the NP *the garage* falling within the PP *to the garage*. The two-place transitive verb *fix* in (29) assigns only two thematic roles to its arguments – an Agent to the NP *Mitzi*, and a Theme to the NP *the car*. The PP *in the garage* is considered a locative adjunct; its "meaning" is not inherent in the verb's representation. Indeed, locative PP's like *in the garage, under the rug*, etc. can be inserted in almost any sentence with any verb.

If virtually any verb can take a particular kind of phrase, then the representations that refer to that phrase need not be stipulated in the verb's lexical entry.

Phrasal geometry also distinguishes between arguments and adjuncts. Adjunct PP's can often be attached at two distinct points, thus making them *structurally ambiguous*. For example, (28) can mean something like "it was the car that was *in the garage* (not the car outside the garage) that Mitzi fixed" in which case the adjunct PP – *in the garage*

– is attached to (i.e., modifies) the Noun Phrase *the car*. But (28) can also mean something like "it was *in the garage* (not outside the garage) where Mitzi fixed the car". In this case the PP modifies and is attached to a node dominating the complete VP (actually, a V') – *fixed the car*. Unlike adjuncts, arguments are rarely so globally ambiguous. Finally, an argument of the verb can either be obligatory or optional. For example, in (28) the third argument of *send* is optional; it can be omitted from the sentence (as in *Mitzi sent the car*) yet the verb carries it implicitly (one has to send something *to someone*). An argument can also be obligatory, as in *Mitzi handed the ball to Joelle*; omitting the PP in this sentence will render it ungrammatical (**Mitzi handed the ball*). The appearance of an adjunct, however, is almost always optional (*Mitzi fixed the car, Mitzi fixed the car in the garage*).

1.6 Summary

We have described some general aspects of one linguistic theory – Government and Binding. The theory is a modular one, including several levels of representation (S- and D-structure, for example), several independent theories (X-bar theory, Theta-theory, trace theory, for example) and constraining principles (the Projection Principle, the Theta Criterion), as well as the lexicon. X-bar theory involves the PS component; D-structure is the underlying representation of a sentence; NP- and *Wh*-movement apply at the interface between D- and S-structures to derive an S-structure representation; trace theory ensures that proper thematic role assignment is met; and the Lexicon contains information – argument structure and the thematic grid – that affects all levels of representation through both the Projection Principle and the Theta Criterion. We now move on to a discussion of sentence processing, employing some of the representational facts we have discussed thus far.

2 Sentence Processing in Neurologically-intact Populations

We might now ask what aspects of these representations, rules, and principles have been found to apply to sentence processing? That is, do these constructs borne from the minds of theoretical linguists have what one might call "processing reality" (at least in terms of the output of the empirical methods most closely associated with psycholinguistics)? In this section we will briefly review work that addresses this question. One of our aims, again, is to show that the language deficits found in aphasia can be best understood when making reference to the normal processing system.

2.1 Accessing verbs and their thematic representations

In a series of psycholinguistic studies, Shapiro and colleagues (Shapiro, Zurif & Grimshaw 1987, 1989; Shapiro, Brookins, Gordon & Nagel 1991) sought to determine whether or not thematic representations would have an affect on verb processing during on-line sentence comprehension. We exploited what we called the "representational complexity" of verbs – complexity defined in terms of the number of different thematic grids each verb allowed. A verb with fewer grids (or sub-entries) was considered less complex than a verb with more grids. For example, our "two-complement" verbs allowed a two-place argument structure with either an (Agent Theme) or (Agent Proposition) grid and our "four-complement" verbs allowed, again, a two-place argument structure but with four grids: an (Agent Theme), (Agent Proposition), (Agent Exclamation), and (Agent Interrogative):

(30)	"Two-complement"	*accept*	(Agent Theme) (Agent Proposition)
	"Four-complement"	*discover*	(Agent Theme) (Agent Proposition) (Agent Exclamation) (Agent Interrogative)

We placed instances of these verb types into similar, simple NP-V-NP-PP sentences like the following:

(31) The child accepted # that the key was missing

(32) The woman discovered # that the key was missing

and presented these to normal listeners via headphones. Immediately after hearing the verb in the sentence, a visual probe (word or nonword) appeared on a computer screen. The subject was required to listen to the sentence for meaning and to decide as rapidly and as accurately as possible whether the probe was a word or nonword. Reaction times (RT's) to this lexical decision were recorded. It was assumed that as the verb became more complex, the time taken to make the secondary lexical decision would increase. And that was indeed what we found. Verbs that accommodated more thematic grids yielded longer RT's than verbs that accommodated fewer grids. For example, RT's to the lexical decision took 676 ms for the two-complement verbs (31) and 731 ms for the four-complement verbs (32) (Shapiro et al. 1987).

We interpreted these data as showing that all possible thematic grids associated with a particular sense of a verb are momentarily and exhaustively activated in the immediate temporal vicinity of the verb, and this activation appears computationally expensive. One further explanation of these RT patterns involves processing resources: More resources are required to access a verb with more associated representations relative to a verb with less information. Furthermore, it turns out that even when sentences are biased toward only one of the possible multiple thematic grids for a verb, still all thematic grids are activated (Shapiro et al. 1989). Thus, lexical access operates in a form-driven, reflexive manner; that is, its initial operation is not penetrated by sentence context information.

Why should all thematic information be momentarily available to the system? Why should the sentence processing system work this way? First, it has no choice. Thematic information (or the lexical-conceptual representations from which it is read off) defines, in a sense, each particular verb in a language, or at the very least it characterizes the distinctions among verbs respected by the system. Thus, once a phonological form is contacted from the lexicon, so to are the thematic representations associated with it. Second, as we shall show in a later section, a verb's lexical properties restricts the hypothesis space the parser will need to work within, and can set up the possible paths it will need to subsequently take. Relatedly, sentence interpretation at least partially relies on the assignment of relational notions like Agent and Theme to the arguments in the sentence. Thematic grid availability at the point where the head is encountered at least ensures such assignment can occur, in principle, on-line.
For example, consider a verb like *think* that only selects a Proposition complement (i.e., it does not select for a direct object NP):

(Proposition)
(33) Joelle thinks......Dillon is cute

Note that when the parser encounters the NP – *Dillon* – verb information can, at least in principle, be used to interpret the argument not as a Theme, Patient, or "canonical" direct object of the verb – which would violate the verb's lexical properties – but as part of the Proposition (note that argument structure can't do this job, since in this case the standard argument structure would simply be an (x,y) in either the Theme or Proposition case).

2.2 Post-access integration effects

In a recent set of experiments (Shapiro, Nagel & Levine 1993) we examined whether or not the parser initially exploits the information contained in a lexical entry once *that information has been accessed.* We set up our experiments with two models of sentence processing in mind: the phrase structure-driven account (also known as the garden-path model), and the lexical guidance account. The phrase structure-driven account, argued by Frazier, Clifton, and others (e.g., Frazier 1978; Frazier & Rayner 1982), claims that the sentence processor uses a set of heuristics that make contact only with phrasal geometry as stipulated by the PS rules of a language. These heuristics, known as "late closure" and "minimal attachment", for example, state principles like "do not postulate any unnecessary nodes", "take the simplest route", etc. Only the lexical category of an item is used during the initial parse of a sentence; no other lexical information is used during the application of these heuristics and thus it is only during re-analysis that other verb properties, like thematic information, come into play. The lexical guidance account, originally argued by Ford, Bresnan & Kaplan 1983) and most recently by Trueswell, Tanenhaus & Kello, in press) claims that lexical properties like subcategorization or argument structure are used during the first-pass parse of a sentence. More than that, this account often claims that verbs *prefer* one complement over others, and that the preferred complement – not necessarily the one conforming to the simplest structure – is the first attempted parse. Consider:

(34) While the baby kicked the babysitter took a nap

(35) The neighbor knew the babysitter took a nap

The phrase structure-driven model would claim, on some accounts, that the post-verb NP – *the babysitter* in (34) – when initially encountered, is first attached as the verb kick's direct object; and in (35) it is first considered the direct object of the verb *know*. When the embedded verb took is subsequently encountered in either sentence, the parser notes that it has been garden-pathed, and thus re-analyzes the sentence, this time taking a look at the verb's lexical properties and realizing that there are other possible analyses. The lexical guidance account would claim that *the babysitter* might or might not be attached as the direct object of the verb *kick* and *know,* but such a decision would be based initially on the verb's lexical properties, which could include information about what complement the verb prefers – either the direct object NP or no overt complement, as in (34), or a direct object NP or a sentential clause, as in (35). It turns out that the evidence is equivocal; many of the studies claiming evidence for either account can be explained away by the other account. For example, the studies supporting the phrase structure-driven account have been reading tasks that chunk information artificially, or omit optional markers like commas and complementizers that just by their omission alone can be argued to interact with the processor in confounding ways (Trueswell et al., in press); this may be the reason why readers are garden-pathed in both (34) and (35). On the other hand, support for lexical guidance almost always is explained away by the phrase structure-driven account by claiming that lexical information is used only after phrase structure heuristics are employed.
However, we found a way to check for lexical preference effects *independently* from phrase structure heuristics. We asked whether there were cases where lexical preferences do affect a purportedly first-pass parse when phrase structure heuristics like minimal attachment, for example, were not relevant – do not even come into play. First, we gathered a set of lexical preferences for several types of verbs, including optionally transitive verbs, dative verbs, and complement verbs. So, for example, we rated whether subjects preferred a verb like *notice* with either a Proposition (*John noticed that the two diamonds were different*) or an Interrogative (*John noticed why the two diamonds were different*). Then, for each individual subject, we placed verbs in both their preferred and non-preferred structures. As an example, consider again the verb *notice.*

(36) (a) John noticed why # the two diamonds were different! – Interrogative
(b) John noticed that # the two diamonds were different – Proposition

Consider also the following pairs that we also used in our experiments:

(37) (a) The baby sitter read the # story to the sick child – Transitive
(b) The baby sitter read to # the sick child – Intransitive

(38) (a) The woman lent a dollar to # the man for a cup of coffee – NP PP (double-object verbs)
(b) The woman lent the man a # dollar for a cup of coffee – NP NP

(39) (a) The young girl donated the clothes to # the Boy Scouts – NP PP-argument (non-alternating datives)
(b) The young girl donated the clothes in # the basement – NP PP-adjunct

For some subjects, for example, the verb *notice* might be preferred with an argument having the semantic realization of a Proposition (36b) while other subjects might prefer it with an Interrogative (36a). And there were subjects who had the opposite preferences. We presented these sentences to normal listeners over headphones. At the point in the sentence where the structure of the verb's complement became evident, a visual *cross-modal lexical decision task* was presented. If lexical preferences are used on-line during the initial parse, then greater interference as shown by increased RT's should be observed in sentences where the complement is non-preferred relative to sentences where the complement is preferred.

In almost all of the cases, RT's were longer when the verb was contained in a sentence with the verb's non-preferred, relative to preferred, complement. These patterns suggest that lexical preferences are used very early, perhaps even initially, during on-line sentence processing. We assumed that if lexical information is used in unambiguous sentences – that is, sentences that do not contain local attachment ambiguities – then surely such information must be used initially in sentences *containing* local ambiguities. After all, the sentence processor has no knowledge of potential ambiguities until after the verb is encountered – beyond the point where preference information is made available to the system.

We also found that in one comparison, that between PP-arguments (39a) versus PP-adjuncts (39b), RT's were longer in the latter case than the former, *ignoring subject preferences*. Consider that in (a) the PP includes an argument of the verb *donate* yet in (b) it is an adjunct. That is, in (b) the PP does not form part of the verb's contribution to the sentence and in (a) it does. There are at least two explanations for this effect. First, it might simply reflect a preference for a verb to have all its arguments around it – to have its theta-grid saturated (i.e., all thematic roles in the grid are assigned to the arguments in the sentence). The processor 'expects' all the arguments to be evident in the syntax, thus when it encounters the head of a PP that is not in accordance with the lexical properties of the verb – in this case a Goal – interference to the system occurs. A second possibility is that there is no ambiguity associated with a prepositional phrase that forms an argument of the verb. Yet consider a locative adjunct PP like *in the basement*, it can either attach to an N' (modify the NP) – *the clothes* – or to the V' – *donated the clothes*. Perhaps the processor is aware that non-argument PP's are, in principle, inherently ambiguous – that is are associated with multiple parses. Thus an increased processing load is observed at the head of an adjunct phrase. However this turns out, once again such a result is evidence that verb information is indeed used on-line and immediately.

2.3 Parsing sentences with moved constituents: Re-activation effects

Thus far we have presented evidence from our laboratory supporting the "processing reality" of certain lexical properties and how such properties interact with the structure and interpretation of sentences. We now ask how the processor deals with trace-antecedent relations during on-line processing, particularly how they are interpreted during sentence comprehension. First, consider that when a trace (or "gap" in psycholinguistic terminology) is postulated, its antecedent (or "filler") is purportedly re-accessed in the trace's immediate temporal vicinity. Swinney, Ford, Frauenfelder & Brensan, reported in Swinney & Osterhaut (1990) presented sentences like the following over headphones to normal listeners:

(40) The policeman saw *the boy$_i$* that the crowd at the party (1) accused *trace$_i$* (2) of the crime.

At either position (1) or (2), a visual lexical decision probe was presented. Sometimes the probes were semantically related to the antecedent (e.g., GIRL) and sometimes they were semantically unrelated control words (e.g., GROUP). In experimental situations where a semantically related word is presented prior to a test word, and RT's to the test word are significantly faster than when it is preceded by an unrelated word, *priming* is said to have occurred – evidence that a lexical representation of the test word has been contacted. In the present case Swinney et al. were interested in whether or not a moved NP is primed – or re-accessed – at its trace. Results showed that at probe position (1), prior to the trace, targets related to *crowd* resulted in significantly faster RT's than did control probes. But at test point (2), in the immediate vicinity of the trace, only targets related to *boy* were primed, suggesting that the antecedent to a trace is indeed re-accessed once the trace is encountered (see also Nicol, in press).

2.3.1 Finding the trace

How does a reader/listener note the presence of a trace in a sentence? A trace is a lexically-unfilled position; there is perhaps nothing in the morpho-syntactic information that signifies its position in the sentence. We (Nagel & Shapiro 1994) recently investigated how listeners might in fact locate a trace during the temporal unfolding of a sentence. In this experiment we asked whether or not *prosodic* information could affect where a listener might postulate a trace. Consider the following sentences:

PAW 821 ms
NUN 735 ms

(47) Which priest$_i$ did the parishioner ask # *trace*$_i$ to give a blessing for her friend Mary?

PAW 728 ms
NUN 716 ms

(48) Which priest$_i$ did the parishioner ask # to give a blessing for trace$_i$ in the seminary?

The verb *ask* is optionally transitive; that is, it selects either for one external argument or two arguments – an external and internal one. In (47) *ask* is contained in a sentence with a direct object, but the direct object – *which priest* – has been moved, leaving behind a trace. In (48) *ask* is used intransitively thus no overt NP or trace is in the direct object argument position. Instead, the object of the preposition has been moved, leaving behind a trace. Note that the morphosyntactic information is the same up to and including the preposition *for*. That is, the sentences differ in terms of the location of the trace, though the antecedent is the same in both cases. We used the cross-modal priming technique. We presented sentences like these over headphones to normal listeners and asked them to make a visual lexical decision to either a probe (e.g., NUN) related to the antecedent *priest* or to a control probe (e.g. PAW). Again, when reaction times to the related probe are significantly faster than to its control, then priming is said to have occurred, which means that the lexical item to which the related probe refers has been accessed.

The results (shown in (47) and (48)) revealed a significant difference between the related and control probes at the trace in sentences like (47); but we did not get such a difference immediately after *ask* – a non-trace position – after (48). This pattern means that *priest* is (re)activated at the real trace in (47) and a trace is not erroneously postulated after the verb *ask* in (48). Note also that since there is no priming for *priest* at the probe position in (48), what we are observing in (47) must be reactivation of *priest*, not continuous activation. Consider also only the control probes. Significantly longer RT's to these probes were observed when they were presented at the trace in (47) compared to the post-verb non-trace position in (48), suggesting the "more work" (reflected in greater processing load) needs to be done when a trace must be computed, connected to its antecedent, and locally interpreted.

Importantly, consider that the only difference between sentences (47) and (48) is the prosodic contour. We have recently found that there are acoustic parameters that underlie the different prosodic contours in sentences like (47) and (48). The duration of the verb plus 'pause time' between off-set of the verb and onset of the beginning of the next lexical item is significantly longer in sentences that contain traces immediately after the verb (47) than in sentences that do not (48). Additionally, the pitch (Fo) declination on the verb is significantly steeper in (47) relative to (48). Thus, there are clear acoustic differences at local points in sentences containing traces relative to those that don't contain traces – all other things being equal – and thus prosody might very well be clueing the listeners in on the location of the trace.

2.4 Summary

In our psycholinguistic investigations we have found that lexical properties, including abstract thematic information, are accessed with the verb during on-line sentence processing. We have also found that antecedents to traces are re-accessed at lexically-unfilled trace positions, and that traces are located, perhaps, by the acoustic information that underlies the prosodic contour of the sentence. We now turn to some of our work in neurolinguistics which exploits the linguistic and psycholinguistic facts we have just presented.

3 Sentence Comprehension in Neurologically-impaired Populations

Our work in this area has sought to explain the performance of brain-damaged subjects by making reference to linguistic theory and to normal sentence processing routines, with the goal of ultimately shedding light on the normal operation of the sentence processing system.

3.1 Accessing thematic information in aphasia

As we have shown earlier, there's quite a bit of evidence suggesting that verbs have a lot to do with both the syntactic and semantic characteristics of a sentence. As an example consider that when we acquire the verb *discover*, we likely gain the real-world fact that *discover* requires two arguments – both a "discoverer" and something that is "discovered". The "something that is discovered", however, can take several forms that display different syntactic and semantic characteristics. For example, you can "discover the answer" – where *the answer* is a direct object; you can "discover that the answer was wrong" – where the clause after the verb has the interpretation of a Proposition; you can "discover what a stupid question it was!" – where the clause after the verb has the interpretation of an Exclamation; and you can "discover why the answer was wrong" – where, again, the material after the verb is a clause but is interpreted as an Interrogative. A lexical entry for *discover*, then, could contain at least the following information:

(49) *discover* **lexical category:** V
phonology (phonemic structure, syllable structure, etc.)...
argument structure: (x,y)
thematic grids:
Agent Theme (...the answer to the question)
Agent Proposition (...that the answer was wrong)
Agent Interrogative (...why the answer was wrong)
Agent Exclamation (...what a dumb question it was!)

Given the richness of the lexicon, the verb and its properties might provide crucial semantic and syntactic information to the sentence processor. And indeed it does. Our work has shown that the normally intact sentence processing system access all thematic information about a verb in the verb's immediate vicinity, setting up possible paths the parser needs to take and allowing the on-line assignment of thematic and semantic roles onto arguments in the sentence.

These linguistic and psycholinguistic facts have important implications for the investigation of the language deficits subsequent to aphasia. For example, it is fairly well-established that the aberrant language performance of some Broca's aphasic patients may have to do with assigning thematic roles onto arguments. Consider:

(50) It was Dillon who kissed Joelle last night

(51) It was *Joelle*$_i$ who Dillon kissed *trace*$_i$ last night

In the cleft-subject sentence (50), the arguments can be said to be in 'canonical' positions. But in the cleft-object (51), the post-verb direct object position is not lexically filled. Instead, the direct object NP has been moved out of the direct object argument position, leaving behind a trace. In an off-line task where a listener is presented with a sentence and has to point to one of two pictures, the Broca's aphasic patient will often perform at-chance when confronted with cleft-object sentences (and passives), yet when confronted with cleft-subjects (and actives), above-chance performance is often observed. Skipping the details here, Grodzinsky (1990) and now others (see, for example, Hickok, Zurif & Canseco-Gonzalez 1993) have offered a descriptive generalization that captures this pattern: The connection between the trace and the moved NP is deleted, thus the moved NP cannot be interpreted normally as the direct object.

However, Grodzinsky's theory is strictly a description of a deficit, one that, admittedly, makes important contact with linguistic theory but makes no contact with any possible processing antecedents to the deficit. We reasoned that perhaps Broca's aphasic patients cannot ultimately interpret these sentences off-line because they do not have – in the first place – normal *access* to the thematic information about verbs in such sentences. For example, consider:

(52)

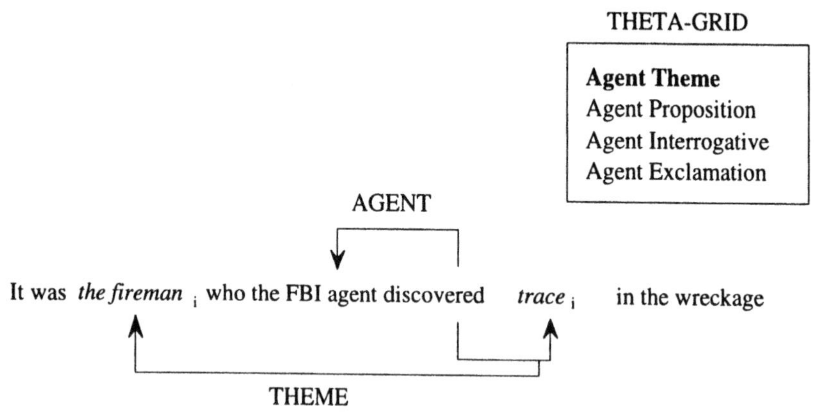

In (52), once the verb is encountered and accessed, so to are its thematic grids – as we have shown in our previous work. Then some selection process picks one of the multiple possibilities, in this case the Agent Theme grid, and the Agent is assigned to the *FBI man* and the Theme is assigned to the direct object argument position. That position is empty so the Theme is essentially passed on to the moved NP *the fireman*. So, logically, if the Broca's aphasic patient can't even access the thematic grid at the point where the verb is encountered, there will be no grammatical method for determining which arguments play which roles, since only the verb itself carries this information. There are independent reasons for suggesting that Broca's aphasic patients might have difficulty with the automatic access of information (see, for example, Swinney Zurif & Nicol 1989).

We (Shapiro, Gordon, Hack & Killackey 1993) ran a few experiments to assess the interaction between verb access and complex sentences. In one experiment (of a series) we compared what we have called "two-complement" verbs to "four-complement" verbs. We inserted the two verb types in this experiment into cleft-subjects and cleft-objects:

(53)	*demand*	(Agent Theme) (Agent Proposition)	*discover*	(Agent Theme) (Agent Proposition) (Agent Interrogative) (Agent Exclamation)

(54) It was the FBI agent who demanded/discovered # the key in the morning

(55) It was *the key* that the FBI agent demanded/discovered # $trace_i$ in the morning

Our Broca's aphasic patients could interpret sentences like (54) – a cleft-subject sentence – but could not interpret sentences like (55) – a cleft-object sentence. We used the cross-modal lexical decision task where we present sentences over headphones and a specific point during the unfolding of the sentence, a visual lexical decision probe – a word or a nonword – is presented on a computer monitor. The reaction times associated with the lexical decision are, again, a measure of processing load. Recall that in our previous work, for example, we found that four-complement verbs – like *discovered* – yielded longer RT's than our two-complement verbs – like *demanded*, but only at the point where the verb was encountered.

Three groups were included in the experiment: a matched group of 10 nomial controls; a group of 6 Broca's aphasic patients; and a group of 4 Wernicke's aphasic patients. The six Broca's aphasic patients presented with non-fluent and telegraphic verbal output and with relative sparing of auditory comprehension at the conversational level. On a sentence-picture matching task presented at the time of the experiment involving 10 each of active, passive, cleft-object and cleft-subject sentences, all six subjects showed above-chance performance on active and cleft-subject sentences, and at-chance performance on passives and cleft-object sentences. Three of the four Wernicke's aphasic patients presented with fluent, relatively empty speech; one presented with fluent speech that appeared conversationally appropriate, though considerable word-finding problems were observed.

First, consider the results from the cleft-subject sentences. Recall that these sentences could indeed be interpreted by our Broca's aphasic patients. For the normal control subjects, the two-complement verbs yielded faster RT's than the four-complement verbs. This pattern offered further empirical support for our claim that multiple thematic grids are accessed with the verb during on-line sentence processing. For the Broca's aphasic patients, the same normal pattern was observed: Two-complement verbs yielded significantly faster RT's than the four-complement verbs. So at least in the sentences that these patients can interpret, they show normal access of a verb's thematic properties. For Wernicke's aphasic patients, however, the difference was not significant; they apparently did not show sensitivity to the thematic properties of verbs.

Now consider the results from the cleft-object sentences. Recall here that these sentences could not be interpreted by our Broca's aphasic subjects. For the normals, the same distinction we observed in the cleft-subjects was observed here. That is, the two-complement verbs yielded faster RT's than the four-complement verbs. For the Broca's aphasic patients, they again showed the nomial pattern. Thus, these brain-damaged subjects indeed show normal access of a verb's thematic properties, *even in sentences that they ultimately do not interpret.* This pattern suggests that the real-time process of accessing a verb and its thematic properties must be *independent* from the difficulties these patients have with comprehending complex sentences. That is, though the time-course of thematic access may be normal with these patients, integrating this information into the temporal unfolding of the sentence may not be. We are presently working on a series of experiments that is attempting to discover where in the processing stream between access and (off-line) integration do these patients break down.

For the Wernicke's aphasic patients, differences between the verb types in the cleft-object sentences were, again, not significant. Since recent linguistic accounts of the lexicon claim that thematic information is part of lexical-conceptual structure or "conceptual semantics" (Grimshaw 1990; Jackendoff 1990), perhaps Wernicke's aphasic patients have a disorder in either representing or, more likely, accessing this information. In this vein consider that there have been several suggestions in the literature that Wernicke's aphasia involves some sort of "semantic deficit" in terms of conceptual features, though no consensus exists on the nature of this disorder (see, for example, Baker 1986). Our present data provide a grammatical angle on this semantic deficit – these patients just don't seem to have normal access to the conceptual representations of lexical items.

These patterns can be compared to a recent series of investigations of syntactic processing in Broca's and Wernicke's aphasia by Zurif, Swinney, Prather, Solomon & Bushell. Zurif et al. examined whether or not their aphasic subjects could normally link a moved NP to its empty argument position, or "trace" in complex sentences. They used sentences similar to the following:

Cleft-subject:

(56) It was the agent who discovered the burglary at the dock on Christmas

Cleft-object:

(57) It was *the burglaryi* that the agent discovered $trace_i$ at the dock on Christmas

Skipping the details here, Zurif and colleagues established that their Broca's aphasic patients did not show the normal link between the trace and its antecedent, that is, they did not normally re-access the antecedent to the trace. Yet different from that found for the Broca's aphasic patients, the Wernicke's aphasic patients in the Zurif et al. studies showed the normal connection between the trace and the antecedent, they did show antecedent re-access. So, summarizing the Zurif et al. and present studies, we find the following: 1) Broca's aphasic patients *do not* normally connect a trace to its antecedent while Wernicke's patients show the normal connection; and 2) Broca's aphasic patients are normally sensitive to a verb's thematic properties; Wernicke's aphasic patients are not (and, by the way, most of the Broca's and Wernicke's patients were the same in both sets of studies).

These patterns are important for a number of reasons. They suggest that the lexical process of accessing a verb's thematic properties and the operation of connecting a trace to its antecedent can be dissociated in brain damage, and perhaps are even independent. They also speak to a recently popular set of accounts of sentence processing collectively known as the "reduced capacity" hypothesis. The basic premise is that sentence processing requires the availability of enough resources to complete the task, the resources stemming from either a single "central processing capacity" (see Frazier & Friederici 1991), or a general attentional pool (see McNeil, Odell & Tseng 1990), or working memory (see MacDonald, Just & Carpenter, in press; Caplan & Hildebrandt 1988). When task and linguistic demands exceed the limited resources available to the Broca's aphasic patients, performance declines. Using this hypothesis, researchers have attempted to explain the inability of these patients to comprehend sentences involving traces as well as sentences with multiple arguments.

What do these patterns say about the capacity limitation hypothesis? First, though accessing a verb's thematic information appears costly, the cost does not exceed the capacity of Broca's aphasic patients to exhaustively access this information. Moreover, the resources necessary to process sentences that contain multiple arguments and trace-antecedent relations does not impinge on the resources necessary to access the verb's lexical properties. This resource independence occurs even though the verb and the trace-antecedent relation must be computed within the same temporal range during the unfolding of the sentence. So, consider (50) again. Notice that accessing the verb and its multiple thematic properties and computing the trace-antecedent relation occur in the same temporal vicinity; in fact, they might be working concurrently. Thus, on this account, in sentences where complex trace-antecedent relations must be computed, accessing the verb's multiple thematic information should suffer. Our results however, suggest otherwise. We suggest that there is not a single resource as these accounts imply, but multiple resources, each dedicated to a particular sub-process.

We now turn to another, recent line of neurolinguistic research that we have taken, one that attempts to connect the facts we have gathered about verbs and syntax to sentence production.

4 Aphasic and Normal Language Production: Lexical Properties and Syntax

Clearly, psycholinguistic investigations have shown that lexical properties, including abstract thematic information, are accessed with the verb during on-line sentence processing and that antecedents to traces are re-accessed at lexically-unfilled trace positions. We might ask then whether these linguistic constructs, too, influence sentence production. Our ultimate goal, once again, is to show that the language deficits found in brain damage can be best understood when making reference to the normal language processing system. In our production work, we move a step closer to this goal.

4.1 An investigation of "sentence memory" in production

We (Shapiro, McNamara, Zurif, Lanzoni & Cermak 1992) recently tested a group of Korsakoff amnesic patients and control subjects on a sentence repetition task to assess the role of analytical deficits on sentence memory performance (see Cermak 1989). We manipulated verb complexity (defined in terms of the number of possible thematic grids a verb accommodated), length of sentence, arguments versus adjuncts, and sentence complexity using actives, passives, and cleft-relative sentences. Recall that on some grammatical accounts passive sentences involve NP-movement and relative clauses involve *Wh*-movement. We found that: 1) amnesic subjects performed more poorly than control subjects; 2) both subject groups were affected by increases in length (particularly when length was increased by the addition of adjuncts relative to arguments), by cleft sentence type, and by verb complexity. That is, adding adjunct PP's (e.g., *...in the park*) to sentences resulted in more repetition errors than adding argument PP's (e.g., *...to the girl*), object relative clefts were more difficult than passives, and more errors at the verb occurred when the verb allowed more possible thematic grids than when it allowed less thematic grids; and 3) amnesic performance was particularly affected when complex sentences – relative to simpler sentences – contained non-argument length increases.

We interpreted these findings in the following way: First, increases in length decreased sentence production performance, but that was only part of the story. All other variables being equal, increases by adjuncts posed significantly more difficulty than increases with arguments because interpretation of adjuncts is not linked to the verb. That is, adjuncts do not match up to any thematic grid associated with the head of a VP, only arguments do (see also Clifton, Speer, & Abney 1981). Second, we assumed that the antecedent search process performed by the parser may proceed differently for NP-versus Wh-movement. For example, consider the (partial) S-structure for the following passive and object relative cleft sentences in (58) and (59):

(58) $[_{S}$ $[_{NP}$ Joelle$]_i$ was kissed $[_{NP}$ *trace*$]_i$ by $[_{NP}$ Dillon$]]$

(59) It was $[_{NP}$ Joelle$]_i$ $[_{S'}$ $[_{COMP}$ who$]_i$ $[_{S}$ $[_{NP}$ Dillon$]$ kissed $[_{NP}$ *trace*$]_i]]$

Note that (58) shows that only one S node is required for the passive, yet in the object cleft (59) both a more dominant S (an S-bar) and an embedded S are required. Just in terms of structural density, then, (59) requires more complex parsing routines than (58). Notice also that a search back for the antecedent of the trace in (59) crosses both an S and S-bar boundary. Berwick and Weinberg (1984) point out that the S-bar in sentences like (59) causes the parser to wait for various structural attachments to occur before the parser can co-index a Wh-element to its trace. On the other hand, the NP trace from the passive can be co-indexed immediately since no S-bar is involved. We suggest that this extra parsing complexity associated with *Wh*-movement contributed to the difficulty subjects experienced when attempting to process these types of sentences.

4.2 Sentence production in Broca's aphasia

We take two lines of investigation here. The first details verbs, their thematic representations, as well other aspects of sentence production in free narrative conditions in both normal and aphasic subjects. And the second involves experimental manipulation of 'complex' sentences – those in which sentence constituents (i.e., arguments of the verb) are moved out of their canonical positions. This research uses an experimental treatment paradigm – that is, single-subject experimental designs – in which subjects are trained to produce certain sentences while other linguistically related sentences are tested for generalization. These designs are particularly well suited for close examination of sentence production patterns. In this work we train subjects to operate on the "underlying" form of sentences and take them through the movement of NP's and their thematic role assignments that eventually derive the surface realization of non-canonical sentences. Through repeated measurement of both trained and untrained sentences throughout the course of training, the relation among the various sentences used in our studies is examined. In this work we (Jacobs 1994; Shapiro & Thompson 1994; Thompson & Shapiro 1994; Thompson, Shapiro, Li & Schendel, in press; Thompson, Shapiro & Roberts 1993; Thompson, Shapiro, Tait, Schneider & Jacobs 1994) have found that many of the representations, rules and principles found to apply to sentence processing also influence sentence production.

4.2.1 Production of verbs and their thematic representations

Using a coding system that we (Thompson, Shapiro, Tait, Schneider & Jacobs 1994) recently developed for analyzing various morpho-syntactic and lexical aspects of production with respect to the structure of the grammar we sought to characterize sentence production in agrammatic and normal speakers. One major aspect of this work was to specify the types of verbs that are most frequently accessed for production and the extent to which these verbs, when accessed, are produced in their various argument structure arrangements. Clearly, it has been shown that verb production often is impoverished in agrammatic speakers (McCarthy & Warrington 1985; Miceli, Silveri,

Villa & Caramazza 1984; Zingeser & Berndt 1990). Further, as we have shown above, verbs influence sentence processing in various ways (e.g., increased processing time is required for more complex verbs; adjuncts increase processing load relative to arguments; thematic grid preferences perhaps guide initial parsing). What we sought to explore here, then, was the relation between verb production and syntax.

Narrative discourse samples were obtained by asking Broca's aphasic patients and normal subjects to retell the story of Cinderella using methods described by Saffran, Berndt & Schwartz (1989). Language samples were segmented into utterances based on syntactic, prosodic, and semantic criteria, entered into a computer for analysis, and coded. Each utterance was coded as either a grammatical sentence, an ungrammatical sentence, or a non-sentence (utterances not containing a matrix verb were considered non-sentences; all others were coded as sentences). Sentences were coded as ungrammatical when required phrasal or clausal constituents were absent, when arguments were produced in the wrong syntactic position, when subject/verb agreement errors occurred, or when other similar errors were noted. All verbs produced in both grammatical and ungrammatical sentences and their accompanying argument structures were then coded.

Verb codes included (a) obligatory one-place (Ob1), (b) obligatory two-place (Ob2), (c) obligatory three-place (Ob3), (d) optional two-place (Op2), (e) optional three-place (Op3), (f) complement verbs (C), and (g) copulas (Cop). Thematic roles attached to arguments, i.e., Agent (x), Theme/Patient (y), and Goal (z), as well as adjuncts (J) – which have been found to be computationally more expensive than arguments – found in each utterance also were coded, as were sentential complements (S') occurring with complement verbs and predication phrases (P) (i.e., NP, adjectival phrase, PP) occurring with copulas (see Appendix). These codes were assigned based on the underlying linguistic representation of utterances with reference to Government-Binding theory (Chomsky 1981, 1986). Because thematic roles that are represented in a verb's lexical entry – Agent, Theme, Goal, etc. – are assigned to argument positions (i.e., NPs) at d-structure, it is at this linguistic level that we assign verb-argument codes. Syntactically legal omissions of arguments were also coded (e.g. truncated passive sentences like "The ball was hit" in which the *by*-phrase is omitted were coded as containing an obligatory two-place verb (Ob2) accompanied by the internal argument (Theme (y), the ball) with a legally omitted external argument (x, Agent)). Misuse or omission of either verbs and/or arguments & adjuncts also were noted in transcript coding.

For each sample the mean length of utterance, the proportion of utterances comprised of grammatical sentences, the mean number of verbs produced, and the proportion of utterances containing verbs was calculated. The frequency of occurrence of each verb type and the proportion of the data accounted for by each verb type then was computed as was the extent to which each verb type was produced with correct argument structure. The number of contexts in which individual arguments and adjuncts were produced correctly also was calculated. For each of these variables, means and standard deviations for normal and aphasic groups were calculated and t-tests were performed to compute differences between group means.

Results of this work has indicated, as expected, that Broca's aphasic subjects use significantly shorter and less complex sentences in their narrative discourse than do normals. Few aphasic utterances were comprised of grammatical sentences (i.e., only 13 % of aphasic utterances were grammatical sentences as compared to normals' 87 %), and proportionately fewer utterances produced by aphasics as compared to normals contained verbs (65 % of aphasic vs. 99 % of normals). These data support previously reported findings that nonfluent aphasic subjects produce primarily short, asyntactic utterances with relatively few verbs (Gleason, Goodglass, Obler, Green, Hyde & Weintraub 1980; Meyerson & Goodglass 1972; Saffran, Schwartz & Marin 1980).

When the data were analyzed for the type of verbs produced by the two subject groups, we found that both aphasic patients and normal subjects produced similar proportions of copulas. However, the aphasic subjects produced significantly more one- and two-place verbs than did normal subjects and, conversely, the normal subjects produced more three-place and complement verbs than did the aphasics. Of interest, however, was the significant finding that within the categories of optional three-place verbs, the aphasic subjects more often produced them in (x,y) form, rarely using the optional third argument (z). Conversely, normal subjects more often produced these optional three-place verbs with all three arguments present. Analysis of complement verb productions revealed similar differences across subjects: Normal subjects more often produced complement verbs with a sentential complement (x, S') whereas aphasic subjects more often produced complement verbs in (x,y) form. These findings are somewhat consistent with distinctions in verb complexity born out in our reaction time studies with both normal and aphasic subjects. Optional three-place verbs and complement verbs – both of which allow a wider range of thematic grid possibilities than do, for example, obligatory one- and two-place verbs – require greater processing time in on-line sentence processing experiments, suggesting the need for greater resources in processing these verbs.

There is one important difference between our on-line sentence comprehension studies (see, for example, Shapiro et al. 1993) and our current production data: Though Broca's aphasic patients appear normal in their access of a verb's lexical properties in comprehension, our production data indicate that aphasic subjects evince a preference for producing primarily simple verbs that require accessing simple argument structure arrangements and that when more "complex" verbs are accessed for production, aphasic subjects retain a preference for producing them in their simplest form. So, not surprisingly, we have not found a simple one-to-one correspondence between comprehension and production.

When we further considered these data with regard to the accuracy of the argument structures produced around verbs, we found that normal subject produced most verb argument structures correctly, regardless of the type of verb produced (98 % of all verbs were produced with correct argument structure). Aphasic subjects, however, did not. That is, significant differences were noted between aphasic and normal subjects in the proportion of verbs produced with correct argument structure for all verbs types in all forms – even for simple two-place forms. Interestingly, however, aphasic subjects evinced more success in accessing correct argument structures for obligatory one- and two-place verbs than for optional two-place, optional three-place, and complement verbs. These data indicated that aphasic subjects have little success in accessing argument structures/thematic information for "complex" verbs, although attempts to do so were apparent in the data.

These findings also are in keeping with expectations based on the lexical properties of verbs: Aphasic subjects were unable to consistently produce the appropriate arguments around simple verbs (those which allow only one argument structure arrangement), and showed even less success in producing appropriate argument structures for more complex verbs (those allowing a wider array of argument structure possibilities). And when these more complex verbs were produced, the most simple argument structures for these verbs were accessed. These findings, therefore, explain, in part, the simple sentence production patterns noted in agrammatic aphasic individuals. Compared to normal subjects, nonfluent aphasic patients do not use the full range of lexical properties available given a particular verb. This restriction, we surmise, is not due to any simple length or "economy of effort" consideration, but is due to a complex mixture of verb and sentence variables that affects the computational complexity of producing sentences. We suggest that this limitation may partially explain the short utterance length that is prevalent in agrammatic aphasia.

4.2.2 Experimental Analysis of Sentence Production in Agrammatic Aphasia

Thus far we have presented evidence that the lexical properties of verbs not only influence interpretation of sentences, but that they also come into play in sentence production. We now ask whether trace-antecedent relations, which have been found to have "processing reality" in on-line experiments, also should be considered with regard to sentence production. Perhaps, for example, the difficulty that Broca's aphasic subjects appear to have in properly assigning thematic roles onto arguments that have been moved out of their canonical positions may also influence production of these non-canonical sentences. That is, because Broca's subjects do not appear to "fill the gap" when it is encountered in the temporal unfolding of sentences (see, for example, Zurif et al. 1993), they too may not have on-time access to co-referenced sentence constituents when attempting to produce sentences. We have explored this possibility in a series of experiments concerned with production of sentences in which NP's have been moved out of their underlying position, leaving behind a 'trace' or gap of that movement.

Our subjects in these experiments were Broca's aphasic subjects who evinced good comprehension of canonical sentences (i.e., actives and cleft-subjects), but performed at-chance or below in comprehending passive, object-cleft, and wh-question constructions. Too, these subjects showed similar performance patterns in both narrative and constrained sentence production tasks. In narrative discourse, their sentences were asyntactic and telegraphic; and in constrained sentence production tasks they evinced ability to produce active, but not passive, object cleft or wh-questions. To test constrained sentence production we used a sentence production priming task in which semantically reversible action pictures were presented in pairs and target sentence types were primed using one picture in the pair. Following the sentence prime, subject were expected to produce the primed sentence type using the semantically reversed picture in the pair.

4.2.2.1 Production of Moved Sentence Constituents: Wh-Movement and NP-Movement

As shown in section 4.1, there are two kinds of movement subsumed under the general rule *move-alpha*, *wh-* and NP-movement. For example, wh-movement derives sentences such as wh-questions (e.g., *Who*$_i$ is the bully hitting *trace*$_i$?) and object clefts (e.g., It was *the boy*$_i$ who the bully hit *trace*$_i$); whereas, NP-movement derives sentences such as passives (e.g., *The boy*$_i$ was hit *trace*$_i$ by the bully). In NP-movement, a noun phrase (NP) is moved from an *argument position* (e.g., in the passive, the direct object position), to another *argument position* (e.g., the subject position), leaving behind an NP-trace. In effect, both the site from which the constituent moves and it's "landing site" are positions projected from the verb's lexical representation. Unlike NP-movement, wh-movement involves displacement of wh-phrases from *argument positions* (e.g., direct object) to *non-argument positions* (e.g., Specifier of COMP), leaving behind a wh-trace. Another difference between NP-movement (the passive) and wh-movement involves the distance between the trace and its antecedent (please see again, (58)-(59)). Again, sentence processing work has indicated that *wh-* and NP-movement may have their own "processing routines". That is, more "work" needs to be done to attach an antecedent to a *wh*-trace (i.e., in *wh*-questions or object clefts) than to an NP-trace (i.e., in a passive sentence) because a *wh*-trace and its antecedent are separated by clausal boundaries (e.g., Berwick & Weinberg 1984). In addition, such a distinction between the movement types shows up in aphasic performance (Caplan & Hildebrandt 1988) and in the sentence production performance of amnesic patients and their controls (Shapiro et al. 1992): Better performance is observed on sentences derived from NP-movement relative to *wh*-movement.

In our sentence production work we, too, have noted this distinction between *wh-* and NP-movement. Our experimental paradigm involves teaching agrammatic aphasic subjects to produce sentences derived from either *wh*-movement (i.e., *wh*-questions and object clefts) or from NP-movement (i.e., passive sentences) and testing generalized production both within and across sentence types. In one of our experiments, for example, we (Thompson & Shapiro 1994) trained aphasic subjects to produce *wh*-questions such as (60) and tested generalization to object-cleft and passive sentences such as (61) and (62). At the same time, we trained other subjects to produce object-cleft sentences such as (61) and tested generalization to *wh*-questions (60) and passives (62).

(60) Who did the girl hit? (*Wh*-question)

(61) It was the boy who the girl hit. (Object-cleft)

(62) The boy was hit by the girl. (Passive)

The treatment applied utilized the active form of sentences trained, assuming that the active form is directly related to the derived form which shares similar thematic roles. For example, in teaching production of either (60) or (61), the related sentence form as shown in (62) was presented:

(63) The girl hit the boy. (Active form)

Using the active sentence form, subjects were taught to recognize the verb, its arguments, and their thematic role assignments. Then instructions concerned with movement of arguments to – in this case – non-argument positions was demonstrated to derive the surface form of targeted sentences. Subjects then were instructed to produce the derived surface representation of target sentences. Additional morphemes required in the surface form also were provided and inserted into sentence frames. Throughout the training period, production of both trained and untrained sentence types was tested using our sentence production priming task and emergent production patterns were recorded.

Results of this experiment indicated that, indeed, the distinction between *wh*-movement and NP-movement processes is honored in sentence production in brain-damaged subjects. That is, two of our three agrammatic Broca's aphasic subjects who participated in this study readily learned to produce sentences derived from *wh*-movement (e.g., *wh*-questions), and with this learning, generalized production of other *wh*-movement derived sentences (i.e., object-clefts) was observed, while no change in production of NP-movement derived, passive sentences were noted. This same pattern of responding was noted for subjects trained to produced object-cleft sentences. That is, teaching object-clefts resulted in emergent production of both object-clefts and *wh*-questions, but not passive sentences.

In another related study conducted in our lab involving four agrammatic Broca's aphasic subjects, we have also found a dissociation between *wh*- and NP-movement derived sentences. That is, when subjects were taught to produce passive sentences using the same heuristic utilized for training *wh*-questions and object-cleft forms as described above, production of object-cleft sentences was not influenced. Similarly, when subjects were trained to produce object-cleft sentences, no change in production of passive sentences was noted (Jacobs 1994).

4.2.2.2 Production of Sentences Involving Argument vs. Adjunct Movement

Another distinction noted in sentence processing work concerns the distinction between arguments of the verb and adjuncts. As noted above, arguments of the verb and adjuncts differentially affect sentence processing in both normal and in brain damaged populations. We exploited this distinction in sentence production – again using an experimental treatment approach – by sequentially training seven of our agrammatic Broca's aphasic subjects to produce either *who* or *what* questions which require similar movement of the argument NP (direct object), or *when* and *where* questions which require adjunct movement (object of a preposition contained in an

adjunct prepositional phrase). We then measured generalization within and across these four *wh*-questions.
Using a set of 20 optionally transitive verbs, eighty active sentence stimuli (NP-V-NP-PP) were developed to help elicit the four question constructions as shown in (64)-(67).

(64) The soldier is pushing the woman into the street.

(65) The boy is kicking the cow in the barn.

(66) The student is helping the doctor during the evening.

(67) The guard is protecting the clerk at the store.

Through application of the rule *move-alpha*, these sentences are related to the *wh*-questions indicated in (68)-(71). *Who*- and *what*-questions are formed by displacement of the verb argument (i.e., object NP) to COMP as depicted in (68) and (69); and *where*- and *when*-questions are formulated by displacement of the NP contained within the adjunct PP as shown in (70) and (71).

(68) Who_i is the soldier pushing $trace_i$ into the street?

(69) $What_i$ is the boy kicking $trace_i$ in the barn?

(70) $When_i$ is the student helping the doctor $trace_i$?

(71) $Where_i$ is the guard protecting the clerk $trace_i$?

Using stimuli such as those in (64) to (67), *wh*-questions as in (68) to (71) were elicited in the following manner: A stimulus sentence (e.g., (64) above) was presented for the subject to read and the following instructions were given: 'You want to know *the person* the soldier is pushing, so you ask?'. The word 'person' was emphasized, rising inflection was used, and a question mark card was placed above the sentence. To elicit *what*-questions using the stimulus sentence in (65) above, the examiner instructed: 'You want to know *the thing* the boy is kicking, so you ask?'. This time, the word 'thing' was emphasized. To elicit *when*- and *where*-questions, the same procedure was used except that subjects were instructed to ask about *the time* or *the place*, respectively. Using this procedure during baseline testing indicated that none of the subjects were able to produce any of the *wh*-questions under study.
As in our previous experiments, subjects were trained (a) to recognize the verb and verb-argument structures of sentences in their active form, (b) to move the proper sentence constituent to formulate *wh*-questions, and (c) to produce the surface form of targeted *wh*-questions. Subjects received this training using only one *wh*-question form at a time (e.g., *who*), while the remaining *wh*-question forms (i.e., *what, where, when*) as well as untrained exemplars of the trained form (i.e., untrained *who*-questions) were tested for generalization using procedures identical to those used in baseline testing. The emergent sentence production patterns, then, provided information regarding the organization of sentence production operations within and across subjects.

Results indicated two distinct patterns of emergent sentence production across the subjects under study. The first pattern was noted in four of the agrammatic subjects who demonstrated acquisition and generalization patterns as expected. That is, when treatment was applied to *wh*-questions requiring movement of the argument NP (i.e., direct object; e.g., *what*-questions), generalized production of untrained *wh*-questions was restricted to those also relying on argument NP-movement (e.g., *who*-questions). Similarly, when treatment was applied to *wh*-questions requiring adjunct movement (e.g., *where*-questions), generalization occurred to untrained *wh*-questions relying on adjunct movement (e.g., *when*-questions). Importantly, argument movement did not generalize to adjunct movement constructions, and vice versa, indicating that the argument/adjunct distinction found in the normal experimental psycholinguistics literature extends to the cross-generalization distinction found between argument and adjunct movement with our aphasic patients.

A second pattern of sentence production acquisition was noted in the other three agrammatic subjects. These subjects evinced generalization across *all wh*-question constructions when treatment was applied to only one of the four, regardless of which *wh*-question was selected for treatment. For example, when *who*-questions were trained (requiring argument NP-movement), improved production was noted for not only *what*-questions, but also was observed for *when*- and *where*-questions. Interestingly, these subjects showed no difficulty with movement of the appropriate sentence constituent. However, they consistently mis-selected the Specifier – producing any one of the four wh-morphemes at random. Therefore, for these subjects, lexical discrimination training (of *wh*-morphemes) was instituted, which resulted in correct wh-question production of all four question types.

Based on our detailed data from this and other studies, we suggest that there may be separate processes underlying the production (and perhaps comprehension) of *wh*-movement constructions, specifically regarding control of syntactic features of *wh*-question formation (i.e., movement of the NP itself) and control of sub-lexical features of *wh*-questions (i.e., *wh*-morpheme selection). Four of our agrammatic patients presented primarily with a syntactic deficit which influenced their *wh*-sentence production – they had difficulty with selecting the proper NP to be moved. Whereas the other three of the agrammatic subjects presented with a selection deficit involving the non-lexical Specifier position – they mis-selected, randomly, among the corpus of *wh*-morphemes under study. We note that this latter finding supports Grodzinsky's (1990) mis-selection hypothesis of agrammatic sentence production.

These findings attest to the contribution that detailed recovery data can make both to understanding the nature of sentence production deficits and to issues regarding normal sentence production. Based on our detailed production data in brain damaged subjects, we suggest following:

1. The lexical properties of verbs – including semantic and thematic information accessed when verbs are encountered in sentence processing – also influences sentence production in agrammatic Broca's aphasic patients. Compared to normal subjects, nonfluent aphasic patients do not use the full range of lexical properties available given a particular verb. This restriction, we surmise, is due to a complex mixture

of verb and sentence variables that affect the computational complexity of producing sentences.
2. The difficulty noted in aphasic subjects' ability to properly assign thematic roles to arguments that have been moved out of their canonical position might also influence production of non-canonical sentences. Our data showing that *wh*- and NP-movement constructions emerge in linguistically predictable ways – that is, the two dissociate in recovery – indicate that agrammatic sentence production patterns may be explained, in part, by limitations concerned with the ways that verb arguments refer to one another when placed in sentence frames.
3. The argument/adjunct distinction found in the normal experimental psycholinguistic literature extends to the cross-generalization distinction found between argument and adjunct movement with our aphasic patients.
4. There may be separate processes underlying the production (and perhaps comprehension) of *wh*-movement constructions, specifically regarding control of syntactic features of *wh*-question formation (i.e., movement of the NP itself) and control of lexical features of *wh*-questions (i.e., *wh*-morpheme selection).

5 Summary

In this paper we have described aspects of the mind/brain data base specific to the language domain. We then showed how linguistic theory can be used as a set of deductions about how normal and disordered sentence processing might operate. Specifically, we have shown that 1) abstract lexical properties (i.e., thematic information; the argument/adjunct distinction) are computed on-line during sentence processing and that they are subsequently used to help determine the structure and interpretation of sentences; 2) the trace-antecedent relation is also computed on-line, allowing the processor to connect (and interpret) non-adjacent positions in a sentence; 3) these lexical and syntactic properties appear to be dissociated, and thus respected, in brain damage; and 4) these linguistic constructs can also be used fruitfully when investigating sentence production patterns in aphasia.

Appendix

Verb, argument, and adjunct codes used for detailing lexical and syntactic aspects of narrative language samples in aphasic and normal subjects.

Obligatory one-place verbs (Ob1), intransitive verbs, requiring and external argument only (Agent), e.g., the verb *work*. [The men $_{\text{Agent(x)}}$] work$_{\text{(Ob1)}}$.

Obligatory two-place verbs (Ob2), transitive verbs, requiring two arguments (an external Agent [x] and a Theme or Patient [y], or a Theme or Patient [y] and a Predication Phrase [P] – Noun Phrase, Prepositional Phrase, or Adjectival Phrase) (x,y; y,P).
e.g., the verb *fix*. [Zack $_{\text{Agent(x)}}$] fixed$_{\text{(Ob2)}}$ [the radio $_{\text{Theme}}$ (y)].
e.g., the verb *look*. That looks$_{\text{(Ob2)}}$ [good $_{\text{Adjectival Phrase (P)}}$].

Obligatory three-place verbs (Ob3), requiring three arguments (an external agent [x], theme or patient [y], goal [z]). Includes both alternating and non-alternating datives (x,y,z; x,z,y).
e.g., the verb *give.* [Joelle $_{\text{Agent(x)}}$] gave$_{\text{(Ob3)}}$ [the ball $_{\text{Theme (y)}}$] [to Zack $_{\text{Goal(z)}}$].
[Joelle $_{\text{Agent(x)}}$] gave$_{\text{(Ob3)}}$ [Zack $_{\text{Goal(z)}}$] [the ball $_{\text{Theme (y)}}$].

Optional two-place verbs (Op2), also known as optional transitives, must take an agent [x], but the theme [y] is optional. Therefore, they may take two possible argument structure arrangements (x) and (x,y).
e.g., the verb *eat.* (We $_{\text{Agent(x)}}$] eat$_{\text{(Op2)}}$.
e.g., the verb *read.* [John $_{\text{Agent(x)}}$] read$_{\text{(Op2)}}$ [the book $_{\text{Theme (y)}}$].

Optional three-place verbs (Op3), must take an external argument and a theme/patient, but the goal is optional, therefore, three argument structure arrangements are possible (x,y), (x,y,z) and (x,z,y). Includes both alternating (i.e, double-object) and non-alternating datives.
e.g., the verb *send.* [John $_{\text{Agent(X)}}$] sent$_{\text{(Op3)}}$ [the paper $_{\text{Theme (y)}}$].
[John $_{\text{Agent(x)}}$] sent$_{\text{(Op3)}}$ [the paper $_{\text{Theme (y)}}$] [to Joan $_{\text{Goal (z)}}$].
[John $_{\text{Agent(xX)}}$] sent$_{\text{(Op3)}}$ [Joan $_{\text{Goal (z)}}$] [the paper $_{\text{Theme(y)}}$].

Complement verbs (c), may be produced with three argument structure arrangements, requiring an external argument (x) and (a) a theme/patient [y] (x,y), or (b) a sentential complement [S'] such as a *wh*-clause, *that*-clause, or an infinitive clause (x, S'), or (c) a predication phrase [P] (x,P).
e.g., the verb *accept.*
[Zack $_{\text{Agent(x)}}$] accepted$_{\text{(c)}}$ [the money $_{\text{Theme (y)}}$].
[Zack $_{\text{Agent(x)}}$] accepted$_{\text{(c)}}$ [that the money was for research $_{\text{(S')}}$].
e.g., the verb *feel.*
[Zack $_{\text{Agent(X)}}$] felt$_{\text{(c)}}$ [tired $_{\text{(P)}}$].

Copulas (cop), a form of *be*, serving as the matrix verb in a sentence, takes a theme [y] and (a) a predication phrase (noun phrase, prepositional phrase, or adjective phrase) [P] (y,P), or (b) a sentential clause [S'] (y,S').
e.g., the verb *is.*
[John $_{\text{(y)}}$] is$_{\text{(cop)}}$ [a boy $_{\text{(P)}}$].
[John $_{\text{(y)}}$] is$_{\text{(cop)}}$ [who I want $_{\text{(S')}}$]

Argument, adjunct codes:

x Subject, Agent
y Direct Object, Theme, Patient
z Indirect Object, Goal
S' Sentential Complement
P Predication Phrase (NP, PP, AP)
J Adjunct (outside the domain of verb structure)

References

Baker, E. (1986): Categorization of natural objects by aphasics and non-brain-damaged adults: An experimental analysis of featural dimensions. Unpublished doctoral dissertation. Clark University, Worcester, MA.

Berwick, R.D. & A. Weinberg (1984): The grammatical basis of linguistic performance: language use and acquisition. Cambridge, MA: MIT Press.

Caplan, D. & N. Hildebrandt (1988): Disorders of syntactic comprehension. Cambridge, MA: MIT Press.

Cermak, L.S. (1989): "Synergistic ecphory and the amnesic patient". In: H.L. Roediger & F.I.M. Craik, eds., Festschrift for Endel Tulving. Hillsdale, NJ: Lawrence Erlbaum Associates.

Chomsky, N. (1981): Lectures on government and binding. Dordrecht: Foris.

Chomsky, N. (1985): Barriers. Cambridge, MA: MIT Press.

Clifton, C., S. Speer & S.P. Abney (1991): "Parsing arguments: phrase structure and argument structure as determinants of initial parsing decisions". Journal of Memory and Language 30.

Ford, M., J. Bresnan & R. Kaplan (1983): "A competence based theory of syntactic closure". In: J Bresnan, ed., The mental representation of grammatical relations. Cambridge, MA: MIT Press.

Frazier, L. (1978): On comprehending sentences: syntactic parsing strategies, Bloomington: Indiana University Linguistics Club.

Frazier, L. & A. Friederici (1991): "On deriving the properties of agrammatic comprehension". Brain and Language 40, 51 - 66.

Frazier, L. & K. Rayner (1982): "Making and correcting errors during sentence comprehension: eye movements in the analysis of structurally ambiguous sentences". Cognitive Psychology 14, 178 - 210.

Gleason, J.B., H. Goodglass, L. Obler, E. Green, M. Hyde & S. Weintraub (1980): "Narrative strategies of aphasic and normal-speaking subjects". Journal of Speech and Hearing Research 23, 370 - 382.

Grimshaw, J. (1979): "Complement selection and the lexicon". Linguistic Inquiry 10, 279 - 326.

Grimshaw, J. (1990): Argument structure. Cambridge, MA: MIT Press.

Grodzinsky, Y. (1990): Theoretical perspective on language disorders. Cambridge, MA: MIT Press.

Hickok, G., E.B. Zurif & E. Canseco-Gonzalez (1993): "Traces in the explanation of comprehension in Broca's aphasia". Brain and Language 45, 371 - 395.

Haegeman, L. (1992): Introduction to Government and Binding Theory. Cambridge, MA: Blackwell.

Jackendoff, R. (1987): "The status of thematic relations in linguistic theory". Linguistic Inquiry 18, 369 - 411.

Jackendoff, R. (1990): Semantic structures, Cambridge, MA: MIT Press.

Jacobs, B. (1994): Linguistically based sentence production treatment: A comparison of the effects of comprehension versus production treatment. Unpublished doctoral dissertation. The University of Florida.

MacDonald, M., M.A. Just & P.A. Carpenter (in press): Working memory constraints on the processing of syntactic ambiguity. Cognitive Psychology.

McCarthy, R. & E.K. Warrington (1985): "Category specificity in an agrammatic patient: The relative impairment of verb retrieval and comprehension". Neuropsychologia 23, 709 - 727.

McNeil, M.R., K. Odell & C.-H. Tseng (1990): "Toward the integration of resource allocation into a general theory of aphasia". Clinical Aphasiology 20, 21 - 39.

Meyerson, R. & H. Goodglass (1972): "Transformational grammars of three aphasic patients". Language and Speech 15, 40 – 50.
Miceli, G., C. Silveri, G. Villa & A. Caramazza (1984): "On the basis for the agrammatic's difficulty in producing main verbs". Cortex 20, 207 – 220.
Nagel, H.N. & L.P. Shapiro (1994): Prosodic influences on real-time sentence comprehension. Paper presented to the CUNY sentence processing conference. New York.
Nicol, J. (in press): "Reconsidering reactivation". In: Altman & Shillock, eds., Cognitive models of speech processing: The Sperlonga Meeting II.
Pesetsky, D. (1983): Paths and categories. Unpublished doctoral dissertation. Cambridge, MA: MIT Press.
Riemsdijk, H. van & E. Williams (1986): Introduction to the theory of grammar. Cambridge, MA: MIT Press.
Saffran, E.M., M.F. Schwartz & O.S.M. Marin (1980): "Evidence from aphasia: Isolating the components of a production model". In: B. Butterworth, ed., Language production (Vol. 1). London: Academic Press.
Shapiro, L.P. & B. Levine (1990): "Verb processing during sentence comprehension in aphasia". Brain and Language 38, 21 – 47.
Shapiro, L.P. & C.K. Thompson (1994): "The use of linguistic theory as a framework for treatment studies in aphasia". In: P. Lemme, ed., Clinical aphasiology, Volume 22.
Shapiro, L.P., N. Nagel & B.A. Levine (1993): "Preferences for a verb's complements and their use in sentence processing". Journal of Memory and Language 32, 96 – 114.
Shapiro, L.P., E. Zurif & J. Grimshaw (1987): "Sentence processing and the mental representation of verbs". Cognition 27, 219 – 246.
Shapiro, L.P., E. Zurif & J. Grimshaw (1989): "Verb representation and sentence processing: contextual impenetrability". Journal of Psycholinguistic Research 18, 223 – 243.
Shapiro, L.P., B. Brookins, B. Gordon & N. Nagel (1991): "Verb effects during sentence processing". Journal of Experimental Psychology: Learning, Memory and Cognition 17, 983 – 996.
Shapiro, L.P., B. Gordon, N. Hack & J. Killackey (1993): "Verb-argument structure processing in complex sentences in Broca's and Wernicke's aphasia". Brain and Language 45, 423 – 447.
Shapiro, L.P., P. McNamara, E. Zurif, S. Lanzoni & L. Cermak (1992): "Processing complexity and sentence memory: evidence from amnesia". Brain and Language 42, 431 – 453.
Swinney, D. & L. Osterhaut (1990): "Inference generation during auditory language comprehension". In: A. Graesser & G. Bower, eds., Inferences and text comprehension. San Diego: Academic Press.
Swinney, D., E.B. Zurif & J. Nicol (1989): "The effects of focal brain damage on sentence processing: An examination of the neurological organization of a mental module". Journal of Cognitive Neuroscience 1, 25 – 37.
Thompson, C.K. & L.P. Shapiro (1994): "A linguistic-specific approach to treatment of sentence production deficits in aphasia". In: P. Lemme, ed., Clinical aphasiology, Volume 22.
Thompson, C.K., L.P. Shapiro, L. Li & L. Schendel (in press): "Analysis of verbs and verb-argument structure: A method for quantification of aphasic language production". In: P. Lemme, ed., Clinical aphasiology, Volume 23.
Thompson, C.K., L.P. Shapiro & M. Roberts (1993): "Treatment of sentence production deficits in aphasia: a linguistic-specific approach to *wh*-interrogative training and generalization". Aphasiology 7, 111 – 133.
Thompson, C.K., L.P. Shapiro, M. Tait, S.S. Schneider & B. Jacobs (1994): Morpho-syntactic and lexical analysis of normal and agrammatic aphasic language production. Paper presented at TENNET V.

Trueswell, J.C., M.K. Tanenhaus & C. Kello (in press): "Verb-specific constraints in sentence processing: Separating effects of lexical preference from garden-paths". Journal of Memory and Language.
Zingeser, L.B. & R.S. Berndt (1990): "Retrieval of nouns and verbs in agrammatism and anomia". Brain and Language 39, 14 – 32.
Zurif, E., D. Swinney, P. Prather, J. Solomon & C. Bushell (1993): "An on-line analysis of syntactic processing in Broca's and Wernicke's aphasia". Brain and Language 45, 448 – 464.

Morphological Deficits in Aphasia: Problems of Representation, Access or Integration?*

Lorraine K. Tyler, London

1 Introduction

A considerable amount of recent work in aphasia has focused on one particular "type" of aphasic deficit known as "agrammatism". Agrammatism is typically characterised in terms of the speech output of the patient. If an aphasic patient produces slow, hesitant, syntactically simple speech which contains very few grammatical morphemes, then this patient is usually given the label "agrammatic". Although there has been considerable debate as to whether agrammatism constitutes a distinct syndrome, this issue remains unresolved (cf. Caramazza 1984). However, the label continues to be used as a useful way of describing the general characteristics of the speech output of certain patients, although it currently carries little explanatory weight.

Agrammatic patients sometimes, although not always, also have impairments in language comprehension, and considerable research effort has been devoted to determining the extent to which their production and comprehension deficits stem from the same underlying deficit. The cluster of impairments associated with agrammatism are generally considered to result from problems with syntax, although the exact nature of the syntactic deficit remains in doubt. Some people claim that agrammatics have impaired syntactic knowledge, while others claim that syntactic knowledge remains intact, but the ability to use it is impaired. Still others claim that agrammatic patients cannot access syntactic knowledge as rapidly and automatically as normal subjects (Haarmann & Kolk 1991; but see Tyler, Ostrin, Cooke & Moss 1994, for a different view).

One of the most popular accounts of agrammatism is that these patients have specific problems with the grammatical morphemes which constitute the closed class (Bradley, Garrett & Zurif 1980; Zurif, Caramazza & Meyerson 1972; Miceli & Caramazza 1988) – both free-standing and bound grammatical morphemes. This is generally seen as arising from their inability to exploit the syntactic function of the closed class, and thus is part of their more general syntactic deficit. Many people have claimed that free-standing grammatical morphemes have a special parsing function in that they mark the onset of constituent phrases, such as noun phrases (marked by determiners) and prepositional phrases (marked by prepositions). It is this parsing function which agram-

* I thank DE and JG for their patience at enduring so many years of testing, Mary Cooke for carrying out many of the studies reported here, and the MRC (UK) for their generous support over the years.

matic patients can not exploit (Cooper & Zurif 1983). Bound morphemes also have a syntactic function; derivational morphemes often change the form-class of the stem to which they apply and this has parsing consequences, and inflectional morphemes can serve to determine the syntactic structure of an utterance, as in: "Jack was *painting...*" where the inflectional affix [*-ing*] in *painting* indicates that the construction is in the active voice, compared with: *"Jack was painted..."* where the affix [*-ed*] in *painted* marks the construction as being in the passive voice (Tyler 1992).

But when agrammatic patients have problems with members of the closed class, it is not inevitably the case that this is because they are unable to exploit their syntactic properties. There are many alternative possibilities, all of which need to be experimentally evaluated before we can draw conclusions about the underlying cause of a patient's deficit. This is the issue I will discuss in the present paper and in doing so I will focus on bound morphemes.

Morphologically complex words may be difficult for patients for a number of reasons, some of which have nothing to do with syntax. First, it may be the case that morphological structure is not represented normally in the mental lexicon. There may be some problem with the representation of the stem-affixal relationship, for example. A second possibility is that morphological structure is represented normally, but the patient may be unable to access it in the normal way. Third, the representation and access of complex words may be unimpaired, but the patient may be unable to combine morphemes into the appropriate complex form. And fourth, all of above processes may be intact, but the patient may be unable to integrate the complex word into the sentential context.

To try to determine which of these possibilities is the source of a patient's problem with complex words, we need to probe different aspects of the processing of complex words. This requires using tasks which tap into these different aspects; tasks which tap into the representation and access of complex words and those that reflect the processes involved in integrating complex words into the sentential context. Standard comprehension tests which are typically used with aphasic patients (such as: acting-out, sentence-picture matching, etc.) are not appropriate to address these sorts of issues. Although these tasks can give us a general idea about whether a patient has problems with complex words, they are not sensitive enough to determine the source of the problem. To do that, we need to use tasks which tap into the real-time processing of complex words, and we need to use these tasks within the context of a well-articulated model of language processing in the unimpaired adult.

The research I will describe in this paper constitutes an attempt in that direction. I will describe a series of experiments which examine the processing of one type of complex word – namely, derived words – when they occur in context and in isolation. All of these studies have been carried out within the context of a model of the normal representation and processing of derived words (Marslen-Wilson, Tyler, Waksler & Older 1994).

All of the studies I will discuss are attempts to determine whether patients have impairments in what we can call the *"computational infrastructure"* of language processing.[1] What I mean by this is the core set of automatic processes which operate upon the speech input as it is heard. When listeners hear an utterance spoken in their native language, they cannot chose to hear it as anything other than a meaningful utterance

– although for this to happen the utterance will have undergone a complex sequence of operations: the speech sounds will have been encoded into individual words, and the semantic and syntactic properties of these words will have been combined into syntactically and semantically well-formed phrases, etc. But listeners do not normally "hear" the utterance as, for example, a string of grammatical formatives. What they hear is the *final* representation – a pragmatically coherent utterance in which many of the details of the intermediate representations have been lost.

Much research on language-impaired patients examines the effects of brain damage only on the final representation – on the top layer of the process. This is the level of the system that most standard tasks tap into – tasks like grammaticality judgements, semantic judgements, sentence-picture matching, acting out with puppets or toys. These tasks – which we call "off-line tasks" – vary in a number of ways, but they all share one important property – they all require the listener to attend to particular aspects of the sentence. Carrying out the task requires the patient to be consciously aware of aspects of linguistic structure – to read information off the top layer. What these tasks can tell us about is the structure of the language system. They cannot, however, tell us about the processes involved in the computation of that information. And yet, for many patients, it may be the case that what looks on the surface to be an impairment in the organisation of the language system may, in fact, be an impairment in the functioning of the computational substrate.

To see whether the automatic processes involved in language comprehension are impaired following brain damage, we have to use "on-line" tasks. I have argued elsewhere (Tyler 1992) that these tasks have certain defining properties. First of all, they *implicitly* tap into linguistic representations and processes. A number of tasks, such as word monitoring and lexical decision, can satisfy the requirement of implicitly tapping mental representations. For example, in the word monitoring task, listeners are asked to press a response key when they hear a pre-specified target word in an utterance. This task becomes an implicit measure of language processing when the monitoring target word occurs immediately after the relevant stimulus, so that the listener's awareness of the properties of the target is not at issue. Rather, we are interested in how monitoring latencies to the target word are affected by what has been heard prior to that word. For example, in the sentence:

> Sally couldn't believe that John used so much butter. He was the most wastage COOK she had ever met.

the target word (COOK) occurs after the derived word *wastage*. It is the processing of the derived word that we are actually interested in. We measure the ease with which listeners process this word with respect to the previous context by obtaining monitoring latencies to the following word COOK. Using the word monitoring task in this way provides an implicit measure of language processing. If instead we had been interested in the subject's processing of the target word COOK, then the task would not be implicit.

The second important property of on-line tasks is that the listener's response must be closely tied in time to relevant stretches of the speech input – otherwise non-linguistic,

post-perceptual, factors can affect the subject's response. We are trying to measure the system's initial response to some input, and if we allow the subjects lots of time to think about what they are doing, then it is difficult to disentangle their initial response from other factors.
In the experiments I will describe in this paper, we use two kinds of on-line tasks: the word monitoring task and the auditory lexical decision task. The first set of studies uses the word monitoring task to see whether our patients have problems with the on-line integration of derived words into the sentential context. The second set of experiments are priming studies, using the lexical decision task, with derived and simple words. These enable us to determine whether agrammatic patients have selective problems with the *representation and access* of derived words. The results from these studies taken together enable us to be much more precise about locating the source of each patient's deficit.
Before outlining the experiments, I will describe the two agrammatic patients that were tested in the studies.

Patients

JG: JG suffered a left temporo-parietal cerebro-vascular accident in November 1980 when he was 55 years old. He was right handed prior to his CVA, but now has a dense right-sided hemiplegia, such that he is unable to use his right arm. JG left school at an early age, and then was employed as a groundsman for thirty years, until the time of his stroke in 1980.
JG has been tested on a number of standardised tests (Ostrin & Tyler 1994; Byng 1988). On the Boston Diagnostic Aphasia Exam (Goodglass & Kaplan 1983), he is classified as a Broca's aphasic with impaired comprehension (auditory comprehension z-score = –.75) and a severity rating of 1. His spontaneous speech is effortful and hesitant as seen below in his description of the Cookie Theft picture:

> The boy is fallin down because the chocolate in in..... then the stool is woompy and the water is a....... taps is on and drippin down. And a...... and the boy girl and the father eh father no the.... yeh far father ha ha ha. And.... a an boy and and still it's carryin on and an an the y' know. There is water and there is runnin an that boy and y know.... this ole boy.

JG's auditory comprehension was tested using the TROG (Bishop 1982), where he scored 70 % correct. His errors in the syntactic conditions are consistently reverse role distractors. Because of the nature of JG's errors on the TROG, namely, difficulty with reverse role but not lexical distractors, we have also tested him on a more extensive sentence-picture matching task – the Birkbeck Reversible Sentence Comprehension Test (Black, Nickels & Byng 1992) – to confirm that he shows the classic asyntactic comprehension pattern. On this test JG scored 36 correct out of a total of 70 (normal range = 55-70). He chose the reverse role distractor 32 times (normal range = 0-13), and the lexical distractor twice (normal range = 0-5).

His performance on the sentence-picture matching task is the asyntactic comprehension pattern which is typical of agrammatics (for additional details, see Tyler 1992).

DE: DE was born in 1954. When he was 16 he suffered a motor-scooter accident which left him with a right-sided hemiplegia. A CAT scan performed in 1978 revealed a large left hemisphere lesion affecting the middle and posterior parts of the frontal lobe and most of the temporal lobe.
On the BDAE, he is classified as an agrammatic with a mild comprehension impairment (z = +.75). Like JG, his speech is slow and effortful. It is severely non-fluent, consisting of one- or two-word utterances, as is shown by his response to the Cookie theft picture from the BDAE:

> Right .... children first... alright...like chair tip over wrong...you got cookies high up...wrong again, right...like ask um...lady right washing um...dry up, right... washing right...right...full up with water...right...turn it off right...wrong...overflowing right...on the floor...everywhere on th floor, and that's it.

On the Birkbeck Reversible Sentence Comprehension Test he showed the classic asyntactic comprehension pattern, scoring 55 correct out of a total of 70 (normal range = 55-70), with 14 reverse role errors (normal range = 0-13), and 1 lexical distractor error (normal range = 0-5). (For additional details, see Tyler 1985, 1992.)
These patients were tested, together with a number of other aphasic patients, over many years on a variety of experiments designed to examine a wide range of real-time language processing abilities. As part of this programme of research, they participated in several studies specifically focusing on morphologically complex words, some of which will be described below. (For data on other experiments on complex words, see Tyler 1992.)

2 The real-time processing of derived and simple words in sentence contexts

2.1 Derived words

The first set of studies used the word-monitoring task to examine the processing of derived words in sentence contexts. We carried out a series of experiments, all of which used materials like:

(1) Charles had a good night out. He went to see a very *enjoyable* OPERA which he'd been looking forward to for weeks.

(2) Charles had a good night out. He went to see a very *enjoyment* OPERA which he'd been looking forward to for weeks.

In these materials, consisting of pairs of sentences, the test sentence was always the second member of the pair. The test sentence contained a target word which the subject had to monitor for (OPERA in the examples), which was immediately preceded by a derived word. In one condition (1) the derived word was contextually appropriate. In the other condition (2), the derived word was inappropriate.

We used the word monitoring task to measure processing difficulty. If monitoring latencies are faster when there is no disruption (1) than when the target follows a linguistic violation (2), then this suggests that in (1) the linguistic information must have been available and necessary for the listener to develop the appropriate representation. Thus, elevated reaction times suggest that constructing the appropriate linguistic representation is made more difficult when that particular type of linguistic information is disrupted in some way. On this logic, if JG and DE have problems processing derived words in contexts then their monitoring latencies should not be faster in sentences like (1) than in sentences like (2).

We constructed 21 sentence-pairs like those above (1 and 2), all of which were pre-tested[2] to ensure that the undisrupted sentences were fully grammatical and the violation versions were judged to be ungrammatical. The target nouns were all common nouns or adjectives of reasonably high frequency. The test items were pseudo-randomly mixed with a set of filler items, each of which contained a target word. We placed timing pulses at the onset of each target word. These pulses, which could not be heard by the subjects, served to trigger a timing device, which was stopped by the subject's key-press response. Two versions of the materials were constructed, such that each test item occurred once in each version.

Apart from the 2 patients, we also ran a group of control subjects whose ages ranged between 62-73 years.[3] Both the patients and controls were tested on both versions, with a month separating each testing session.

We found that the monitoring latencies of control subjects were significantly slower when the target word was preceded by a derived word which was contextually inappropriate, compared to when the derived word was appropriate (see Table 1). In contrast, neither of the patients showed a significant difference between the two conditions (see Table 1).

We obtained essentially the same pattern of results when we tested DE and JG in another word monitoring study, where we manipulated the relationship between the stem and suffix of a derived word. In our first study, the relationship between the stem

Table 1 Mean Monitoring RTs (msec) for the elderly controls, DE and JG

	Elderly controls	DE	JG
Appropriate	291	247	374
Inappropriate	354	254	357
Difference	63*	7	–17
	95 % confidence limits: 53-73 msec		

*: $p < .05$

and affix was always phonologically transparent. That is, the addition of a suffix did not induce any phonological changes in the stem (e.g. *happy/happiness*). In a second study, we manipulated phonological transparency such that we had pairs of derived words like *consumable,* which is phonologically transparent with respect to its stem consume, and *consumption,* which is phonologically opaque in that the addition of the affix [*-tion*] induces phonological changes in the stem [*consume*]. These words were placed in sentences like the following:

(5) It was really amazing. John could *consume* CHOCOLATES at an incredible rate.

(6) *It was really amazing. John could *consumable* CHOCOLATES at an incredible rate.

(7) *It was really amazing. John could *consump*tion CHOCOLATES at an incredible rate.

In both (6) and (7), the derived word is contextually inappropriate. If our patients have problems processing a derived word in context, irrespective of its phonological transparency or opacity, then their monitoring reaction times in (6) and (7) should not be significantly different from those in the baseline condition (5).
We found that elderly control subjects were faster to monitor for the target word CHOCOLATES in (5) than in (6) or (7), whereas both DE and JG showed no significant difference between any of the three conditions. On the basis of these studies, we can conclude that normal subjects are immediately sensitive to the contextual appropriateness of a derived word, and that this sensitivity reveals itself in their monitoring performance. In contrast, both patients appear to be insensitive to the appropriateness of derived words during the immediate processing of an utterance.

2.2 Simple words

However, before we can claim that our patients have particular problems with derived words, we need another piece of information. We need to know whether they are specifically insensitive to derivational suffixes or whether they have a general problem with word-endings. It might be the case that the patients have problems discriminating between the ends of any type of words which share a great deal of initial phonological overlap – e.g. *caravan/caramel* – and that their problem processing derived words in context is just part of this more general difficulty.
To address this issue, we[4] chose pairs of simple words which shared the same amount of initial overlap and final deviation as the derived words. The derived words which we had used in our studies shared, on average, the first two syllables, and deviated in their final syllable (e.g. *maturity-maturation*). We chose simple words with a similar amount of overlap and deviation (*caramel-caravan*). The question we asked was whether our patients could distinguish between them on basis of word-final deviation.
For this study, we constructed 20 stimuli like those in (3) and (4)

(3) Fiona has just returned from Africa. She spent years studying a *cannibal* TRIBE and now plans to write a book.

(4) Fiona has just returned from Africa. She spent years studying a **canopy* TRIBE and now plans to write a book.

Just as for the experiment using complex words, these stimuli consisted of sentence-pairs. The second sentence of each pair contained a target word (TRIBE in the example) which was immediately preceded by a morphologically simple test word which was appropriate for the context (3). In the second condition (4), the test word (*canopy*) was contextually inappropriate. All sentences were pretested to ensure that the appropriate sentences were judged acceptable, and the inappropriate sentences became unacceptable on or before the target.[5]

The 20 test pairs were divided into two lists, each containing half the appropriate and half the inappropriate sentences, such that each target word occurred only once per list. The test pairs were scrambled among 45 fillers which were designed to obscure both the test manipulation and the position in the sentence where the target word occurred.

In addition to our patients, we tested 10 elderly controls. These subjects showed significantly slower word monitoring latencies in the inappropriate condition (384 msec.) compared to the appropriate condition (322 msec).[6] Just like the controls, JG was sensitive to the manipulations in this experiment. His mean RT in the appropriate condition (212 msec) was significantly faster than his mean RT in the inappropriate condition (289 msec). On average, his RTs to targets in the inappropriate sentences are 26 % longer than his RTs to the appropriate targets. Similarly, DE was also sensitive to the contextual appropriateness of a simple word. His mean monitoring latency in the appropriate condition (270 msec) was significantly faster than his mean latency (319 msec) in the inappropriate condition.

3 Interim conclusions

The word-monitoring studies with complex words established that our two agrammatic patients have problems with the real-time processing of derived words when they occur in sentence contexts. This could not be attributed to a general problem discriminating between words when they share a great deal of phonological overlap, since the patients had no problems distinguishing between simple words which overlap and deviate in the same ways as the derived words. Therefore, their difficulty with derived words appears to constitute a special problem with morphological endings. The question is why? Is it because they are unable to integrate the derived word into the sentential context or is it the case that the representation and access of these words are impaired in some way?

To address this question we carried out a priming study which was based on our model of the representation of derived words (Marslen-Wilson et al. 1994). It is against this model of the normal representation of derived words that we test the patients' performance, therefore I will first briefly describe the model and the major findings from which it was derived.

3.1 The normal model

Our research with unimpaired subjects was concerned with the structure of the *lexical entry* for English derived words, rather than the access representation. By "lexical entry" I mean the abstract, modality-independent representation of a word's phonological, morphological, syntactic and semantic properties. In a series of six experiments, we asked whether the lexical entry for derivationally suffixed words (e.g. *happiness, maturity*) is morphologically structured or not (i.e. [Stem+affix]), and how this relates to the semantic and the phonological transparency of the relationship between the stem and the affix. By *semantic transparency,* we mean the extent to which the meaning of a complex word is derivable (i.e. composed) from the meaning of its constituent morphemes. Thus, the derived word *happiness* is semantically transparent in that its meaning is composed of its two morphemes *happy + ness.* In contrast, the derived word *department* is semantically opaque in that the meaning of the constituent morphemes, when combined together, does not produce the correct meaning. By phonologically transparent we mean the degree to which there is a change in the phonetic realisation of the stem (and possibly the affix) when it occurs in a morphologically complex word. Pairs of words like *vain/vanity* are examples of phonologically opaque forms whereas *mature/maturity* are phonologically transparent.

In these studies, we used a *cross-modal immediate repetition priming* task where the subject hears a prime word, and immediately at its offset, sees a visual probe and makes a lexical decision to the probe. The prime word is either related to the visual probe in one of a variety of ways, or it is an unrelated control word. We chose this task because it avoids certain modality-specific effects and taps into the lexical entry rather than into the access representation. In addition, the task reflects the immediate consequences of hearing a complex word.

We carried out six experiments using this task in which we looked at the various types of relationship between stems and derived forms:

- We varied semantic transparency by having stem-derived pairs which were semantically transparent (*happiness-happy*) and pairs which were opaque (*depart-department*).
- We varied the morphological relationship between the pairs of words by having stem-derived pairs (*happy-happiness, decision-decide*) and derived-derived pairs (*maturity-maturation*).
- We varied the phonological relationship between the morphologically related words by using phonologically transparent (*happiness-happily*) and phonologically opaque pairs (*decide-decision; consume-consumption*).

We found that only certain types of morphologically related words primed each other. So, for example, stem-derived pairs which are semantically transparent like *happy-happiness* primed each other, as did derived-stem pairs like *maturity-mature.* However, semantically opaque pairs like *depart-department* did not prime. This held true inde-

Figure 1 The normal model of the representation of (a) semantically transparent derived words and (b) semantically opaque derived words (after Marslen-Wilson et al. 1994)

A) Semantically transparent derived words

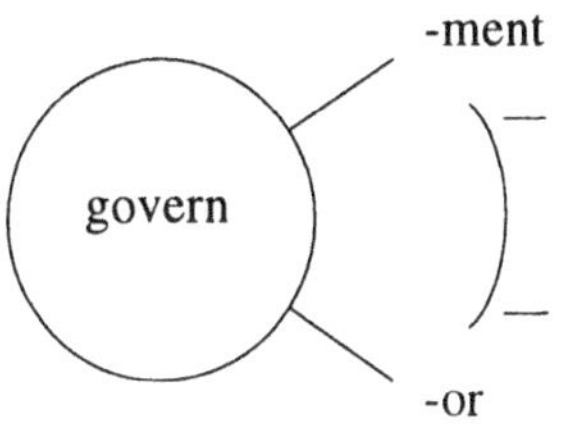

B) Semantically opaque derived words

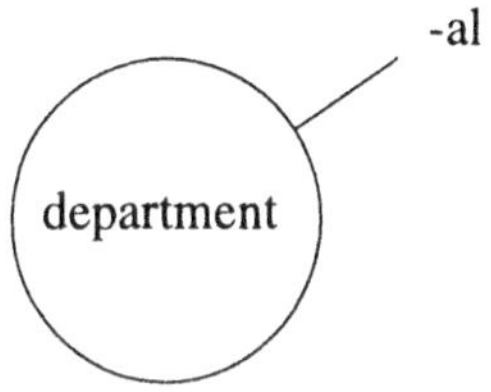

pendent of the degree of surface transparency in the phonological relationship between the stem and the affix in the derived word. Moreover, derived-derived pairs did not prime, whether they were semantically related (e.g. *confession-confessor*) or unrelated (e.g. *succession-successful*). This argues against a purely semantic explanation of morphological priming effects.

These results led us to propose two different types of representation for derived words – one for semantically transparent and the other for semantically opaque forms. We claim that transparent forms are represented as a free stem with a connection to its associated affix. In contrast, a semantically opaque form, like *department,* is represented at the level of the lexical entry as if it were morphologically simple. It can enter into combination with other morphemes (as in *interdepartmental* or *departmental*) but itself has no internal structure. It does not share a stem morpheme with words like *departure,* which has a separate representation consisting of a free stem [*depart*], linked to the affix [*-ure*]. This model is graphically represented in Figure 1.

The absence of priming between derived-derived suffixed pairs is accounted for in terms of inhibition between suffixes within the same lexical paradigm – that is, attached to the same stem (see Figure 1). So, hearing a semantically transparent form like *government* activates *govern* and the derivational suffix [*-ment*]. At the same time it inhibits other suffixes, such as [*-or*]. This means that when a suffixed word is heard it will momentarily inhibit the combination of the stem with its other suffixes. This has the effect of slowing recognition to a subsequently presented suffixed word, even though the same stem is activated. In contrast, when the stem is presented following a suffixed word, there will be no inhibition and so recognition of the stem will be facilitated. Similarly, when the stem functions as the prime, this will change the state of the shared stem morpheme, but it will not affect the state of any of its links to suffixes. Thus, when a suffixed word follows as a target, the effects of stem activation will facilitate recognition without any counter-balancing inhibitory effects.

This model provides an account of the representation of derived words; we need a model like this, which makes the representational structure explicit, to be able to evaluate whether our patients have problems with the representation of derived words.

4 Patient priming study

We carried out a priming study with our patients to address the issue of whether their representation and access of derived words is unimpaired. The priming task, like the word monitoring task, can be used as an implicit measure of language processing. In the priming task, subjects are presented with pairs of words and they make a lexical decision to the second member of the pair. Thus, the subject's attention is not focused on the relationship between the word-pairs; rather it is focused on making the lexical decision response. In addition, subjects produce fast lexical decision latencies. Thus, this task satisfies the two main criteria for being able to tap into the on-line processes involved in language comprehension which I mentioned earlier: implicit and fast response times.

The priming study for the patients used some of the crucial conditions extracted from the original series of studies with normals. However, because agrammatic patients often have problems reading, we modified our original paradigm so that instead of it being a cross-modal lexical decision task, it was an auditory-auditory lexical decision task. Subjects heard pairs of words and made a lexical decision to the second member of the pair.[7]

We extracted four crucial conditions from the original experiments with normals. There were two test conditions: Condition 1 consisted of derived-derived suffixed words which were semantically opaque (*department-departure*) and condition 2 used derived-derived suffixed words which were semantically transparent (*confessor-confession*). If the representation of derived words is unimpaired in our patients, then they should show the normal pattern – i.e. no priming for the two derived-derived conditions.

We also included two control conditions. One consisted of synonym pairs like *idea-notion*, which were semantically but not morphologically related.[8] We needed a condition of this type, which reliably produces priming in patients (Ostrin & Tyler 1993; Tyler, Ostrin, Cooke & Moss 1994) to ensure that the task produces priming effects in our patients. Our final condition consisted of pairs of words which were phonologically but not morphologically related. This was included as a control for purely phonological priming. Since the morphologically related pairs overlapped by an average of 2 syllables, we selected word-pairs for this condition in which the pairs also shared a 2-syllable

Table 2 Mean lexical decision RTs (msec) for the elderly controls in the auditory-auditory priming study

Condition	Test	Control	Diff
Opaque (*department/departure*)	956	977	11
Transparent (*maturity/maturation*)	938	968	30
Synonyms (*idea/notion*)	840	933	93*
Phonological (*caramel/caravan*)	935	949	14

*: significant at $p < .01$

overlap (e.g. *caravan/caramel)*. Moreover, they also deviated from each other by a full syllable, in just the same way as the morphologically related pairs.[9]

Our elderly control subjects showed a pattern of results consistent with our earlier research. That is, there was no significant priming for either of the derived-derived conditions, nor for the phonological controls. But there was significant priming for the synonyms. The results for the elderly controls, as a group, are given in Table 2.

We also analysed each control subject's data individually, and found that no subject produced priming in the phonological control condition and one subject showed a marginal priming effect in the opaque derived condition. All subjects showed faster RTs to primes compared to controls in the synonym condition, and one showed priming in the transparent derived condition (see Table 3). These results confirm the major findings from our original studies (Marslen-Wilson et al. 1994) and show that even in this intra-modal task, phonological overlap between prime and target does not, by itself, produce priming in normal subjects.

Our agrammatic patients produced a different pattern of results from the controls, and from each other. JG produced significant priming for the synonyms, just like the normal subjects, showing that he is unimpaired when it comes to processing the meaning of simple words. Like normals, he also shows no priming for the phonological controls. However, unlike the controls, he showed significant priming for both the opaque and transparent derived pairs (see Table 4).

There are various possible explanations for this pattern of results. One is that JG only accesses the stem of a derived word – whether it is transparent or opaque. It is through the activation of the stem *depart* that *department* primes *departure,* for example. However, this account leads to the claim that brain damage causes a word which has no morphological structure (*department*) to be treated as if it were morphologically structured. We think this is implausible, although we have no direct evidence against it. A more plausible hypothesis is that brain damage has not affected the representation of complex words; rather it has affected the processes involved in their access.

Table 3 Auditory-auditory priming study: Individual control ANOVAs

Subject	D/D Opaque	D/D Trans	Synonym	Phonological
Subject 1	ns	ns	*	ns
Subject 2	ns	ns	*	ns
Subject 3	ns	ns	*	ns
Subject 4	ns	ns	*	ns
Subject 5	ns	ns	*	ns
Subject 6	ns	ns	*	ns
Subject 7	ns	*	*	ns
Subject 8	ns	ns	*	ns
Subject 9	*	ns	*	ns

*: significant at $p < .05$ or above

Table 4 Mean lexical decision RTs (msec) for the patients in the auditory-auditory priming study

Condition	Patients					
	DE			JG		
	Test	Control	Diff	Test	Control	Diff
Opaque (*department/departure*)	928	1019	91*	839	895	56*
Transparent (*maturity/maturation*)	955	945	–10	805	851	46*
Synonyms (*idea/notion*)	907	992	85*	685	750	65*
Phonological (*caramel/caravan*)	813	885	72*	907	897	–10

*: significant at $p < .05$ or above

Assuming that the recognition of a spoken word involves processes of activation and decay, when listeners hear a spoken word, they initially access a number of candidate words beginning with the same sound sequence. This initial activation of a large set is followed by the gradual decay of candidates which do not continue to match the sensory input (cf. Marslen-Wilson & Welsh 1978; Marslen-Wilson 1987; McClelland & Elman 1986). Thus, when listeners hear either *department* or *departure,* in both cases the stem *depart is* initially activated (together with other words sharing the same initial sound sequences). For JG, the subsequent processing of the stem and its potential affixes are disrupted, possibly as a result of less effective inhibition between affixes within a derivational paradigm. In the case of transparent derived forms, reduced inhibition results in all of the forms within the derivational paradigm remaining more highly activated. Thus, when JG hears the transparent form *happily,* both *happily* and *happiness* are activated. Instead of *happiness* being inhibited (as in the normal case) it remains active so that when it is subsequently presented as a target, its recognition is primed. When normal listeners hear an opaque form like *department,* activation of the stem *depart* will start to decay as soon as evidence becomes available (i.e. at the [m] *in department*) that the word that is being heard is neither the stem nor any of its derivations. For JG, less effective inhibition within a derivational paradigm results in slower decay of candidates activated by the input, so that when *departure* is presented as a target word following *department,* his lexical decision response is facilitated.

Interestingly, this problem seems to be confined to complex words, since simple words which share a great deal of initial phonological input (*caramel/caravan*) do not prime for JG, just as they don't for the normal controls. Thus, the pattern of activation and decay for simple words seem to be unimpaired. So, for JG, his problems with derived words stem – at least in part – from impairments in the processes involved in their access.

In contrast, DE showed significant priming for the opaque derived-derived pairs, the synonyms and the phonological controls. He did not show priming for the transparent derived-derived pairs (see Table 3). I will discuss the complex words first.

The absence of priming for the transparent derived-derived pairs suggests that semantically transparent complex words are represented for DE, as for the normal subjects, in terms of stems connected to associated affixes which mutually inhibit each other. Thus, derived words inhibit each other, and derived-stem pairs prime through activation of a common stem. So, these results suggest that DE's representation of semantically transparent derived words is unimpaired. If this is indeed the case, then we would expect DE to show priming for derived/stem pairs which are semantically transparent (*happiness-happy*; *confessor-confess*), just like normal subjects. In a second auditory-auditory priming study, this is exactly what we found – significant priming for transparent derived/stem (*happiness-happy*) pairs (RT test = 825 msec; RT control = 900 msec).

Turning to simple words, unlike the controls, DE showed priming for the semantically opaque derived words, which we have claimed on the basis of our research with normals (which I described earlier) are morphologically simple. He also showed priming for the phonological controls, which are also simple words. These results can best be explained within an activation-based model of word recognition (cf. Marslen-Wilson 1987). We assume something like a cohort model where multiple word-candidates are activated on the basis of the initial portion of the speech input and a single word-candidate eventually emerges as the best fit with the input. We suggest that although the initial process of activation is unimpaired in DE, the competitors which become active in the process of recognising a word do not decay for him as rapidly as they do for normal listeners. Thus, when normal listeners hear the word *caravan,* the word *caramel* is also momentarily activated. However, when the words separate at the consonant [v] in the word *caravan*, activation of the competitor *caramel* starts to decay; thus, *caravan* and *caramel* do not prime each other. We suggest that for DE the competitor remains active for longer and thus functions as a prime for the subsequent presentation of the target. This continuing presence of an active competitor is likely to be the result of the slow decay of activation. This may be a general problem for DE, affecting all words, but it will tend to show up most strongly for words which share a great deal of phonological overlap and which deviate from each other fairly late in the word.[10]

5 General Conclusions

What can we say about these patients' abilities to process derived words? Have we been able to locate the source of the morphological processing deficit in these patients by using a combination of real-time tasks which probe different aspects of the representation, access and integration of derived words? I would argue that we have. First, DE: On the standard off-line aphasia tests, DE clearly had problems processing derived words. But we had no idea from those studies where his problems should be located – whether in representation, access or integration processes. It was only by using various tasks which are sensitive to the real-time processing of speech that we were able to locate the source of his deficit.

We found in the priming studies that the representation and access of derived words seems to be unimpaired – so that can not be the source of his problem with derived words. By comparing the priming and word-monitoring data, we see that his problems with derived words can be located in the processes involved in integrating derived words into the sentential context. Moreover, we know that this is a problem which is peculiar to derived words and does not extend to simple words. What we do not yet know, however, is whether his problems processing derived words in context is primarily due to his inability to exploit the syntactic properties of derived words when comprehending an utterance. To answer this question requires further experiments.

Turning to JG, we see that his problems with derived words stem from a different cause. He does have problems with their representation and this shows up both in the priming studies and in his word-monitoring performance. So, on the basis of the priming and word monitoring studies, we can conclude that the reason why JG has problems with derived words is not because of their syntactic role in sentence interpretation. JG, then, is at least one agrammatic patient who does not conform to the typical characterisation of agrammatic patients.

One important general implication of the contrasting pattern of results for JG and DE is that what looks on the surface to be the same type of problem can, in fact, stem from different underlying causes. Both patients showed the same profile when tested on standard off-line tests and in the word-monitoring studies, leading to the conclusion that they had problems processing complex words. If we had stopped testing at that point, we would have concluded that they both had the same underlying deficit. It was only by developing experiments which tapped into a range of real-time sentence processing operations that we could locate the source of each patient's deficit, to pin-point the processing operations which were impaired.

Over the years, we have carried out in-depth studies of the language impairments of many different types of aphasic patients. All of the patients we have tested, whatever their syndrome classification, show some degree of difficulty with complex words. This may, on the face of it, seem surprising given the commonly-held view that problems with members of the closed class differentiate agrammatic patients from other types of aphasic patients. But, upon reflection, this may not be so surprising after all since most studies of closed class deficits have focused upon agrammatic patients. Patients of other types – who do not present with agrammatic production – are rarely tested to see if they exhibit similar deficits as the agrammatics. Thus, perhaps it is not surprising that there is little data on the ability of non-agrammatic patients to comprehend members of the closed class. On the rare occasions when non-agrammatic patients are also tested, evidence emerges that agrammatics may not be the only patients who have problems with the closed class. Studies by Bates & Wulfeck (1989) and Tyler (1992) show that, at least for some types of closed class morphemes, non-agrammatic patients are as severely impaired as agrammatics. Morphology seems to be vulnerable to brain damage across a wide range of patients.

One possible explanation for this derives from our model of the representation of derived words described earlier. If this is correct, then complex words are computed "on the fly", as speech is being processed. They are not represented as whole word-forms in the way that simple words are. Stems and affixes are combined as a complex word is being heard. It may be this additional computation (over simple words) which poses problems for many patients.

Notes

1 See Tyler (1993): Language and the Brain. Inaugural Address. Manuscript, Birkbeck College, March 1993.
2 See Tyler & Cobb (1987) for additional experimental details.
3 See Tyler & Cobb (1987) for results for mid-age controls, whose average age was 37 years (range: 34-41 years).
4 This experiment was carried out with Ruth Ostrin.
5 For additional details about the pre-tests, see Ostrin & Tyler (1994).
6 The mean difference between the two conditions was 62 msec (range: 27-109 msec.)
7 There was a 200 msec ISI between prime and target.
8 We established by means of pre-tests that these pairs were not associates. This was to maintain comparability with the morphologically related pairs, which in general were not associatively related.
9 For additional methodological details, see Tyler & Ostrin (1994).
10 We are assuming that there is no inhibition between word candidates (cf. Marslen-Wilson 1987), but only between members of a derivational paradigm (Marslen-Wilson et al. 1994). This explains why the complex words do not show the same pattern of priming as the simple words.

References

Bates, E. & B. Wulfeck (1989): "Crosslinguistic studies of aphasia". In: B. MacWhinney & E. Bates, eds., The crosslinguistic study of sentence processing. New York: Cambridge University Press.

Black, M, L. Nickels & S. Byng (1992): "Patterns of sentence processing deficits: Processing simple sentences can be a complex matter". Journal of Neurolinguistics 6, 79 – 101.

Bishop, D. (1982): The TROG: Test for the reception of grammar. Medical Research Council, UK.

Bradley, D., M. Garrett & E. Zurif (1980): "Syntactic deficits in Broca's aphasia". In: D. Caplan, ed., Biological studies of mental processes. Cambridge, Mass: MIT Press.

Byng, S. (1988): "Sentence processing deficits: Theory and therapy". Cognitive Neuropsychology 5(6), 629 – 676.

Caramazza, A. (1984): "The logic of neuropsychological research and the problem of patient classification". Brain and Language 21, 9 – 20.

Cooper, W. & E. Zurif (1983): "Aphasia: Information processing in language production and reception". In: B. Butterworth, ed., Language Production, Vol. 2. New York: Academic Press.

Goodglass, H. & E. Kaplan (1983): The Assessment of Aphasia and Related Disorders. Philadelphia, PA: Lea & Febiger.

Haarmann, H.J. & H. Kolk (1991): "Syntactic priming in Broca's aphasics: Evidence for slow activation". Aphasiology 5(3), 247 – 263.

Marslen-Wilson, W.D. (1987): "Functional parallelism in spoken word recognition". Cognition 25, 71 – 103.

Marslen-Wilson, W.D., L.K. Tyler, S. Waksler & L. Older (1994): "Morphology and meaning in the English mental lexicon". Psychological Review 101(1), 3 – 33.

Marslen-Wilson, W.D. & A. Welsh (1978): "Processing interactions and lexical access during word recognition in continuous speech". Cognitive Psychology 10, 29 – 63.

McClelland, J. & J. Elman (1986): "The TRACE model of speech perception". Cognitive Psychology 18, 1 – 86.

Miceli, G. & A. Caramazza (1988): "Dissociation of inflectional and derivational morphology". Brain and Language 35, 24 – 65.

Ostrin, R. & L.K. Tyler (1993): "Automatic access to lexical semantics in aphasia: Evidence from semantic and associative priming". Brain and Language 45, 147 – 160.

Ostrin, R. & L.K. Tyler (1994): "Dissociations of lexical function: Semantics, syntax and morphology". Cognitive Neuropsychology (in press).

Tyler, L.K. (1992): Spoken Language Comprehension: An experimental approach to disordered and normal processing. Cambridge, Mass: MIT Press.

Tyler, L.K. & H. Cobb (1987): "Processing bound grammatical morphemes in context: The case of an aphasic patient". Language and Cognitive Processes 2, 245 – 263.

Tyler, L.K. & R. Ostrin (1994): The processing of simple and complex words in an agrammatic patient. Neuropsychologia (in press).

Tyler, L.K., R. Ostrin, M. Cooke & H. Moss (1994): "Automatic access of lexical information in Broca's aphasics: Against the automaticity hypothesis". Brain and Language (in press).

Zurif, E., A. Caramazza & R. Meyerson (1972): "Grammatical judgements of agrammatic aphasics". Neuropsychology 10, 405 – 417.

On-line Integration of Grammatical Information in Wernicke's and Broca's Aphasia

Kerry Kilborn, Glasgow

Introduction

Normal sentence comprehension depends on the listener's ability to compute structural as well as meaning-based information, and to relate the ongoing analyses of these two global information sources in language to each other quickly and efficiently (Marslen-Wilson & Welsh 1978; Marslen-Wilson & Tyler 1980; Tyler 1985, 1988; Marslen-Wilson 1987, 1989). Normal comprehension can fail, at least partially, in two ways. First, if the representation of either type of information is lost, then the integration process will be unable to function normally. Second, the representation of grammatical information may remain intact, but a temporal lag in the computation of syntactic and/or semantic information may result in a failure to construct a coherent, integrated meaning.

One principal feature of language behavior in patients with Wernicke's aphasia is an impairment of comprehension (Holland & Reinmuth 1986). Comprehension deficits have also been described for agrammatic Broca's aphasics (Zurif, Caramazza & Myerson 1972). However, the functional locus of such impairments in either type of aphasia is not well understood. Proposals have included a selective loss of function in the syntactic parser (Berndt & Caramazza 1980; Grodzinsky 1986); in the closed class vocabulary (Goodglass & Menn 1985; Bradley, Garret & Zurif 1980); via phonological processes (Kean 1980). More recent evidence, based on on-line experiments, suggests that the comprehension deficit observed in aphasia may be computational in nature (Baum 1988, 1989; Blumstein, Milberg, Dworetzky, Rosen & Gershberg 1991; Friederici & Kilborn 1989; Shankweiler, Crain, Gorrell & Tuller 1989; Tyler 1988). That is, grammatical information is not totally lost, but the ability to access and exploit grammatical representations as language processing unfolds in real time is impaired.

In a series of studies, Blumstein, Milberg and colleagues (Blumstein et al. 1991; Milberg, Blumstein & Dworetzky 1987; Blumstein, Milberg & Shrier 1982; Milberg & Blumstein 1981) have demonstrated that Wernicke's aphasics show semantic facilitation in lexical decision tasks. Hagoort (1990) has also shown semantic priming effects in Wernicke's aphasics, and concluded in agreement with the latter authors that lexical-semantic representations are not lost and that the network structure of the semantic lexicon is not compromised. Given the relative sparing of much syntactic ability in Wernicke's aphasics, and the apparent intactness of the semantic lexicon, one aim of this study was to investigate whether the comprehension deficit normally observed in Wernicke's aphasia can be accounted for in terms of a breakdown in the real-time integration of syntactic and semantic information.

Swinney, Zurif & Nicol (1989) and Hagoort (1990) report findings that suggest that while lexical-semantic processes appear to remain intact, Wernicke's aphasics do not combine contextual information with syntactic representations in real time. Such findings argue that the comprehension deficit observed in Wernicke's aphasia may be due to the lack of integration under on-line processing constraints (however, see Tyler (1988) for one report of a fluent aphasic who, although differing from normals in processing subcategorization constraints on verbs, was generally able to construct global representations).

A second aim of this study was to compare the performance of fluent Wernicke's aphasics and normal controls with that of agrammatic Broca's aphasics on the same task. Patients displaying the characteristic profile of agrammatic Broca's aphasia are prone to have difficulty in the output of the syntactic and morphological features of language. It has now been well documented that these patients may also suffer from a comprehension deficit. Yet some retention of the ability to comprehend language suggests that different sources of grammatical information are available and are brought together to aid in comprehension at some level. Friederici and Kilborn (1989; see also Kilborn and Friederici (in press) and Friederici 1983, 1985) have suggested that the agrammatic comprehension deficit is at least partly due to a degradation of automaticity in accessing syntactic information at the moment it is needed during normal processing. This results not in the total breakdown of grammatical processing, but in a pervasive temporal mismatch which occurs when incoming grammatical forms are being mapped onto functions in order to construct a meaning representation. Aberrant temporal processing may have a more devastating effect on those parts of language which are normally subject to automatic procedures: unstressed, relatively contentless, highly frequent morphological forms which perform much of the syntactic "work" in any language.

A concrete model of normal spoken word recognition, the Cohort Model, provides a context in which to consider just how the continuous interaction of sensory and contextual information contribute to comprehension. Marslen-Wilson (1989) cites the repeated finding that humans are capable of early selection in lexical access: A spoken word can be identified in its utterance context before enough acoustic-phonetic information to identify the word on that basis alone has been perceived (within about 200 msec from word onset). To explain this, Marslen-Wilson argues that two sets of constraints – sensory-based (the match between incoming acoustic-phonetic signal and word forms) and contextually-based (the match between lexical content and the ongoing utterance and discourse context) – interact to converge on a unique word identity. The speed of these constituent processes requires a system architecture built around a "functional parallelism" (Marslen-Wilson 1987): Sensory information is used to access and assess multiple word forms, while concurrent selection procedures based on contextual constraints operate. Early selection reflects the integration of the domains of form and content during real-time language processing.

In this study, an on-line sentence processing task based on the word monitoring paradigm of Marslen-Wilson and Tyler (1980) was used to examine whether Wernicke's aphasics are able to integrate different global information sources during auditory sentence comprehension. In brief, subjects monitor for identical target words in three types of prose: (1) Normal prose (syntactic and semantic relations are maintained); (2) Syntactic prose (syntactic form is maintained but content words are replaced to produce semantically anomalous sentences (called "anomalous prose" by Tyler (1985, 1988)); and (3) Random prose (neither semantic nor syntactic structures are maintained (called "scrambled prose" by Tyler (1985, 1988)). Numerous earlier studies (e.g., Cole & Jakimik 1980; Cole & Perfetti 1980; Marslen-Wilson & Tyler 1980; Kilborn 1992) have shown that word recognition is facilitated when the listener is able to combine the acoustic-phonetic information in the auditory word form with contextual information, including phonological, lexical, syntactic, semantic, pragmatic, prosodic, and conceptual sources (see Frauenfelder & Tyler 1987 for an overview). Thus, words heard in sentences constrained by normal semantic and syntactic relations are recognized faster than words in syntactically intact but semantically anomalous sentences. Listeners are slowest to recognize words heard in random strings, where no linguistic or real world contextual constraints apply.

If, as suggested earlier, the temporal relations that normally apply to mapping sensory and contextual information are disrupted in agrammatism, then we would expect that an agrammatic Broca's aphasic would have difficulty managing the flow of information from different sources during on-line processing.

Tyler (1985) studied the ability of D.E., who was classed as a Broca's aphasic, to construct a global structural representation across the span of a sentence during comprehension. Tyler used a task similar to the one reported in Marslen-Wilson and Tyler (1980) and used here. Tyler (1985) reported that D.E. performed similarly to controls in that word monitoring latencies were faster in normal prose than anomalous prose, and faster in anomalous than in scrambled prose. However, D.E. did not show a word-position effect found in normals. In normals, Tyler has found that RTs decrease across normal and anomalous prose sentences, but remain constant across a scrambled prose string. This pattern, according to Tyler, reflects the build-up of a structural representation across the sentence, and not merely a serial position effect. D.E. showed no decrease in anomalous prose, from which Tyler concluded that the locus of the agrammatic processing deficit is in the real-time analysis of the speech input. In particular, D.E. does not develop a normal syntactic structural representation.

The word-monitoring paradigm provides very general contrasts between syntactic and semantic information sources used during on-line processing. The current study extends the use of this approach by comparing groups of Broca's and Wernicke's aphasics with age-matched control subjects. In addition, most earlier studies using this paradigm have been carried out in English. The current study looks at on-line processing in German.

Subjects

Six Wernicke's aphasics and seven agrammatic Broca's aphasics from the Max-Planck-Institut Berlin Laboratory patient pool participated voluntarily in the experiment. Each patient was a native speaker of German. All aphasic patients were administered the German version of the Aachen Aphasia Test (AAT) (Huber et al. 1983, 1984). Patients were selected on the basis of the Token Test (TT) and comprehension subtest components of the AAT. The Token Test is a selection test which strongly correlates with the severity of aphasia. The comprehension subtest measures comprehension of single words and sentences in auditory and visual mode without a need for expressive language. Each subject was classified as presenting with a mild or moderate Wernicke's or Broca's aphasia according to the comprehension subtest and Token Test.
A further seventeen neurologically normal control subjects were recruited from the Berlin area. All were native German speakers, had normal vision and hearing, and were approximately matched to the aphasic groups for age and education levels.

Materials

Three blocks of 40 sentences were constructed. ***Normal*** sentences maintain syntactic and semantic relations as usual. ***Syntactic*** sentences were constructed by replacing open class (content) words in the Normal sentences, with pseudo-randomly selected words of the same form class (i.e., nouns replace nouns, verbs replace verbs, etc.), matched for length and frequency. Thus, Syntactic sentences have intact structural relations, and are of the same length and complexity as Normal sentences, but have no plausible semantic interpretation. ***Random*** sentences were constructed by first making an additional set of Syntactic strings, then randomizing the order of words within each sentence while keeping the target position constant. Random sentences thus maintain neither semantic nor syntactic relations, but do contain the same proportion of content and function words as Normal and Syntactic sentences. All sentences were 9 to 12 words. Half of the targets occurred in **early** positions (the first half of the sentence), and half in **late** positions (second half).

Prose Type	Visual Target	Auditory Sentence
Normal	*RULES*	Playing hockey without observing the **rules** is extremely dangerous
Syntactic	*TRAIN*	Checking gravel without walking the **train** is perfectly yellow.
Random	*TRIP*	Is ducks without securely the tired **trip** blocking illegal.

All materials were spoken by a female speaker in a sound-proofed booth and recorded on a Revox A 700 tape recorder. The speaker was careful to read each sentence type at a normal speaking rate, and with fairly flat intonation. The speaker was not aware of target items when the sentences were recorded. All recorded materials were digitized at a sampling rate of 20 kHz and stored in a VAX 750 computer, and target-sentence pairs were constructed such that the target was heard first, followed by 2 seconds of silence, followed by the onset of the sentence containing the target item. Using a waveform editor to examine the sentences visually and auditorily, a trigger pulse was placed concurrent with the onset of the target item in each stimulus sentence. Three audio cassette tapes, corresponding to each prose type, were constructed with sentences in random order. For the experiment, an Uher stereo cassette player was used. The stimulus materials were recorded onto the right channel, and the timing pulse on the left channel. Sennheiser HD 224 headphones (one each for the subject and the experimenter) were used to present the stimuli binaurally from the right channel, while the pulse on the left – inaudible to the subjects – started a millisecond timer. A Miro GD laboratory computer equipped with a pulse-read unit was used to record reaction times during the experiment.

Procedure

Each subject was tested individually. A single trial consisted of the visual presentation, in capitals, of a target noun for 3 seconds. One second later, an auditory sentence containing the target word was played via headphones. Subjects responded by pressing a button as quickly as possible when the target was detected. Different prose types were presented in blocks across separate sessions, with order of presentation counterbalanced across subjects. Subjects were instructed to watch the video screen and to read each target word carefully when it appeared, and to then listen for the appearance of the word target when they heard it in the following auditory sentence. As soon as they detected the word, subjects pushed a button on a single-push button pad. Subjects were told that there would be no "trick" sentences; every visual target was paired with an auditory sentence containing that word.

Results

Reaction times exceeding subject means by 2 standard deviations were replaced with subject grand means, a relatively conservative estimate of missing data. This procedure resulted in a replacement rate of 6.9 % for Broca's aphasics, 3.1 % for Wernicke's aphasics, and less than 1 % for age-matched controls. These data were entered into separate 3 (Normal × Syntactic × Random) × 2 (early × late targets) analyses of variance with prose type and position as within-subject variables. Table 1 summarizes response latencies in each cell of the design for each group (see Appendix 1 for a table listing RT scores for each aphasic subject).

Table 1 Mean word recognition latencies and standard deviations by Prose Type and Position for the Control, Broca's aphasics, and Wernicke's groups

	Normal Prose	Syntactic Prose	Random Prose
Controls			
Prose Type Mean	290	355	413
SD	68	81	72
Early Targets	321	396	458
SD	64	90	68
Late Targets	258	314	369
SD	57	46	41
Broca's aphasics			
Prose Type Mean	456	495	583
SD	103	84	76
Early Targets	471	507	594
SD	94	87	64
Late Targets	441	484	571
SD	117	87	90
Wernicke's aphasics			
Prose Type Mean	480	454	574
SD	147	70	109
Early Targets	507	460	587
SD	185	86	122
Late Targets	453	448	562
SD	107	58	103

Age-matched control subjects

Age-matched control subjects responded fastest to targets in Normal prose, followed by Syntactic prose, and were slowest to identify targets in Random prose. The main effect of sentence type was significant, $F(2,32) = 87.9$, $p < 0.001$. Scheffé confidence intervals were calculated around the mean of each sentence type, revealing significant differences at the $p < 0.01$ level between each condition. The data indicate clearly that structural information, independent of meaning, facilitates word recognition. When meaning is available as well, additional facilitation is observed. This main effect is illustrated in Figure 1.

Figure 1 Main effect of Prose Type in normal control subjects

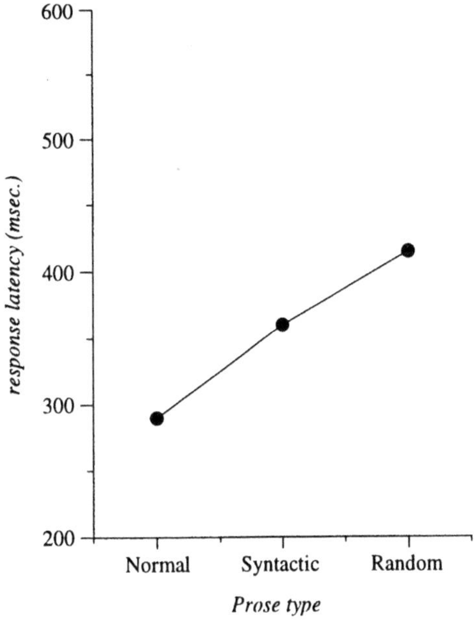

Figure 2 Main effect of Word Position in normal control subjects

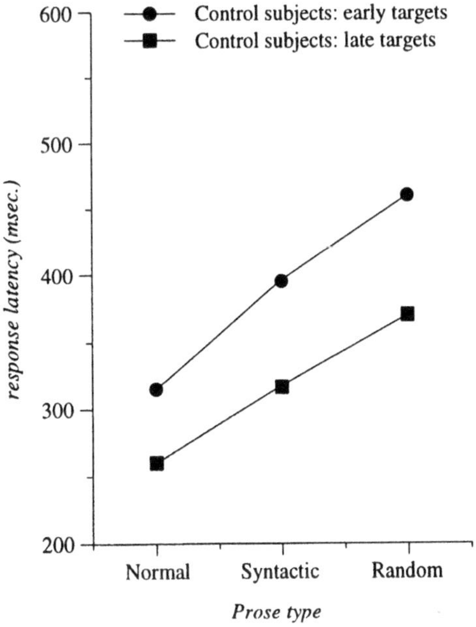

There was also a significant main effect of word position in control subjects: Early targets were detected more slowly than late targets ($F(1,16) = 60.8$, $p < 0.001$). This effect is illustrated in Figure 2. The interaction of position with prose type was not significant ($F(2,32) = 1.3$, $p > 0.05$). A Scheffé test reveals that the main effect of position was significant at each prose type ($p < 0.05$). This contrasts with findings from Marslen-Wilson & Tyler (1980), who report an interaction such that the position effect diminished in Random prose. We will return to this point in the discussion.

Broca's aphasics

A significant main effect of prose type was observed in Broca's aphasics, $F(2,12) = 15.7$, $p < .001$. This effect is shown in Figure 3. Word monitoring latencies were significantly faster in Normal than Syntactic prose, and faster in Syntactic than in Random prose (Scheffé < 0.05). This finding indicates that agrammatics as well as controls are integrating different global information sources quickly during on-line sentence processing.

Although the Broca's patients show a trend toward a position effect (see Figure 4), this main effect did not reach significance ($F(1,6) = 2.9$, $p = .1$). There was no prose type by position interaction ($F(2,12) = .09$, $p = .1$).

Figure 3 Main effect of Prose Type in Broca's aphasics

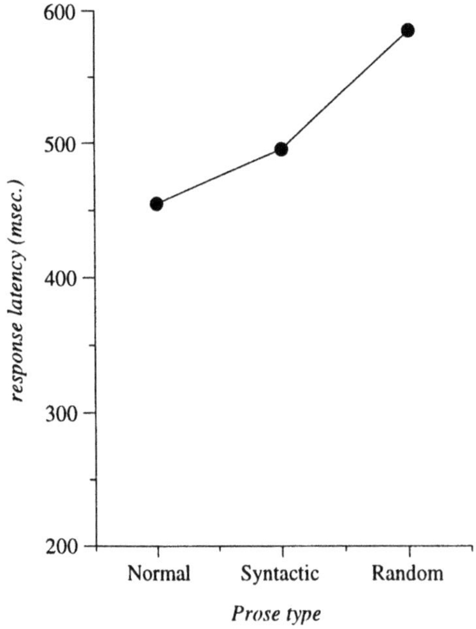

Figure 4 Main effect of Word Position in Broca's aphasics

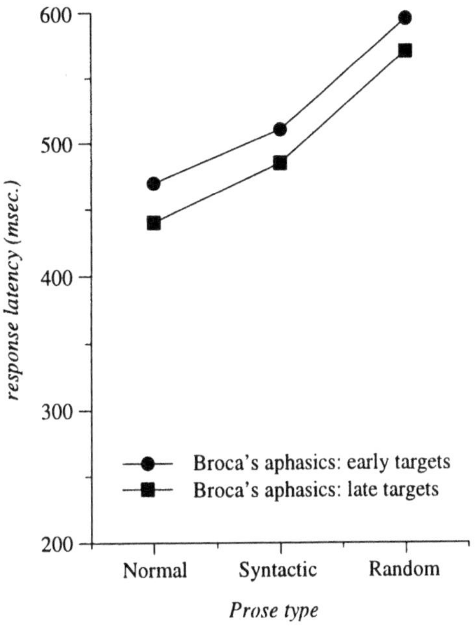

Wernicke's aphasics

Wernicke's aphasics also showed a main effect of prose type $F(2,10) = 4.8$, $p < 0.05$. This effect is shown in Figure 5. Planned comparisons between conditions revealed that Wernicke's subjects responded slower to targets in Random than to Syntactic or Normal prose types. However, Wernicke's patients did not show this same difference between Syntactic and Normal conditions. The small difference (26 msec) in favor of Syntactic strings was not significant ($p > .05$).

In contrast with the controls, the Wernicke's group showed no main effect of position ($F(1,5) = 1.4$, $p = .3$), but there was a significant position by sentence type interaction, $F(2,10) = 4.2$, $p < .05$. Inspection of Figure 6 reveals clearly the source of this interaction. There was no difference between early and late targets in Random and Syntactic strings, but in Normal sentences there was a significant (Scheffé $> .05$) advantage of 64 msec for late over early targets. When both syntactic and semantic information are present, Wernicke's aphasics perform differently than when only syntactic information is present. The position by sentence type interaction suggests that Wernicke's aphasics may indeed attempt to integrate different global information sources, but this attempt is costly in terms of processing resources.

Subsequent ANOVAs with group (control group versus each aphasic group respectively) as a between-subjects factor revealed a significant interaction of group by prose type for the Wernicke's patients alone: ($F(2,42) = 5.5$, $p < .01$). Wernicke's aphasics, although easily able to perform the task, and exhibiting overall response latencies in the same

Figure 5 Main effect of Prose Type in Wernicke's aphasics

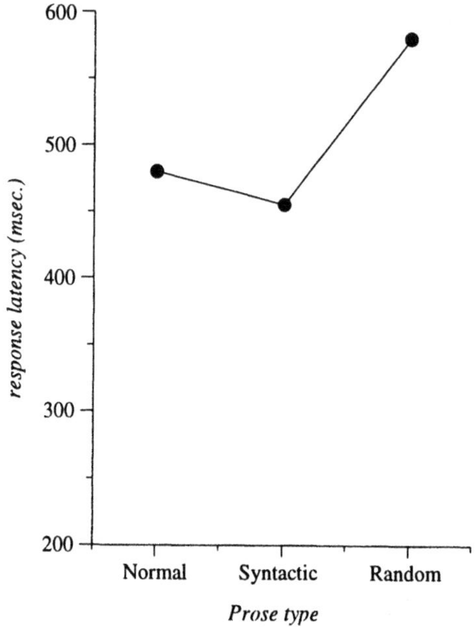

Figure 6 Interaction of Word Position by Prose Type in Wernicke's aphasics

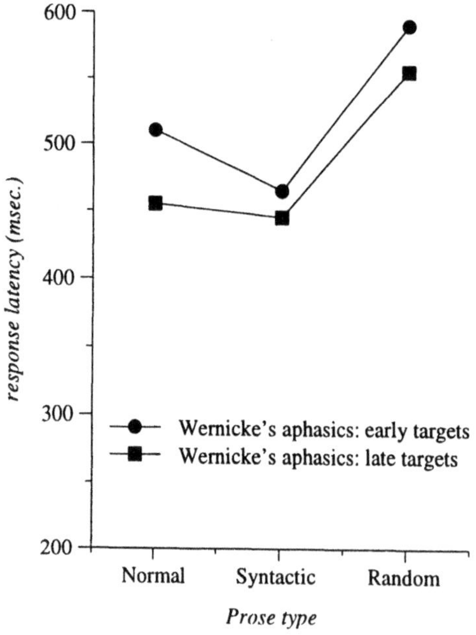

neighborhood as the Broca's aphasics, show a qualitatively different pattern of processing than either Broca's or normals: Wernicke's patients show facilitation in Syntactic relative to Random strings, but no additional facilitation is derived from the availability of richer contextual information in Normal sentences. Wernicke's aphasics do use form-based information to help in accessing the lexicon during sentence processing, but fail to integrate content with form in real time.

Discussion

Performance by normal controls indicates that structural information from different sources can be independently utilized to aid in word recognition during on-line processing. The slowest responses were obtained in Random word strings, where neither semantic nor syntactic information is available for integration. Reaction times were significantly faster in Syntactic than in Random strings, where sentences were structurally intact but semantically anomalous. In Normal sentences, where both semantic and syntactic features are present, reaction times are faster yet, reflecting the rapid integration of these two global information sources.

It is worth noting that, in contrast with the findings reported by Tyler (1985, 1988), normals did not show an interaction of word position with prose type. Early targets produced slower responses than late ones, but this main effect held in all prose types. Although this study was carried out in German, it does replicate findings from one other study which also used single sentences in English (Kilborn 1992). The main difference between the current study and those carried out by Tyler is that the latter author used sentence pairs, with the target occurring in the second sentence, while in this experiment each trial consisted of a single sentence. In a single sentence, less context is available overall, which provides less opportunity to build up a semantic and structural representation on-line. The goal of this experiment was to explore whether aphasics integrate global information sources in real time. The use of single sentences is adequate to this purpose, and has the added advantage of decreasing the task demands on subjects, a considerable problem in interpreting results from typical cross-modal language processing experiments, and one that is especially acute in work with language-impaired populations (see Kilborn 1991, for a discussion). The consistent main effect of word position in this study can be interpreted as reflecting a non-linguistic task effect. How much this effect contributed to the findings in other studies using this type of paradigm is an open question (see Montgomery, Scudder and Moore 1990 for one approach to reducing the effects of age-related non-linguistic processing factors).

Agrammatic Broca's aphasics, though slower overall, display a pattern of performance on this processing task nearly identical to that of non-impaired controls. While such patients frequently do demonstrate a lack of automaticity in processing especially syntactic information on other tasks (Baum 1989; Blumstein et al. 1991), the facilitation observed in Syntactic over Random, and in Normal over Syntactic sentences, suggests that both meaning and structure are available during processing and can be integrated fairly quickly.

Note, however, that the relatively slower response latencies mean that, on average, aphasic subjects identify targets after the "uniqueness point" has been reached; indeed, most responses in this group fall somewhere during the presentation of the word which follows. While early selection may characterize word recognition most of the time (Marslen-Wilson 1989), Bard, Shillcock & Altmann (1988) have shown that about 20 % of words are not recognized before their endpoints. For these Broca's aphasics, it may be the case that all of the processes which converge to produce the observed facilitation of response latencies in Normal over Syntactic, and Syntactic over Random sentences, are affected to the same degree by focal brain damage of the sort that produces agrammatic symptoms. If so, then the processing system, though functioning in a highly interactive manner normally, would be seen to respond in a unitary fashion to damage. Clearly, however, dissociations in some tasks indicate that selective impairments of core processing subsystems do occur. Task differences may account for part of this discrepancy; when a task is designed to tap into processing as it takes place in real time, even subtle effects may emerge which are not so apparent in paradigms less sensitive to real-time constraints (Friederici & Kilborn 1989).

The claim that a highly interactive system can respond to a selective deficit at some level in a more or less unitary way is not a claim that there are no functional or structural divisions within the language processing system (divisions which may or may not relate to divisions of language along traditional theoretical linguistic lines). Rather, we might observe global slowing – but preservation of overall patterns – of processing due to an ability of different processing subsystems to adapt to changes in the timing and perhaps the nature of the information relayed by other divisions of the language processing system, i.e., a slowdown (but not complete cessation) in a syntactic processor may cause a delay (but not complete failure) of integration of that information with semantic information. Thus, in a processing system in which all components must interact under the timing constraints imposed by the demands of normal communication, an apparently selective deficit may be due to the occurrence of a temporal mismatch in the integration of information in real time.

Fluent Wernicke's aphasics also benefited from the structural information in syntactically intact but semantically anomalous sentences. This is consistent with the linguistic abilities normally cited in these patients: Fluent, connected speech with phrases of normal melody and length (Murdoch 1990). Wernicke's patients did not exhibit the additional degree of facilitation observed in controls and in Broca's patients in processing meaningful sentences. However, faster responses to late than to early targets in Normal sentences by Wernicke's aphasics indicates that both information sources may come into play when they are available. Taken together, the data point to a lack of integration: Semantic and syntactic information may be computed, but the fluent aphasic patient is unable to combine the two types of linguistic input in real time.

There is independent evidence that the pattern observed in the performance of Wernicke's aphasics in this study – a failure to integrate sensory and contextual information in real time – may not be due to a selective deficit in one or another part of a fluent aphasic's processing system. A similar pattern of performance has been reported for normal second language learners performing a similar task in their non-native language (Kilborn 1992), and for normals under different conditions of cognitive load, including a listening to sentences through an auditory noise mask, and a visual speeded reading version of the same task (Kilborn 1987). In addition, Montgomery, Scudder & Moore (1990) report that language-impaired children performing an identical word monitoring task with Normal, Syntactic, and Acoustic (i.e., "Random" in this study) sentences showed the greatest difference from a control group in monitoring latencies in Normal sentences. The similarity in performance among these disparate groups – who do not share an underlying deficit – suggests that comprehension deficits in Wernicke's aphasia may be accounted for in part by a computational deficit rather than loss, and that such a deficit can be understood in terms of a general reduction in computational resources.

Blumstein et al. (1991) concluded that "the language impairments in Broca's and Wernicke's aphasics reflect processing disorders that cut across the linguistic components of the grammar, i.e., the lexicon and the parser ... the language impairments of aphasics are not selective with respect to a particular linguistic representation ... specifically they reflect impairments to those processing routines used to access this information" (p. 418). Hagoort (1990) replicated these effects, and concluded in a similar vein, "aphasic deficits, at least those in Broca's and Wernicke's aphasics, are more due to an impairment in one of the processing components than to a loss of stored knowledge representations" (p. 168). Despite citing computational operations as the locus for comprehension deficits in both Wernicke's and Broca's aphasia, Blumstein et al. add that the similarity in performance they found do not reflect the same underlying disorder.

The results of this study are consistent with this view. The good performance by Broca's aphasics, despite overall slowness, suggests that the deficit in this form of non-fluent aphasia can be characterized as procedural in nature. Lexical and grammatical forms are largely spared, as are some of the functions these carry out. However, normal comprehension requires that forms are mapped onto functions in real time, and seldom, as was the case in this experiment, with clear, single sentences, and few other distracting discourse processes to interfere with sensory and contextual integration. The Wernicke's aphasics, in contrast, differed from both the Broca's group and the control group. For these fluent aphasics, the locus of the deficit is also procedural, though perhaps due to a different underlying disorder, it is manifested in a lack of integration of different global information sources in real time.

References

Bard, E.G., R. Shillcock & G. Altmann (1988): "The recognition of words after their acoustic offsets in spontaneous speech: Effects of subsequent context". Perception and Psychophysics 44(5), 395 – 408.

Baum, S.R. (1988): "Syntactic processing in agrammatism: Evidence from lexical decision and grammaticality judgement tasks". Aphasiology 2, 117 – 135.

Baum, S.R. (1989): "On-line sensitivity to local and long-distance syntactic dependencies in Broca's aphasia". Brain and Language 37, 327 – 338.

Berndt, R. & A. Caramazza (1980): "A redefinition of Broca's aphasia: Implications for a neuropsychological model of language". Applied Psycholinguistics 1, 225 – 278.

Blumstein, S.E., W.P. Milberg, B. Dworetzky, A. Rosen & F. Gershberg (1991): "Syntactic priming effects in aphasia: An investigation of local syntactic dependencies". Brain and Language 40, 393 – 421.

Blumstein, S.E., W.P. Milberg & R. Shrier (1982): "Semantic processing aphasia: Evidence from an auditory lexical decision task". Brain and Language 17, 301 – 315.

Bradley, D.C., M.E. Garret & E.B. Zurif (1980): "Syntactic deficits in Broca's aphasia". In: D. Caplan, ed., Biological studies of mental processes. Cambridge, MA: MIT Press.

Cole, R.A. & J. Jakimik (1980): "A model of speech perception". In: R.A Cole, ed., Perception and production of fluent speech. Hillsdale, NJ: Erlbaum, 133 – 163.

Cole, R.A. & C.A. Perfetti (1980): "Listening for mispronounciations in a children's story: The use of context by children and adults". Journal of Verbal Learning and Verbal Behavior 19, 297 – 315.

Frauenfelder, U. & L.K. Tyler (1987): "The process of spoken word recognition: An introduction". Cognition 25, 1 – 20.

Friederici, A.D. (1985): "Levels of processing and vocabulary types: Evidence from on-line comprehension in normals and agrammatics". Cognition 19, 133 – 166.

Friederici, A.D. (1983): "Aphasics' perception of words in sentential context: Some real-time processing evidence". Neuropsychologia 21, 351 – 358.

Friederici, A.D. & K. Kilborn (1989): "Temporal constraints on language processing: Syntactic priming in Broca's aphasia". Journal of Cognitive Neuroscience 1, 3, 262 – 272.

Goodglass, H. & L. Menn (1985): "Is agrammatism a unitary phenomenon?" In: M.L. Kean, ed., Agrammatism. Orlando: Academic Press.

Grodzinsky, Y. (1986): "Language deficits and the theory of syntax". Brain and Language 27, 135 – 159.

Hagoort, P. (1990): Tracking the time course of language understanding in aphasia. Doctoral dissertation, K. Universiteit Nijmegen.

Hagoort, P. (1989): "Decay of syntactic information in language comprehension of agrammatic aphasics". Journal of Clinical and Experimental Neuropsychology 11, 357.

Heeschen, C., J. Ryalls & P. Hagoort (1988): "Psychological stress in Broca's versus Wernicke's aphasia". Clinical Linguistics & Phonetics 2, 309 – 316.

Holland, A.L. & O.M. Reinmuth (1986): "Aphasia in adults". In: G.H. Shames & E.G. Wiig, eds., Human communication disorders, 2nd edition. Columbus, OH: Charles E. Merrill.

Huber, W., K. Poeck, K. Weniger & K. Willmes (1983): "Der Aachener Aphasia Test". Göttingen: Hogrefe.

Huber, W., K. Poeck & K. Willmes (1984): "The Aachen Aphasia Test". In: F.C. Rose, ed., Progress in aphasiology. New York: Raven Press.

Kean, M.L. (1980): "Grammatical representations and the description of language processing". In: D. Caplan, ed., Biological studies of mental processes. Cambridge, MA: MIT Press.

Kilborn, K. & A.D. Friederici (in press): "Cognitive penetrability of syntactic processing in Broca's aphasia." Neuropsychology.

Kilborn, K. (1992): "The on-line integration of grammatical information in a second language". In: R.J. Harris, ed., Cognitive processing in bilinguals. Amsterdam: Elsevier.

Kilborn, K. (1991): "Selective impairment of grammatical morphology due to induced stress in normal listeners: Implications for aphasia". Brain and Language 41, 275 – 288.

Kilborn, K. (1987): Sentence processing in a second language: Seeking a performance definition of fluency. Unpublished Ph.D. dissertation, University of California, San Diego.

Marslen-Wilson, W.D. (1989): "Access and integration: Projecting sound onto meaning". In: W.D. Marslen-Wilson, ed., Lexical Representation and Process. Cambridge: MIT Press.

Marslen-Wilson, W.D. (1987): "Functional parallelism in spoken word recognition". Cognition 25, 71 – 102.

Marslen-Wilson, W.D. & A. Welsh (1978): "Processing interactions and lexical access during word recognition in continuous speech". Cognitive Psychology 10, 29 – 63.

Marslen-Wilson, W.D. & L.K. Tyler (1980): "The temporal structure of spoken language understanding". Cognition 8, 1 – 71.

Milberg, W.P., S.E. Blumstein & B. Dworetzky (1987): "Processing of lexical ambiguities in aphasia". Brain and Language 31, 138 – 150.

Milberg, W.P. & S.E. Blumstein (1981): "Lexical decision and aphasia: Evidence for semantic processing". Brain and Language 14, 371 – 385.

Montgomery, J.W., R.R. Scudder & C.A. Moore (1990): "Language-impaired children's real-time comprehension of spoken language". Applied Psycholinguistics 11, 273 – 290.

Murdoch, B.E. (1990): Acquired speech and language disorders: A functional-neuroanatomical approach. London: Chapman and Hall.

Shankweiler, D., S. Crain, P. Gorrell & B. Tuller (1989): "Reception of language in Broca's aphasia". Language and Cognitive Processes 4 (1), 1 – 33.

Swinney, D.A., E.B. Zurif & J. Nicol (1989): "The effects of focal brain damage on sentence processing: An examination of the neurological organization of a mental module". Journal of Cognitive Neuroscience 1, 25 – 37.

Tyler, L.K. (1985): "Real-time comprehension processes in agrammatism: A case study". Brain and Language 26, 259 – 275.

Tyler, L.K. (1987): "Spoken language comprehension in aphasia: A real-time processing perspective". In: M. Coltheart, G. Sartori & R. Job, eds., The cognitive neuropsychology of language. London: Lawrence Erlbaum Associates.

Tyler, L.K. (1988): "Spoken language comprehension in a fluent aphasic patient". Cognitive Neuropsychology 5, 375 – 400.

Tyler, L.K. (1989): "Syntactic deficits and the construction of local phrases in spoken language comprehension". Cognitive Neuropsychology 6, 333 – 356.

Zurif, E.B., A. Caramazza & R. Meyerson (1972): "Grammatical judgments of agrammatic aphasics". Neuropsychologia 10, 405 – 417.

The Neurological Organization of Lexical and Structural Operations in Sentence Comprehension: Findings and Methodological Considerations*

David Swinney, San Diego; Edgar Zurif, Boston

Introduction

Lexical processing plays a transparently necessary and central role in language comprehension. In what follows, we discuss the connections between lexical activation and lexical integration in the construction of interpreted syntactic representations during sentence comprehension. We provide a basis for inferring how different brain regions support this connection, and we discuss some methodological issues relevant to this type of investigation. Throughout, our concern is with the distinction between rapid-acting, time-constrained processes and relatively temporally unconstrained processes that, together, constitute language comprehension.

Our starting point here is one that Prather, this volume, covers in far greater detail and depth. We repeat just the critical points to support our later observations. These points center on the consistently reported observation that Wernicke's aphasic patients, but not Broca's aphasic patients, demonstrate roughly normal automatic lexical access functions (Milberg & Blumstein 1981; Milberg, Blumstein & Dworetsky 1987; Prather, Zurif & Love 1992; Prather, Shapiro, Zurif & Swinney 1991; Prather, Zurif, Stern & Rosen 1992; Swinney, Zurif & Nicol 1989). This general observation stems primarily from studies of lexical priming, which is the facilitation found for the processing of a word in the presence of a semantically or associatively related word (see, e.g., Meyer, Schvaneveldt & Ruddy 1975; Neely 1977). Thus, Wernicke's but not Broca's aphasic patients demonstrate the normal pattern of facilitation from semantically and associatively related contexts on, for example, a lexical decision made to a letter string.

This said, we note that Wernicke's patients are not entirely normal in their access of word meaning. While existing data suggest normal initial contact with lexical representations takes place for Wernicke's patients, they do not rule out the possibility of something like a "coarse-coding" – a less-than-precise apprehension of a word's mean-

* The writing of this manuscript and some of the research reported herein were supported in part by AFOSR grant 91-0025 and an award from the Alexander von Humboldt foundation to the first author and NIH grants AG 10496 and DC 00081 and support from the W.M. Keck Foundation to the second author. Please address all correspondence to David Swinney, Department of Psychology-0109, University of California, San Diego, La Jolla, CA 92093.

ing. Similarly, we note that Broca's aphasic patients are not completely insensitive to priming relationships. Rather, for Broca's patients priming seems to be temporally protracted. Lexical activation, as revealed by priming tasks, appears to operate with a slow 'rise-time' – i.e., at a slower-than normal temporal course (Friederici & Kilborn 1989; Prather, Zurif & Love 1992; Prather, Zurif, Stern & Rosen 1992; Swinney et al. 1989; Prather, this issue).

It should be noted here that some investigators have a different view of lexical activation in Broca's aphasia than the one we have presented here. In particular, Ostrin & Tyler (1993) and Hagoort, Brown & Swaab (1994) claim that Broca's patients can carry out lexical access in a normally rapid automatic manner. However, a brief consideration of the paradigms used to collect the evidence for the claim we make, as compared to that of Ostrin & Tyler (1993) and Hagoort et al. (1994), will help the reader evaluate the relative merits of these opposing claims.

The most direct evidence of slowing in Broca's patients (non-normal 'automatic' information rise times during lexical access) stems from the two Prather et al. studies (Prather, Zurif, & Love 1992; Prather et al. 1992). In these two studies the patients were presented with words (to make lexical decisions to) in a continuous list (where each word follows the previous, and decisions are made to each). Such presentation breaks down the paired-dependencies that occur in word-pair priming presentation paradigms, and to a certain extent mimics the unbroken succession of words in sentences. Importantly, this list technique has been independently shown to yield automatic (as opposed to strategy-driven) activation in neurologically intact subjects (Shelton & Martin 1992). In contrast, both Ostrin and Tyler (1993) and Hagoort et al. (1994) used a word-pair priming presentation paradigm that incorporated neither a distraction manipulation nor relatedness variations. In this, prime and target are functionally and perceptually grouped. Without a distracter manipulation this paradigm standardly elicits 'controlled' or strategy-driven processing (not automatic priming) and without relatedness variations there is no way of checking on whether controlled or automatic processing was obtained. Setting words together in pairs (or in triplets) typically appears to suggest to subjects that the words 'go together', and it fosters both expectations of relatedness and post-access checking strategies (e.g., Shelton & Martin 1992). Importantly, these aspects of word processing are not obviously or directly relevant to lexical processing as found in sentence or discourse (or, continuous list) contexts. So it appears likely that initial lexical activation is not normal in Broca's aphasia, and indeed, that the 'rise time' of information from lexical items encountered during sentence comprehension is delayed compared to neurologically intact individuals.

We feel that it is reasonable to postulate that slower-than-normal availability of lexical information will ramify throughout the comprehension system, affecting not only deeper lexical processing, but later structural and discourse processes that depend on the 'normal' temporal availability of information for rapid (on-line) function. In what follows we focus on how an impoverished (delayed) lexical data base might disrupt the construction of dependency (co-reference) relations in real time – that is on the linking of 'moved' constitutents to their canonical positions during the course of sentence comprehension (see Swinney & Fodor 1989 for reviews of these issues as studied in normal populations). This co-reference operation is one that is implemented under strict time constraints, and, in light of the Broca's aphasics delayed lexical-information rise time, we have postulated that there may be related consequences for these automatic aspects of structural processing.

The processing of sentential dependency relations in aphasia

One descriptive generalization in aphasia research that seems fairly well agreed upon is that most aphasic patients show sentence-level comprehension impairments, particularly for non-canonical structures (Caplan & Hildebrandt 1988; Grodzinsky 1990; Kean 1985; Zurif & Swinney 1993). A striking feature of such structures is that they often involve long-distance dependencies. Consider for example, the sentence, "THE POLICEMAN SAW THE BOY THAT THE CROWD AT THE PARTY ACCUSED_ OF THE CRIME." To interpret this sentence, the noun BOY must be understood to be the direct object of the verb ACCUSED, which in English canonically follows the verb. In some linguistic theories (e.g. Chomsky 1981) the direct object in such a sentence is represented as having been "moved" from its canonical position. This representation, in consequence, incorporates a dependency relation between the surface position of the direct object and the canonical site from which it was "extracted". A number of studies of sentence processing, employing a range of on-line techniques, examining neurologically unimpaired adults have shown that the direct object is immediately and automatically reactivated by the listener at the site of "extraction" – i.e., immediately following the verb (e.g., Swinney & Fodor 1989; McElree & Bever 1989; Tanenhaus, Boland, Garnsey & Carleson 1989).

As noted, both Broca's and Wernicke's aphasic patients have difficulties understanding sentences involving such dependencies – which involve situations in which one element in the sentence must be recovered or interpreted with respect to a reference-seeking or reference-licensing element. The accounts that have been put forward to account for this problem, however, have differed for the two populations. On the one hand, accounts for this difficulty on the part of Broca's aphasics have typically been characterized syntactically; for example, Broca's aphasic patients show much poorer comprehension for object-gap constructions than for subject-gap constructions, a fact which can be captured syntactically. On the other hand, Wernicke's aphasic patients show no such structural distinction, and more typically make lexical semantic-based errors on tests of comprehension involving these constructions.

In what follows, we show that the more general problem involving lexical access and activation that we foregrounded earlier may account for these distinct forms of language breakdown found in Broca's aphasia and Wernicke's aphasia. Our research provides a processing basis for this distinction. It shows that the two groups diverse at an early stage of processing. The Broca's (but not Wernicke's) aphasic patients show lexical access/activation problems that directly connect to their failure to establish syntactically governed dependency relations. More generally, by employing an on-line experimental technique, our study provides a real-time account of language disruption in terms of broadly localizeable, elemental, processing units. (A pertinent fact in this regard is that the lesion sites that underlie Broca's aphasia are distinguishable from those that underlie Wernicke's aphasia).[1]

Studies of gap-filling with Broca's and Wernicke' aphasic patients

As just mentioned, dependency relationships have processing consequences for the processing in 'neurologically unimpaired' populations. As establishing such relationships is done on-line, immediately at the site of 'extraction' form movement, it is clear that this is an operation that is implemented under strict time constraints and one that is unlikely to accommodate slower-than-normal lexical activation. This being so, it seemed to us reasonable to hypothesize a connection between the Broca's aphasics' slowed lexical processing and their syntactic limitation. Specifically, we hypothesized that the Broca's inability to interpret antecedent-trace relations might be a failure to reactive or integrate 'moved' constituents at the normal time in the processing sequence – in time, that is, to fill gaps in the structural relationship left by their displacement.

We have examined this hypothesis by assessing the time-course of reactivation of antecedents to moved positions (known as 'gap-filling' in psycholinguistic parlance) in Broca's patients and Wernicke's patients in two experiments (Zurif, Swinney, Prather, Solomon & Bushell 1993; Swinney, Zurif, Prather & Love 1993, respectively). In the first of these we used subject-relative constructions such as:

> "The man liked the tailor$_i$ with the British accent ^{*1} who (t)$_i$^{*2} claimed to know the queen."

As shown by this example, movement from subject position is hypothesized in many linguistic characterizations. (We use the (t), following standard linguistic notation, to indicate a 'trace' in the position from which the element (tailor) was hypothesized to have 'moved'. We chose this construction because of the perspective it offered both within and across aphasic groups. Broca's patients show relatively normal comprehension for this construction, but Wernicke's patients are unpredictable, more often than not showing chance comprehension (e.g., Grodzinsky 1984; Shankweiler, personal communication, February 1992). So for Broca's patients these sentences provided the strongest test of our suggestion that they could not carry out normal syntactic (co-reference, dependency) analysis in real time. This would allow us to determine if slower-than-normal lexical activation disallowed normal 'gap-filling' even for sentences correctly comprehended and, further, would also allow us to determine if, in such circumstances, Broca's patients were abnormally reliant on non-grammatical strategies. With regard to the Wernicke's patients, this construction allowed us to determine whether the reverse scenario held: that, even though they would often ultimately fail to understand these sentences, their initial access to (and information rise time from) lexical entries would be normal and hence they would demonstrate a 'structural reflex' and appropriately 'fill' the gap by reactivating the appropriate antecedent at the appropriate time during processing.

Our assessment of gap-filling and the range of possibilities just outlined, employed the cross-modal lexical priming (CMLP) paradigm (Swinney, Onifer, Prather & Hirshkowitz 1979). In this, subjects listened to a sentence over earphones (delivered uninterruptedly and at a normal speaking rate) and at one point, while listening to the sentence, were required to make a lexical (word/nonword) decision for a visually presented letter string flashed on a screen in front of them. (To accommodate the right-sided weakness of Broca's patients, all subjects "button-pressed" with their left hand when making their decisions.) We sought to discover whether a letter-string probe forming a word related to the moved constituent (the antecedent) was primed at the site of the 'gap' (indicated by the (t) in the sample sentence). Such priming would indicate that the moved constituent was reactivated at the gap (thus providing the prime for the lexical decision).

For each of our experimental sentences, we recorded lexical decision times either for antecedent-related probes or for letter string probes that were semantically unassociated control words. For the example given above, the probes were "clothes" (the probe for the antecedent, "tailor") and "weight" (the control probe).

As indicated by the superscripts ^{*1} and ^{*2}, priming was examined at two points – at the gap indexed by the trace (superscript ^{*2}) and at pre-gap position (superscript ^{*1}). The latter served as a baseline; it allowed us to distinguish structurally governed reactivation at the gap site from any residual activation due simply to the earlier appearance of the antecedent ("tailor"). Of course, in each instance, priming was determined by comparing the lexical decision time for the related probe to that for the unrelated probe.

One of the key reasons for our use of the CMLP task to study on-line processing is that the lexical decision, itself, does not require that the subject consciously seek a relation between the visual probe and anything in the orally presented sentence (as is the case, for example, in experiments utilizing a probe-latency task or an off-line technique). Rather, at least until the visual letter string is presented, the subject is simply listening and trying to understand the sentence. (Subjects are further encouraged by the random presentation of comprehension questions between trials.) Once the visual probe is presented all such normalcy ends, of course. But this happens only after the point of theoretical interest concerning sentence processing has passed.

Our findings for this experiments are presented in Table 1. As can be seen, the Wernicke's patients reliably filled gaps (as did our neurologically intact subjects who were used to pretest the sentences). This can be seen by evidence of significant priming for the related (as contrasted with the control) 'probe' at the 'gap' site; the 'reactivated' antecedent acted to prime the lexical decision to the related word presented at that point in the sentence. The Broca's patients did not show any evidence that would lead us to believe that they filled the gap at this point in processing. (There was no significant priming to the related antecedent.) Our initial interpretation, then, is that it appears that the brain areas respectively implicated in Broca's and Wernicke's aphasia have different functional commitments – the former appears to be crucial for the real-time construction of intra-sentence dependency relations in a way that the latter is not.

Our second study on this topic employed object-relative sentences. Given the Broca's patients' failure to fill gaps for subject-relatives (sentences that they understand), we

Table 1 Amount of Priming (Reaction Time to Control Probes Minus Reaction Time to Related Probes) in milliseconds for subject-relative constructions

POSITION	baseline (pregap)	gap
WERNICKE'S PATIENTS	44	125*
BROCA'S PATIENTS	-20	-68

* Significant priming ($p < .03$)

had little expectation that they would show gap-filling for object-relatives (sentences that they fail to interpret). However, our interest in using object-relatives had to do mostly with Wernicke's patients (who also show less-than-normal comprehension for such sentences). We wanted to broaden the base of our observations of this group's gap-filling capacity, particularly because reactivation in subject-relatives might have been affected by the relativizer "who" in that construction and also because movement within subject-relatives has the special property of being "string-vacuous" (e.g., Clements, McCloskey, Maling & Zaenen 1983) in that such movement does not reorder any of the elements of the sequence. We felt re-ordering was a critical aspect of the 'movement-from-canonical-position' aspect of dependency relations that we were interested in, and thus, this second study featured object-relative sentences of the type:

"The priest enjoyed the drink$_i$ that the caterer was^{*1} serving $(t)_i^{*2}$ to the guests."

We used the CMLP task, and again, we checked for priming both at the gap (superscript ^{*2} and at a baseline, pre-gap position (superscript ^{*1}). For the example given, "wine" was the probe for "drink" and "boat", the control probe.

As can be seen from Table 2, the Broca's patients again did not show significant priming at either probe site. (They did, however show some (nonsignificant) advantage for related probes (relative to control probes) at the baseline position. In effect, for this group there was no sign of structurally determined reactivation of the antecedent, only a sign of some residual activation – the consequence, likely, of having processed the earlier appearance of the constituent in a slowed-down fashion. As for the Wernicke's patients, they once more showed priming at the gap and only at the gap, and again, this pattern corresponded to that shown by the neurologically intact subjects with whom we pretested the material.

A number of conclusions may be drawn from the data of these two studies. The first is that cerebral tissue implicated in Wernicke's aphasia is not crucial for the establishment of intrasentence dependency relations. However compromised their understanding of language is, the problem does not turn on a failure of the sort of structure building charted here.

By contrast, the brain region implicated by Broca's aphasia does appear to be necessary for this operation of syntactically governed reactivation. Our data show that Broca's aphasic do not construct syntactic representations normally in real time.

Table 2 Amount of priming (Reaction Time to Control Probes Minus Reaction Time to Related Probes) in milliseconds for object-relative constructions

POSITION	baseline (pregap)	gap
WERNICKE'S PATIENTS	3	108*
BROCA'S PATIENTS	122	-9

* Significant priming ($p < .02$)

Presumably, therefore, they must rely on other processes to achieve the level of comprehension they show in conversational settings. Such processes may involve semantic and/or pragmatic cues, and, indeed, the experimental sentences used in this study provided such cues. (Where such cues are not present Broca's show rather poor comprehension (see, e.g., Ansell & Flowers 1982; Caplan & Futter 1986). We hypothesize that, in fact, these cues, when presented to a temporally-less demanding level of analysis (as one might find, for example, at discourse-level processing) may well allow comprehension to proceed even in the face of temporally constrained, structure building failures such as we have charted here for this population. Wernicke's patients also have problems with such sentences when they are semantically and pragmatically unconstrained. But, as we show here, these ultimate failures turn on disruptions at different points in the processing chain, not at that involving temporally demanding information integration.

We suggest here that the disruption shown by Broca's can be rooted to general slowing of availability of information typically derived from lexical activation and integration. What we have shown here is the way in which this problem ramifies to the syntactic level. In this view, the brain region implicated in Broca's aphasia is not the locus of syntactic representations per se, but rather appears to provide the resources that sustain the normal (automatic) operating characteristics of the lexical and structural processing systems (namely, rapid-temporal-processing). That is, we suggest that neurological specialization within the language system turns not on where different general knowledge sources (e.g. syntax, semantics) are localized, but rather on the anatomical distribution of fairly elemental processing resources such as those involved in rapid temporal integration of language information, as seen in lexical access and structural integration.

Some Final Methodological Issues

The work we have presented here carries with it certain methodological assumptions. Claims about the nature of language processing must be investigated in the framework of paradigms that examine sentence or discourse processing, and not just the processing relations that hold between isolated words. While isolated (or pair or triplet) word studies do, indeed, reflect something of how relations between words can be exploited, the extra-sentence-processing characteristics they bring divorces such findings from valid interpretation with regard to sentence-discourse processing. This is not to say that only work in sentence contexts can reveal important language processing characteristics. Indeed, the issue is one of whether the non-sentential task allows for extra-sentential strategies to affect processing of the material. Thus, while continuous lexical decision tasks prevent pair-wise strategies from developing, paired-presentation of words, obviously, does not.

Next, it needs to be pointed out that, while on-line studies are critical to the investigation of sentence/discourse comprehension, not everything that involves reaction time or speeded response is a valid on-line measure of such processing. Thus, for example, speed to detect grammatical deformations likely bears little relationship to what goes on in language comprehension. Further, most off-line techniques are simply not capable in principle (and fact) of distinguishing the types of moment-by-moment details that are needed to build models of ongoing processing. By off-line measurements we refer to those that merely study (or ask evaluation of the final 'percepts' of language processing – as in sentence enactment, sentence-picture matching, truth-value judgment grammaticality or acceptability judgment tasks. Their worth in helping us think about representational limitations is indisputable. But they have not been particularly valuable in helping us explain these limitations in processing terms.

Linebarger, Schwartz & Saffran's (1983) interpretation of their grammaticality-judgment data can be used to illustrate this last point. Their finding is that Broca's patients carry out quite complex syntactic judgments, showing in this respect a sensitivity to structure and to grammatical categories (e.g., empty categories) that they are unable to exploit for comprehension. Linebarger et al. (1983) take this to indicate that the Broca's comprehension problem is not at the level of syntactic processing, but at a later processing stage – at the stage of thematic role assignment or mapping. However, these off-line grammatical judgment data do not at all militate this interpretation. It is one thing to notice the absence of an empty (trace) position in a deformed sentence; quite another, to link the trace with its antecedent in real-time – to fill the gap indexed by the trace during the strict time constraints imposed on the structure-building process. As simply one of many possibilities, it is entirely possible that performance in the first (off-line) instance is based on a local "checking" procedure – a post-sentence problem solving process in which locally available antecedents are checked against any open (unfilled) verb arguments. This kind of top-down, strategic intervention is likely to be far removed from gap-filling – from the normal reactivation of an antecedent at its post-verb cannonical position in real time (e.g., Swinney & Fodor 1989). Thus, although the off-line judgments charted by Linebarger et al. (1983) indicate the Broca's patient's sensitivity to empty categories, the data do not help us fill in details from a real-time processing perspective. In particular, they do not help us distinguish processing at the syntactic level from processing at a later stage. To isolate such stages we need to apply on-line techniques – techniques that can be brought to bear on ongoing processes at any temporal point in processing of a sentence, and which add as few extra-language processing characteristics (demand characteristics) of their own as possible. It is only with such tasks that we will be able to further a detailed analysis of the functional commitment of brain resources to language processing.

Note

1 While there is considerable variation in lesion extent, particularly for Broca's aphasia which is associated with large superficial and deep lesions, including the posterior portion of the third frontal gyrus, the anterior insula and adjacent and deeper areas, the fact is that the modal lesion site for this form of aphasia is different from that for Wernicke's aphasia, where the greatest involvement is inferior to the Sylvian fissure, implicating especially areas located in the posterior superior portion of the first temporal gyrus (Benson 1985; Vignolo 1988; Mohr 1976).

References

Anseil, B. & C. Flowers (1982): "Aphasic adults' use of heuristic and structural linguistic cues for analysis". Brain and Language 26, 62 – 72.

Alexander, M., M.A. Naeser & C.L. Palumbo (1990): "Broca's area aphasias: aphasia after lesions including the frontal operculum". Neurology 40, 353 – 362.

Bock, K. (1991): "A sketchbook of production problems". Journal of Psycholinguistic Research (Special Issue on Sentence Processing) 20, 141 – 160.

Caplan, D. & N. Hildebrandt (1988): Disorders of syntactic comprehension. Cambridge, MA: MIT Press.

Caplan, D. & C. Futter (1986): "Assignment of thematic roles by an agrammatic aphasic patient". Brain and Language 27.

Chomsky, N. (1981): Lectures on government and binding. Dordrecht: Foris.

Clements, G., J. McCloskey, J. Maling & A. Zaenen (1983): "String-vacuous rule application". Linguistic Inquiry 14, 1 – 17.

Friederici, A. & K. Kilborn (1989): "Temporal constraints on language processing: syntactic priming in Broca's aphasia". Journal of Cognitive Neuroscience 3, 262 – 272.

Goodglass, H. & L. Menn (1984): "Is agrammatism a unitary phenomenon?" In: M.-L. Kean, ed., Agrammatism. Orlando, FL: Academic Press.

Grodzinsky, Y. (1990): Theoretical perspectives on language deficits. Cambridge, MA: MIT Press.

Hagoort, P., C. Brown & T. Swaab (1994): On the nature of lexical-semantic processing impairments in aphasia. Paper presented to TENNET, Montreal, Quebec.

Hickok, G., E. Zurif & E. Canseco-Gonzalez (1993): "Structural description of agrammatic comprehension". Brain and Language 45, 371 – 395.

Kean, M.-L. (ed.) (1984): Agrammatism. Orlando, FL: Academic Press.

Kolk, H. & M. Weijts (1994): "Judgments of semantic anomaly in agrammatic patients". Brain and Language (in press).

Kolk, H., M. van Grunsven & A. Keyser (1984): "Parallelism in agrammatism". In: M.-L. Kean, ed., Agrammatism. Orlando, FL: Academic Press.

Linebarger, M., M. Schwartz & E. Saffran (1983): "Sensitivity to grammatical structure in so-called agrammatic aphasics". Cognition 13, 361 – 393.

Mauner, G., V. Fromkin & T. Cornell (1993): "Comprehension and acceptability judgments in agrammatism: disruptions in the syntax of referential dependency". Brain and Language 45, 340 – 370.

McElree, B. & T.G. Bever (1989): "The psychological reality of linguistically defined gaps". Journal of Psycholinguistics Research 18, 1, 21 – 36.

Meyer, D., R. Schvaneveldt & M. Ruddy (1975): "Loci of contextual effects on visual word recognition". In: P. Rabbit & S. Dornic, eds., Attention and performance, vol. V. New York: Academic Press.
Miceli, G., A. Mazzucchi, L. Menn & H. Goodglass (1983): "Contrasting cases of Italian agrammatic aphasia without comprehension disorder". Brain and Language 19, 65 – 97.
Milberg, W. & S. Blumstein (1981): "Lexical decision and aphasia: evidence for semantic processing". Brain and Language 14, 371 – 385.
Milberg, W., S. Blumstein & B. Dworetsky (1987): "Processing of lexical ambiguities in aphasia". Brain and Language 31, 138 – 150.
Mohr, J. (1976): "Broca's area and Broca's aphasia". In: H. Whitaker & H.A. Whitaker, eds., Studies in neurolinguistics, vol. 1. New York: Academic Press.
Naeser, M.A., C. Palumbo, N. Helm-Estabrooks, D. Stiassny-Eder & M.L. Albert (1989): "Severe nonfluency in aphasia: role of the medial subcallosal fasciculus and other white matter pathways in recovery of spontaneous speech". Brain 112, 1 – 38.
Neely, J.H. (1977): "Semantic priming and retrieval from lexical memory: roles of inhibitionless spreading activation and limited-capacity attention". Journal of Experimental Psychology: General 106, 226 – 254.
Ostrin, R. & M. Schwartz (1986): "Reconstructuring from a degraded trace: A study of sentence repetition in agrammatism". Brain and Language 8, 328 – 345.
Ostrin, R. & L. Tyler (1993): "Automatic access to lexical semantics in aphasia: Evidence from semantic and associative priming". Brain and Language 45, 147 – 159.
Prather, P., E.B. Zurif & T. Love (1992): The time course of lexical access in aphasia. Paper presented to the Academy of aphasia. Toronto, Ontario.
Prather, P., E.B. Zurif, C. Stern & J. Rosen (1992): "Slowed lexical access in non-fluent aphasia: a case study". Brain and Language 43, 336 – 348.
Shapiro, L., E.B. Zurif & J. Grimshaw (1987): "Sentence processing and the mental representation of verbs". Cognition 127, 219 – 246.
Shapiro, L. & B. Levine (1990): "Verb processing during sentence comprehension in aphasia". Brain and Language 38, 21 – 47.
Shapiro, L., B. Gordon, N. Hack & J. Killackey (1993): "Verb-argument structure processing in complex sentences in Broca's and Wernicke's aphasia". Brain and Language 45, 423 – 447.
Shapiro, L., E.B. Zurif & J. Grimshaw (1989): "Verb processing during sentence comprehension: contextual impenetrability". Journal of Psycholinguistic Research 18, 223 – 243.
Shelton, J. & R. Martin (1992): "How semantic is automatic semantic priming?" Journal of Experimental Psychology: Learning, Memory, and Cognition 18, 1191 – 1210.
Swinney, D. & J.D. Fodor (eds.) (1989): Journal of Psycholinguistic Research (Special Issue on Sentence Processing) 18, (1).
Swinney, D. & L. Osterhout (1990): "Inference generation during auditory language comprehension". In: A. Graesser & G. Bower, eds., Inferences and text comprehension. San Diego: Academic Press.
Swinney, D., W. Onifer, P. Prather & M. Hirshkowitz (1979): "Semantic facilitation across sensory modalities in the processing of individual words and sentences". Memory and Cognition 7, 159 – 165.
Swinney, D., E.B. Zurif, P. Prather & T. Love (1993): The neurological distribution of processing operations underlying language comprehension. Manuscript, Dept. of Psychology, University of California, San Diego.
Swinney, D., E.B. Zurif & J. Nicol (1989): "The effects of focal brain damage on sentence processing: An examination of the neurological organization of a mental module". Journal of Cognitive Neuroscience 1, 25 – 37.
Tanenhaus, M., J. Boland, S.M. Garnsey & G. Carleson (1989): "Lexical Structure in Parsing Long-Distance Dependencies". Journal of Psycholinguistics Research 18, 37 – 50.

Zurif, E.B. & D. Swinney (1993): "The Neuropsychology of Language". In: M. Gernsbacher, ed., Handbook of Psycholinguistics. Orlando, FL: Academic Press.
Zurif, E.B., D. Swinney & J.A. Fodor (1991): "An evaluation of assumptions underlying the single-patient-only position in neuropsychological research". Brain and Cognition 16, 198 – 210.
Zurif, E.B., D. Swinney, P. Prather, J. Solomon & C. Bushell (1993): "An on-line analysis of syntactic processing in Broca's and Wernicke's aphasia". Brain and Language 45, 448 – 464.

Automatic Semantic Activation for Lexical Perception: Normal and Disordered Processing*

Dieter Hillert, Douglas F.H. Burrington, Gautam A. Gupta, Manchester

1 Introduction

In everyday conversation a speaker intentionally produces a message and the hearer (or the speaker) can decide which part of the speech s/he wishes to pay attention to in order to integrate the information into some kind of higher-order belief contexts. From the viewpoint of modern psycholinguistic approaches such conscious and executive control of language processing does not relate to automatic processing mechanisms which are characteristic of components of the language processor *per se*. Thus, the distinction between controlled and automatic cognitive processing is fundamental to linguistics and psychology (e.g., Posner & Snyder 1975; Schneider & Shiffrin 1977).
A controlled process reflects an intentional activity and seems to work serially and relatively slowly, that is, attention can be paid only to a few aspects at a time in the so-called working memory. However, a controlled process is highly dynamic and adaptable to the requirements of new task conditions. In contrast, an automatic process works reflex-like and in parallel without sharing processes with other resources. Therefore, an automatic process is quite efficient but static in nature, that is, informationally encapsulated or cognitively impenetrable. That the human's brain develops such "wired-in" subsystems might be a matter of a genetically-driven program. This model is evidenced by specific breakdowns of mental processing when certain neurological tissues are damaged. Thus, neuropsychological evidence suggests that specific neurological substrata are responsible for informationally encapsulated automatic processing. In the case of aphasia, a specific breakdown in automatic language processing might reflect patterns of a genetic predisposition to language.
In this paper we are concerned with automatic semantic activation during lexical perception and with how these activation patterns are impaired in the case of aphasia. The following sections will consider first a psycholinguistic theory of lexical perception which takes into account how semantic entries are automatically accessed and integrated into a higher-level format of conceptual representations. Second, psycholinguistic

* This research was supported by a fellowship of the Alexander von Humboldt Foundation (Feodor Lynen program VB2-FLF) to the first author. He is grateful to Allen I. Selverston for his invitation to work at the University of California, San Diego, and to Elizabeth Bates, Jeffrey L. Elman and David Swinney for providing facilities in the Departments of Cognitive Science, Psychology and Linguistics.

evidence will be reviewed tapping in real-time (on-line) into the temporal course of lexical semantic processing during single word or sentence comprehension. Thus, we focus our research in this context on automatic semantic processing investigated with the lexical priming technique. Those response patterns found in off-line experiments requiring explicit semantic control, like similarity judgments, are not discussed but are addressed when their features might be relevant to the characterization of automatic semantic processing. Finally, experiments investigating on-line lexical semantic access in *Broca's aphasia* and *Wernicke's aphasia*[1] will be critically reviewed. In the light of previously illustrated theoretical and empirical results we then can specify whether disorders of lexical processing in aphasia are caused by deviations of normal semantic activation patterns.

In this way we will introduce in the next section a theory of real-time lexical perception that addresses controversial issues currently under discussion. The preference for the paradigm selected does not imply that other methodological approaches are considered as being irrelevant to the question under discussion. The cognitive demands of off-line tasks require responses depending largely on general cognitive processes or strategies and do not reflect the automatic nature of language processing. For example, off-line tasks (e.g., DeRenzi & Vignolo's Token Test 1962) measuring strategies of problem solving require conscious awareness to a significant degree (Neely 1977). Results which have been found in off-line tasks may be irrelevant to the interpretation of on-line RTs; however, they might be inasmuch relevant as they control conscious processes of identical stimulus material. Theoretical as well as empirical results have been discussed in the light of the off-line method and it has been shown that such an approach is methodologically inappropriate and may imply a solipsistic research strategy (Hillert 1990, 1995). A completely different research program might involve the investigation of possible impairments according to the extent to which the relationship between automatic and conscious processing is regarded as a continuum.

The phenomenon of aphasia is doubtless a case of language impairment caused by specific levels of language processing. Thus, one might find evidence for preserved semantic automatic processing while conscious semantic processes might be impaired and *vice versa* without being able to specify what conscious processing is all about. Thus, the primary goal of the investigation of language processing in aphasia must concern itself with representations already acquired and not learned post-traumatically. Another aspect concerns the importance of a theoretical framework which permits us to tap in real-time into specific levels of representations and processes. This approach assumes that the data evaluated are as little contaminated as possible by compensatory strategies on the part of well-preserved representations of the general cognitive system. According to the evaluation of semantic processing in Wernicke's aphasia a theory must specify the status of different types of meanings (e.g., meanings stated on the lexical, sentential, text or discourse level) and how particular levels of meanings might be affected in the real-time processing of language production and comprehension.

The present review refers primarily to data which are mostly averaged by the overall performance of a whole aphasic group. Because of this methodological weakness (Caramazza 1984, 1986) the interpretation cannot consider that patients' performance in different diagnostic groups might be quite similar for some tasks (e.g., Wernicke's aphasics: Tyler 1988) and conversely, that patients of the same diagnostic group might behave quite differently in some tests (e.g., agrammatic patients: Goodglass & Menn 1985).

2 Lexical Perception

Lexical perception involves many different types of representation and process to translate a speech signal into a meaning representation of what is being said. There is a linguistic level of representation independent of motoric and phonetic representations which maps speech input onto lexical forms (phonological representations) and lexical forms onto lexical content (semantic and syntactic entries). There is a conceptual level of representation which constrains a representation of the proposition underlying a sentence on the basis of linguistic information. The proposition or an interconnected set of propositions generates the text level reflected by atomic and molecular structures (micro- and macrostructures). The integration into a higher-level representation of some kind may involve general knowledge (e.g., common sense or visuo-spatial information) and may constrain the generation of a discourse representation (cf. Garrett's 1992; Levelt 1989). The following general stages of language comprehension may be (a) motor representation to speech representation, (b) speech representation to lexical forms, (c) lexical forms to lexical content, (d) lexical content to proposition, and (e) proposition to discourse representation.
In this context we are mainly concerned with the transformations (c) and (d), that is, we focus on the question of how lexical semantic entries are accessed during sentence comprehension by lexical form and how they are integrated into a propositional format. The process of lexical perception generally consists of three distinct stages: *access, selection* and *integration.* Unfortunately, these concepts are often defined in different ways (Tyler & Frauenfelder 1987; Tanenhaus & Lucas 1987). Lexical access can itself be divided into distinct phases: The *first phase* links the sensory (acoustic-phonetic) input with corresponding phonological entries which in turn activate the corresponding semantic-syntactic entries. In the context of speech production this process is regarded by some as consisting of two discrete stages (e.g., Butterworth 1989; Kempen & Huijbers 1983; Levelt 1992) whereas others prefer to view it as an interactive process (e.g., Dell 1986; Stemberger 1983). This distinction is considered largely irrelevant in most lexical perception models, since access of lexical information implies the activation of phonological *and* semantic-syntactic entries. The *second phase* in speech perception refers to the selection of the most appropriate lexical candidate corresponding to the perceived lexical item. As will be shown later, opinions vary widely on this subject. Lexical identification is the result of this selection phase, that is, the hearer determines at this point which word s/he has perceived. The "uniqueness point", which need not necessarily coincide with the actual point of word identification, can be localized mainly before the perception of the whole word and is subject to semantic-syntactic constraints. In the *third phase,* the integration phase, the selected word is assigned to the meaning context of the whole utterance. In the discourse model mentioned above this assignment takes place at the conceptual level. The question of how the various units of information

are made available is answered in greatly diverging ways in numerous models of lexical perception. The majority of models do not put forward any hypothesis which would allow an empirical distinction between lexical selection and lexical integration. Below we will describe the most frequently and controversially discussed models of word identification which are dealt with in the literature. They can be characterized by their position on a scale ranging from completely interactive at one end to completely autonomous at the other (Tanenhaus, Dell & Carlson 1987).

Autonomous models (Cairns 1983; Fodor 1983; Forster 1976, 1979; Seidenberg 1985; Tanenhaus, Carlson & Seidenberg 1985) describe modules which function independently of one another, that is, the output of a module is produced without the influence of any other module. Lexical access is an autonomous process which can be regarded as a "data-driven" process which determines lexical access and selection. Top-down information (e.g., sentential or conceptual context) can only influence word identification post-lexically, that is, after completion of lexical access. Fodor generally posits autonomous processes for all cognitive input systems in contrast to the operations of the belief system. The language processor *per se* is regarded as being such an input system. Forster's search model implies that the process of access and of selection occurs in an autonomous fashion. Autonomous models have the common feature that they describe relatively more or less static systems containing information lists. Sensory input activates data-driven bottom-up search processes within a list, which in turn allow discrete output without the influence of other lists.

Interactive models on the other hand argue that information of different kinds can exert a direct influence on the analysis of output processes. Morton's (1969, 1979) logogen model, for example, implies that conceptual context can directly influence the early phase of lexical access. In other words, context itself selects lexical candidates through increased activation and the attainment of a specific threshold value before sensory input is even processed. In connectionist models (e.g., McClelland & Rummelhart 1981; McClelland & Elman 1986) word nodes are activated by connection with lower representation such as perceptual features and phonemes and by connection with higher representations such as conceptual context. In Rummelhart and McClelland's model the conceptual context can have both positive and negative effects; that is, the effects are positive in the sense that they increase an activation level by excitation and negative in that they decrease an activation level by inhibition.

The cohort model which will receive particular attention in our work (Marslen-Wilson & Welsh 1978; Marslen-Wilson 1984; Marslen-Wilson & Tyler 1980) accounts for both autonomous and interactive processes. Access to phonological entries and/or to possible lexical candidates within a cohort is autonomous and only accounts for information which matches the sensory input. Thus, lexical access is up to this point a bottom-up process which is completely automatic and unconscious. Interactions caused by context can only take place at the selection phase. In the original model (Marslen-Wilson & Welsh 1978; Marslen-Wilson & Tyler 1980) lexical selection is an all-or-nothing procedure; that is, incompatible units are immediately eliminated from the cohort. In a later version (Marslen-Wilson 1987) missing sensory input leads to a reduced degree of activity. Word identification follows at the end of the selection phase, that is, when only one candidate remains. This occurs when a word has already been recognized at the uniqueness point (cf. Forster 1989; Norris 1986).

In lexical decision tasks the experimental subject decides whether or not a word/lexical item presented either in written or spoken form is a word of his/her language. Should a semantically or conceptually related word be presented, then word identification takes place more quickly (e.g., *salt-pepper*) than when a word which is not semantically or conceptually related (e.g., *cloud-pepper*) is presented. The question arises as to whether this priming effect is of a semantic (intra-lexical) or of a conceptual (inter-lexical) nature. In Meyer & Schvaneveldt's (1971; cf. Schvaneveldt, Meyer & Becker 1976) classic study relatively robust priming effects (about 80 msec) were found with the word pairs *doctor-nurse* or *rat-chesse.* These faster decision times are not necessarily a result of semantic factors but could be attributed to conceptual processes. For example, the concepts *doctor* and *nurse* share features such that certain conceptual aspects of *nurse* are activated as a result of priming. This explanation, also known as the "conceptual mediation hypothesis" argues against autonomous access to lexical meanings (cf. Tanenhaus & Lucas 1987; Tanenhaus, Carlson & Seidenberg 1985).

Autonomous theories offer an alternative explanation of this effect by arguing that the semantic lexicon simply reflects the structure of our experiences (cf. Fodor 1983; Forster 1979; Seidenberg & Tanenhaus 1986); this means that words and concepts which are often produced together like *oil-vinegar* or *black-white* also correspond to fixed represented semantic relations within the lexicon. In other words, these relations enhance the efficiency of lexical access, since no "hypotheses" are generated which incur a processing overhead in terms of time and capacity. These intra-lexical connections are, however, only of limited use within the framework of sentence processing since semantically related words are not often produced together in the same sentence (Forster 1979). Differentiating between autonomous and interactive processes does not contribute to the choice of processing level at which lexical priming takes place. Effects which clearly violate the autonomy hypothesis can be interpreted as internal processes of the lexicon.

Assumptions regarding "automatic" and "controlled" lexical processing are closely linked with but not identical to the differentiation between autonomous and interactive processes. Automatic processes take place unconsciously, relatively fast and without conscious control. In cognitive terms they are therefore impenetrable and static and largely data-driven or bottom-up. On the other hand, controlled processes of which the speaker/hearer can be aware of are dynamic and flexible and relatively slow in comparison with automatic processes (Posner & Snyder 1975; Schneider & Shiffrin 1977; Shiffrin & Schneider 1977).

Interactive processes can be either automatic or controlled, whereas autonomous processes are automatic in nature (Flores d'Arcais 1988; Forster 1979; Friederici 1988; Seidenberg, Tanenhaus, Leiman & Bienkowski 1982). It should be noted, however, that automatic processes must not necessarily be processed autonomously: Automaticity can be assumed to be a necessary condition for autonomy but not *vice versa.* For example, cognitive processes seem to become autonomous during the language acquisition phase through repeated processing. Friederici (1988) suggests that both aspects are therefore functionally independent of each other when autonomous processing has

stabilized itself. Evidence for this hypothesis is provided by the speech of agrammatic Broca's aphasics: Automatic access to function words is impaired in comparison to content words, where function words are processed autonomously, that is, independently of semantic factors. This approach can only be compared in part to that of Blumstein, Milberg & Shrier (1982), for instance, since they assume a deficit in Broca's aphasia of automatic processing of syntactic as well as of semantic information.
The order in which both processing modes may occur is, however, worth investigating. Generally it is assumed that only automatic processes take place in the early phase of lexical access. It is, however, certainly possible that as early as this stage both automatic and controlled processes take effect in parallel. Attempts to split the semantic identification process of a word into its component stages of processing have been made in a number of experiments. Here we deal exclusively with the oral identification process (cf. Neely 1990 for an overview of written word identification).
With respect to the "autonomy hypothesis" two factors seem to be relevant: (a) multiple activation and (b) phrase-sensitivity. With respect to the "selective access hypothesis" three factors are discussed: (a) context sensitivity, (b) dominance specificity, and (c) feature specificity. Autonomous lexical access represents the "standard position" which states that there is a multiple activation of semantic-syntactic entries (lemmas) in the early stage of lexical access. Thus irrespective of the type of sentence context all meanings of a word are simultaneously activated, driven by automatic bottom-up processes. During lexical access the speed and the information activated remain constant. Lexical selection and lexical integration take place post-lexically and may include controlled lexical processes. Selective access takes place post-lexically at a time determined by sentential relevance. In the modified version autonomous processing occurs within the syntactic phrase of the ambiguous word.
Selective lexical access is, in contrast to multiple access, context-sensitive, and context-irrelevant meanings are not activated. A modified version states that access takes place selectively and has, moreover, access to the more dominant or frequent meaning of the ambiguous word. It follows that access to the subdominant meaning takes longer than to the dominant meaning which must be inhibited. Another version states by analogy that selective access occurs when the sentence context suggests specific semantic features pertaining to the dominant homophone's meaning.

3 Normal Lexical Semantic Activation

In phoneme control tasks experimental subjects are required, for example, to press a button as quickly as possible when they hear a word beginning with a specific sound in an acoustically presented sentence. It is believed that the time taken to recognize a phoneme reflects a measure of the *difficulty* of local processing. Foss (1970; cf. Hakes 1972; Swinney & Hakes 1976) for example asked experimental subjects to recognize certain phonemes which followed ambiguous and unambiguous words (e.g., *The farmer/merchant put his straw/hay beside the machine*). In both of these sentences the target phoneme was /b/. Response times make clear the fact that phoneme control for ambiguous words (straw) is longer than for unambiguous words (*hay*); this is also the case with context-relevant sentences (e.g., *The farmer put his...*). The result therefore supports the first hypothesis, that of multiple lexical access. There are, however, methodological flaws which cast doubt on the experiments carried out. Mehler, Segui & Carey (1978) show that the time differences emerging from the experiments can be attributed to lack of control over word length: ambiguous words were shorter than unambiguous words so it is not surprising that phoneme recognition is faster in the case of ambiguous words. Sentence completion tasks, however, point towards multiple access. MacKay (1966) found that subjects take longer to complete a phrase with an ambiguous word (*After taking the right turn at the intersection, I...*) than one with an unambiguous word (*After taking the left turn at the intersection, I...*). The modified multiple access theory of phrase access is supported by Bever, Garrett and Hurtig (1973). The above effect is stronger when sentence completion takes place within the phrase (here *at* versus *I*).

The dichotic sentence perception test carried out by Lackner & Garrett (1972; MacKay 1973) also supports the idea of multiple access. In these experiments the subject hears two different sentences simultaneously in the right and left-hand channels of headphones and is instructed to only pay conscious attention to one of them. When the subjects only paid attention to the ambiguous sentence *The spy put out the torch as our signal to attack,* the verb *put out* in the other sentence was disambiguated (*The spy extinguished/displayed the torch in the window*). The subjects' description of the consciously processed sentence varied according to the meaning suggested by the second sentence. This observation demonstrates that both possible meanings of the verb are activated. Other experimental results support the selective access hypothesis. Hogaboam & Perfetti (1975) claim that access is frequency-sensitive, that is, initially access to the dominant meaning takes place followed by access to the subdominant meaning. In their written experiment on word control experimental subjects were asked to decide whether a word was presented in final position of the sentence was ambiguous or not. The sentence contexts suggested either the dominant (e.g., *The jealous husband read the letter*) or the subdominant meaning of a homograph (e.g., *The antique typewriter was missing a letter*). In a sentence context which conveyed the subdominant meaning recognition time for homographs was faster. The following interpretation was given preference. Initially the dominant meaning of the ambiguous word is activated independently of the sentential context, and in a later stage lexical entries are compared with the sentence meaning. If the dominant meaning and the sentence meaning do not match, then the search process continues and selective access to the subdominant word meaning occurs followed by comparison of contexts. Unfortunately the results reflect a conscious decision process and do not reflect the time-course of real-time lexical access.

All the experimental results discussed in this section provoke similar methodological objections. First, the experimental techniques addressed so far do not tap into processes of the mental lexicon since they do not examine lexical entries, but rather phonemes or conceptual categories. Thus, the effects seem to be pre-lexical and post-lexical in nature. Second, the techniques do not provide us with a way of bringing out the temporal course of lexical access, in particular the intuitively plausible distinction between lexical access and selection. In order to tap in real-time into natural language processes an experiment should ideally take a measurement during the phase within which real-time speech processes occur. Today, the best approach to this aim seems to be offered by the cross-modal priming technique. Auditory stimuli are presented together with visual stimuli, either simultaneously or in quick succession. It is possible to determine the processing load at a given time in real-time processing of, for example, an acoustically presented sentence either by means of (visual) lexical decision or by naming tasks. The processing of homophones in sentence context has been investigated using the cross-modal priming paradigm in a number of experiments.

Conrad (1974) was the first to use a cross-modal variant of the *Stroop* naming task. There were longer naming times for colours when the words exhibited a meaning relation with a homophone. Clearly, both homophone meanings were being activated. In this experiment the visually presented target words (in colour) were immediately followed by the homophone (zero-msec inter-stimulus interval = zero-ISI). In the follow-up study conducted by Oden & Spira (1983) a 500-ISI was used and it was shown that activation of homophone meaning is influenced by context. It must, however, be stressed that lexical access takes place within a period of 200 msec (Marslen-Wilson & Tyler 1980; Seidenberg et al. 1982; Tanenhaus, Leiman & Seidenberg 1979). For this reason we may assume that Oden & Spira's results reflect post-lexical integration processes. The same objection applies to the interpretation of lexical priming effects measured without sentential context because these studies used a 500-ISI (Meyer & Schvaneveldt 1971; Schvaneveldt, Meyer & Becker's 1976). Swinney (1979) introduced a variant of the priming technique developed by Conrad. At a specific point in a spoken sentence (e.g., immediately after a homophone: zero-ISI) the experimental subject makes a lexical decision in relation to visually presented words. These target words which appeared on a monitor in Swinney's experiment at zero- and 1500-ISI, were associated with either the first or second meaning of the homophone. For example, the homophone was presented in the following context:

Rumor had it that, for years, the government building had been plagued with problems. The man was not surprised when he found several spiders, roaches, and other bugs |*| *in the corner* |*| *of his room.* The words *spiders* and *roaches,* which primed the more dominant meaning of the homophone *bugs* (e.g., the insect meaning rather than the espionage meaning), were left out in the case of a neutral context. In the above sentence the target words with related meaning *ant, spy* and the control word *sew* were presented visually on a monitor for lexical decision at the positions marked by asterisks. The following results were obtained. A zero-ISI priming for *ant* as well as *spy* was found independent of contextual variants. This process of multiple access which was also phrase sensitive (cf. Blutner & Sommer 1988: modified theory), finished at a 1500-ISI (after *corner*) since the decision time for *ant* was faster than for *spy* in the suggested sentential context (see above). Swinney, Onifer, Prather & Hirshkowitz (1979) measured a similar effect in the case of the isolated presentation of homophone and target word. Seidenberg et al.'s (1982) results do not, on the other hand, lend themselves to such unambiguous interpretation. In contrast to Swinney's studies, cross-modal naming tasks were carried out rather than cross-modal decision tasks. The possible influence of the following contexts was examined: syntactic context (*They all rose* versus *She bought a rose;* target word: *flower*), conceptual context (semantic bias: *You play the spade* versus

You buy the spade; card) and semantic context (semantic associate: *The farmer bought the straw* versus *Joe bought the straw; hay*). At zero-ISI multiple access was always detected with the exception of one context type and at 200-ISI context-sensitive effects occurred under all conditions. The only instance of selective access at zero-ISI was caused by semantic context. Seidenberg et al. assume that this effect is intra-lexical and therefore does not contradict the multiple access theory. The relevant semantic connections were *farmer...straw; hay* (cf. Schvaneveldt et al. 1976). Simpson's (1981) results argue in turn for a dominance-sensitive and context-sensitive selective access process to homophones. In a neutral context the subjects had faster decision times for dominant target words (e.g., those displaying a meaning relation with the dominant homophone) than for subdominant target words. If, however, the context suggested either the dominant or subdominant meaning irrespective of relevant dominance then faster reaction times occurred only for meaning-relevant context. This result appears to reflect frequency-sensitive access, that is, when no specific meaning is suggested by sentential context the dominant meaning is always activated. It should, however, be noted that Simpson's experiments were conducted with a 120-ISI. It is therefore possible that during this time span (at a zero-ISI) irrelevant meaning is deactivated. Onifer & Swinney, who were unable to duplicate Simpson's results at zero-ISI, refer to this argument.

In contrast to Seidenberg et al.'s interpretation of an intra-lexical effect and of the multiple access theory, numerous experiments provide evidence for contextual influence on specific aspects of a prime's meaning. This type of feature priming was developed by Schwanenflugel & Shoben (1985; cf. Schwanenflugel & Lacount 1988) and used within the cross-modal priming paradigm by Tabossi and his co-workers (Moss & Marslen-Wilson 1993; Tabossi, Colombo & Job 1987; Tabossi 1988a, 1988b). A selective effect was established at a zero-ISI for ambiguous and unambiguous words.

Tabossi found multiple access when from a semantic viewpoint the sentential context seems to be neutral with respect to the homophone (*port*) in the example (*The man had to be at five o'clock at the port* |*| *for a very important meeting*) (N.B. gloss of Tabossi's Italian sentence), and when the target words marked |*| were associated either with the dominant or subdominant homophone meaning (*sea* versus *alcohol;* control word *hand*), or else when the targets displayed characteristic features (*safe* versus *red;* control word *short*). Selective access was, however, found to occur when the dominant sentential context itself contained a characteristic feature (e.g., *The violent hurricane did not damage the ships which were in the port* |*|, *one of the best equipped along the coast*). Lexical decision about a target word which is associated with this dominant feature context (SEA; 643 msec) was noticeably faster than with a target word associated with the subdominant homophone meaning (*alcohol;* 688 msec) or with a control word (*hand*; 682 msec).

The potential objection that lexical decision tasks could involve post-lexical processes does not apply to Tabossi's studies since they were all conducted with the same set of homophones and target words. Another previously discussed aspect is, however, worthy of more attention. Did Tabossi's studies investigate the processing of possibly conceptual features which are not represented intra-lexically? If this is the case, then this argument against the standard position of the multiple access theory is invalidated.

Let us now look at the results of Swinney (1979) and Seidenberg et al. (1982) more closely. It is important to know why the effect interpreted by Seidenberg et al. as intra-lexical has not been found in Swinney's experiment. If intra-lexical connections reflect our subjective experience structures (Fodor 1983) then taxonomic relations such as for example co-hyponymy are generally not represented in the lexicon. Therefore, it is possible that selective access will take place with Seidenberg et al.'s stimulus material but not with Swinney's. Let us recall the meaning relations of *spiders, roaches, bugs* and *ant.* The essential difference between the sets of stimulus material is that Swinney's context is made up of co-hyponyms and Seidenberg et al.'s more of free associations. A sentential context, which, among other things, consists of intra-lexical relations can be assumed to activate only certain semantic features of the homophones such that selective access can be expected. If we take into account the theory that relations such as co-hyponymy, as used by Swinney, reflect inter-lexical (conceptual) relations, then we should not expect selective access. Although the response times in Swinney's (1979) experiments argue in favour of multiple access, it should be borne in mind that mildly context-sensitive effects were nonetheless found: RTs were faster (but not significantly) when meaning-related words like *spider-roaches* were perceived in sentential context before the target word *ant* (cf. Onifer & Swinney 1981).

As has already been shown, the type of information being accessed can be a decisive factor in the question of contextual influence on semantic access (Gerrig 1986; Williams 1988). Onifer & Swinney's (1981) prime/target relations were, for example, cases of near-synonymy (*sage-wise*), antonymy (*cold-hot*), hyponymy (*bug-insect*), attribute relations (*scale fish*) or thematic relations (*pool-swim*). The finding of multiple access in Onifer & Swinney's study supports the theory that no specific meaning aspects of a homophone are activated by sentential context. As Tabossi's studies, however, indicate, selective access can occur when certain semantic features are activated by the sentential context. The kind of relationship existing between prime and target appears, however, not play any essential role in this process. There are various factors which support the view that artificial factors have less influence on linguistic performance in naming tasks than in lexical decision tasks. First of all, naming constitutes a more natural task, since lexical decision implies a binary classification component (words vs. non-words). Lexical decision is then possibly not completely independent of controlled influences (cf. Balota & Chumbley 1990). Moreover, lexical decision, in contrast to naming, is influenced by the factors of *familiarity* and *meaningfulness* of the target word (Balota & Chumbley 1984, 1985).

Backward priming may have led to errors in the results of experiments on multiple access (cf. Koriat 1981; Kiger & Glass 1983). This could, for example, hold for homophone processing in cross-modal decision tasks using a zero-ISI. At zero-ISI, that is, when the meanings of the homophones (prime) and the visually presented target words are both accessible, the semantically related target word can function as a context for the homophone, which in turn primes the target word. We cannot expect selective access if we take such conditions into account, since the target word primes backwards both homophone meanings regardless of sentential context. Glucksberg, Kreuz & Tho (1986) controlled this possible effect by presenting non-words as target items and actually concluded that the multiple access effects found by Onifer & Swinney (1981) could be attributed to backward priming. Glucksberg et al. used non-words bearing a resemblance to actual words (e.g., PETLS {petal} as target item, SLETP as control item and *flower* as homophone) and they established that lexical decision time only became longer when the target item was related in meaning to the homophone which the sentential context suggested. A number of subsequent studies, however, show that multiple access cannot be the result of backward priming (Burgess, Tanenhaus & Seidenberg 1989; Jones 1989; Tanenhaus, Burgess & Seidenberg 1988). When compared to lexical decision tasks we find that backward priming does not occur at all in naming tasks (Seidenberg, Waters, Sanders & Langer 1984).

Moreover, the ISI factor is relevant since lexical selection took place in a time span of about 200 msec. Results which have been found with an ISI of more than zero may reflect post-lexical processes. It is also problematic if the target words are not presented in the middle of the perception process but rather at the end of a sentence: with longer words post-lexical effects in particular occur between the identification point of the homophone and its physical end (for unambiguous words see Zwitserlood 1989).

To sum up: When the context suggests the dominant meaning of the homophone, then both selective and multiple access can occur. Selective access takes place under the condition that specific semantic features of the homophone are activated by the sentential context. The type of features appear to be irrelevant because selective access also takes place in the case of intra-lexical relations between prime and target word. This finding can only be compared to a limited extent with effects which can be discerned between prime and target word in isolation since they do not appear to occur post-lexically. When, on the other hand, the context only weakly suggests the dominant meaning of the homophone multiple access takes place for all or both meanings of the homophone. This applies equally to neutral or subdominant contexts.

It is generally assumed that context effects proceed in a top-down fashion (either consciously or unconsciously) and thereby lead to faster processing of sensory input. This can be assumed in the case of selective access to certain semantic features. A bottom-up activation of the contextually irrelevant meaning cannot be assumed, since there are no significant differences in RTs between control words and contextually irrelevant target words. Future studies should take the identification point of each individual word into account and control the temporal course of lexical processing through a variety of "stimulus onset asynchronies" (SOA). In addition to statistically founded degrees of relationship between prime and target word the way in which feature-specific context may be controlled should be investigated (e.g., intra-lexical relations in sentential context which suggest subdominant homophone meaning). The response patterns demonstrate that *surface* and *deep* semantic processes can be differentiated from one another. Access to a homophone in sentential context can be assumed to be multiple when *shallow* semantic processing is required and selective access may be measured in the case of *in-depth* semantic processing.

4 Disordered Lexical Semantic Activation

A number of experimental studies show that certain factors influence semantic activation for lexical comprehension in Wernicke's aphasics as well as in Broca's aphasics, for example: (a) *reduced memory span* (e.g. Martin 1987; Ostrin & Schwarz 1986; Saffran & Marin 1975; Lesser 1976), (b) *frequency of occurrence* (e.g., Howes 1964; 1967), (c) *task-specific demands* (e.g., Gerwirth 1984; Rinnert & Whitaker 1973), (d) *interaction with phonological factors* (Baker, Blumstein & Goodglass 1981; Milberg, Blumstein & Dworetzky 1988), or (e) *overall significant correlation* and *not an item-to-item correlation with production disorders* (e.g., Butterworth, Howard & McLoughlin 1984; Gainotti 1976; Gainotti, Caltagirone & Ibba 1975; Gainotti, Miceli, Caltagirone, Silveri & Masullo 1981).

In the present context we are concerned with the question whether semantic access or selection is impaired in Wernicke's aphasics and Broca's aphasics. As already outlined, it is essential to define precisely the fuzzy term *semantics* and to differentiate between methods of evaluation used to examine mental processing in aphasia. For the present purpose, that is, for the interpretation of lexical disorders in aphasia, the approach selected is comparable to Fodor's (1983) ideas. Semantic entries like lexical meaning relations represented in an automatic fashion or lexical argument structures are regarded as part of the language input module; other types of knowledge representations such as encyclopedic information are irrelevant to the specification of possible linguistic processing disorders in Broca's aphasics and Wernicke's aphasics. Because of the diagnostic divergence between both groups, we assume that semantic processes are also differently affected. Let us look at Wernicke's aphasics' and Broca's aphasics' performance in several on-line tasks requiring access and integration of lexical semantic information.

In general, Wernicke's aphasics have particular difficulties in processing content words like nouns, verbs, adjectives, adverbs or prepositions as head of a phrase, and Broca's aphasics seem to be impaired in processing clitics like bounded morphemes (affixes) or function words. Content words are dynamic in nature, that is, according to social requirements or personal motivation, an infinite number of new content words might be created; they therefore carry extensional and/or intensional meaning. In contrast, clitics are static in nature, that is, only a certain number of clitics exist, and their meanings are only relevant for sentential processing. Thus, one might expect that when Wernicke's aphasics have to process content words for comprehension this is not so with clitics, and by contrast Broca's aphasics should not show semantic impairments when asked to perform on content words.

However, numerous off-line studies reported in the literature seem to support the issue that the so-called "semantic deficit hypothesis" applies not only to Wernicke's aphasics but also to Broca's aphasics (see for a review for example Caplan 1989, chapter 12; Caramazza, Berndt & Brownell 1982; Hillert 1992; Lesser 1978). Therefore the question arises why Broca's aphasics show semantic impairments, although their comprehension of content words seems not to be deficient in an everyday language situation. As already mentioned, Hillert (1992, 1993) argues that an inadequate experimental approach has produced some artificial results. Control subjects sometimes performed as poorly as Broca's aphasics; for example, high error scores on the semantic relationship "coordination" in word-picture matching tasks were found for both high-comprehension aphasics (comparable to Broca's aphasics) and for control subjects in Goodglass & Baker's (1976) study. Thus, from the viewpoint presented here, the status of semantic processing in aphasia is quite unclear because the response patterns in off-line studies seem to reflect a non-analyzable outcome of different compensatory strategies. It was therefore necessary to investigate the possibility of applying a methodological paradigm which permits us to establish whether lexical meanings are still available or whether the time-course of semantic access or integration reflects a processing deficit. For this reason aphasic lexical access has been examined by the priming paradigm already reviewed.

As we have said, semantic activation caused by lexical priming implies automatic as well as controlled processes (Neely 1977; Posner & Snyder 1975). In considering the fact that lexical decision takes place in the time span of less than 200 ms (Marslen-Wilson & Tyler 1980), it has been suggested that automatic semantic access to a word occurs within this short span. Furthermore, it is certainly quite plausible to assume that automatic semantic access occurs even in a even smaller period if high-frequency words or a word's uniqueness point is considered (< 100 ms). This aspect, however, has hardly been considered when semantic priming has been investigated in aphasia. One reason for this may be that RTs of aphasic patients are sometimes extremely long and, therefore, experiments using a zero-ISI involve a too-rapid presentation. Before we return to this point we will critically review most of the lexical priming studies conducted with Wernicke's aphasics and Broca's aphasics.

In the following sections results from several lexical semantic priming studies are summarized in terms of absolute RTs and of the priming level (Hillert 1994). By priming level we mean RTs on semantically related words minus RTs on non-semantically related words. As we will see, however, differences between studies are influenced by variations between a number of experimental factors: (a) sensory modality, (b) stimulus types, (c) ISI, and (d) diagnostic group (cf. Prather, this volume).

At first Milberg & Blumstein (1981) adopted the single-word priming paradigm developed by Meyer & Schvaneveldt (1971) to investigate semantic processing in aphasia (cf. Table 1). They asked six Wernicke's aphasics, five Broca's aphasics, and one conduction aphasic to decide lexically on nouns which are related either semantically (coordinate associates like *dog-cat* or superordinate associates like *apple-fruit*) or non-semantically related to a preceding noun. These noun pairs were presented with an ISI of approximately 2000 ms. In contrast to the poor performance in off-line semantic judgments, Wernicke's aphasics as control subjects show significant priming effects (280/50 ms).[2] Broca's aphasics and one conduction aphasics show a priming effect (90 ms) with only a tendency to significance. It is important to consider the length of RT in relation to the priming level. Wernicke's aphasics' RTs are almost twice as long as those of control subjects (1550/2450 ms) and Broca's aphasics'/conduction aphasics' RTs seem to be half way between Wernicke's aphasics and normal speakers' RTs (1850 ms). Because deficits of spoken lexical perception might be bypassed by graphemic representations, Blumstein, Milberg & Shier (1992) presented auditorily the noun pairs used in Milberg & Blumstein (1981) but with a shorter ISI of 500 ms. The outcome is that not only 7 Wernicke's aphasics but also 3 Broca's aphasics, 5 conduction aphasics, 4 transmotoric aphasics, and 4 global aphasics showed significant priming effects. Although the overall RTs ratio between the diagnostic groups is not as divergent as in Milberg & Blumstein's study, Wernicke's aphasics had again the longest RTs.

Neither study confirms the results found in off-line studies. According to Milberg and Blumstein's interpretation, the performance of Wernicke's aphasics seems to remain preserved when automatic access of semantic information was examined while, on the other hand conscious semantic processing – required in off-line tasks like similarity judgments – seems to be severely impaired. This may be one reason for their language comprehension deficit. In considering the findings of Milberg & Blumstein (1981) and Blumstein et al. (1982) automatic semantic access seems not to remain constantly preserved in Broca's aphasics. Moreover, because Blumstein et al. examined only 3 Broca's aphasics, there is no clear line of evidence which throws light on the automatic access deficit found in Milberg & Blumstein's experiment. Indeed a further study reports data which seem to reflect a disorder of automatic processing in Broca's aphasics.

In exploring less low-level associate representations of words which may be irrelevant in sentential processing Milberg, Blumstein & Dworetzky (1987) conducted a more demanding task by using a modification of Schvaneveldt, Meyer & Becker's (1976) triplet paradigm, that is, the target sets consisted of two primes and a target. Four priming conditions are examined with a 500-ISI. In the concordant condition the first prime and target shares one meaning with the ambiguous second prime (e.g., *coin-bank-money*); in the discordant condition the first prime's meaning and the target's meaning shares different meanings with the second prime (e.g. *river-bank-money*). In the neutral condition the first prime is unrelated to the ambiguous second prime, while the target is related (e.g. *desk-bank-money*) and in the unrelated condition (baseline condition) the second prime is unambiguous and all three words are unrelated to each other (e.g. *nurse-fish-money*). Much like normal speakers, Wernicke's aphasics showed significant priming effects (110/33 ms) although their overall RT were significantly longer (779/2010 ms). Broca's aphasics showed no significant priming with word triplets and therefore the results found in Milberg & Blumstein (1981) with noun pairs seem to be confirmed. At this point we still have to question the hypothesis that one feature of Broca's aphasics' deficit may best be described by a disorder of automatic access to semantic information. For example, a more demanding task condition, such as with word pairs rather than with word triplets, might require a larger memory load. Considering the well-known fact that Broca's aphasics particularly suffer from reduced verbal short-term memory span, it is therefore premature to interpret the findings as clear evidence of an automatic access disorder.

According to Schvaneveldt et al.'s (1976) hypothesis of lexical spreading activation there exists selective semantic access to different meanings of an ambiguous word. Milberg et al. concluded that automatic selective access is still preserved in Wernicke's aphasics. As outlined before, however, ISI factors have not been systematically controlled; that is, the selective access found might refer to post-lexical effects rather than to automatic spreading activation within the semantic network. Moreover, the distinction between intra-lexical and inter-lexical relations has not been considered. Thus, it might

be the case that not only ISI factors but also the stimulus material used meant that what was studied was not automatic access but rather post-lexical strategies.
This criticism may be supported by the results of Katz (1988) who examined the performance on a subset of Milberg et al.'s (1987) stimulus material by using noun pairs instead of noun triplets: Broca's aphasics showed within a 500-ISI significant priming as normal speakers (160/44) but their RTs were again almost twice as long as those of normal speakers. This finding seems to support the view of continued functioning of automatic access in Broca's aphasics. In another study Hagoort (1993) replicated Milberg et al.'s study by using 100-, 500- and 1250-ISI. Again in 100- and 500-ISI conditions Wernicke's aphasics showed similar priming effects to normal speakers. With a 1250-ISI they show in contrast to normal speakers that a significant priming effect has not been measured, which indicates that either automatic semantic processing has a faster decay in Wernicke's aphasics or that processing is influenced by impaired controlled semantic processing (cf. next section). The fact that Wernicke's aphasics had an estimated average of 2100 msec latencies, then influence of controlled post-lexical effects must be taken into account.
Other studies were more concerned with the question how different semantic relationships are automatically accessed and processed. Chenery, Ingram & Murdoch (1990) confirmed Goodglass & Baker's (1976) off-line findings on several semantic relationships between words and pictures. In addition two types of semantic relations function associates (e.g. *eat-knife*) and superordinate associates (e.g. *cutlery-knife*), have been examined with the auditory priming technique by using a 500-ISI. On both types of relations low comprehension aphasics (comparable with Wernicke's aphasics) and high comprehension aphasics (comparable with Broca's aphasics) did not show impaired processing. Similar, Ostrin & Tyler (1993; cf. Fischler 1977) used a 250-ISI to examine priming differences between associate and semantic relations with Broca's aphasics, elderly normal speakers and young normal speakers (cf. Prather, this volume). According to Fischler (1977) normatively associative relations (e.g. *knife-saw*) might be represented in an automatic fashion within the lexicon (intra-lexical relations) reflecting speech habits and semantic relations (e.g. *room-space*) require classifications according to logical criteria (cf. Wundt's 1907 distinction between "inner" and "outer" associations). Although variance of priming level was found between the four Broca's aphasics tested (associatively: 108-484 ms; semantically: 56-399 ms), no significant deficits have been found between associative and semantic relationships. Compared to elderly normal speakers and young normal speakers, who did not significantly differ in their performance either, Broca's aphasics' RTs show greater variance. In conclusion, the activation of different types of meaning relations seems not to be selectively impaired during automatic activation.
Let us look at another study investigating access in sentential context during language comprehension. Swinney, Zurif & Nicol 1989 (cf. Onifer & Swinney 1981; Swinney et al. 1979) investigated with the CMLP technique the automatic activation of a word's meanings in sentences which biased the interpretation towards the more frequent (dominant) meaning and the less frequent (subdominant) meaning. For example, subjects heard a sentence like *The gardener was responsible for watering every plant // on the enormous estate* and were asked to make lexical decisions on letter strings that

Table 1

Semantic priming in aphasia: Relationship between ISI, priming level, and RT by considering modality of presentation and stimulus types (BA = Broca's aphasics, WA = Wernicke's aphasics, GA = global aphasics, LC = low-comprehension aphasics, TCM = transcortical-motoric aphasic, CA = conduction aphasics, HC = high-comprehension aphasics, CS = control subjects, y = young, e = elderly; in paranthesis: number of subjects or single-case study; N = noun, V = verb; * significant, → tendency to, underlined priming level or RTs: salient results).

Modality	**ISI**	**Stimuli**	**Subjects (n)**	**Priming (ms)**	**RTs (ms)**
Milberg et al. (1981)					
visual	2000	N-N	CS (6)	50*	1550
			WA (6)	280*	<u>2450</u>
			BA (5) I LA (1)	<u>90</u> (→*)	1850
Blumstein et al. (1982)					
auditory	500	N-N	CS (15)	P-Studie (*)	655
			WA (7)	355*	1650
			BA (3) I TCM (4)	220*	1475
			CA (5)	100*	1275
			GA (4)	140*	1550
Milberg et al. (1987)					
auditory	500	N-N-N	CS (20)	33*	779
		(concordant)	WA (7)	110*	<u>2010</u>
			BA (6)	<u>5</u>	1480
Katz (1988)					
auditory	500	N-N	CS (5)	44*	779
			BA (5)	160*	1297
Swinney et al. (1989)					
cross-modal	ø	S1-N1	CS (4)	170*	732
		S2-N2		72*	791
		S1-N2		112*	905
		S2-N2		232*	841
		S1-N1	WA (4)	122*	1833
		S2-N2		155*	1378
		S1-N2		148*	1822
		S2-N2		135*	1798
		S1-N1	BA (4)	107*	1222
		S2-N2		127*	1449
		S1-N2		<u>-15</u>	1348
		S2-N2		<u>2</u>	1556
Hagoort (1990)					
auditory	500	N-N-N I V	CS (12)	59* I 49*	697 I 736
	100	(concordant)		59* I 40*	637 I 693
	1250			62* I 41*	685 I 725
	500		WA (5)	56 I 103 II*	839 I 874
	100		WA (4)	96 I 48 II*	827 I 859
	1250		WA (4)	<u>39 I 75</u>	837 I 870

Table 1 continued

Modality	ISI	Stimuli	Subjects (n)	Priming (ms)	RTs (ms)
	500		BA (12)	59* ǀ 10	700 ǀ 780
	100		BA (7)	131* ǀ 04	764 ǀ 894
	1250		BA (7)	74 ǀ -9	786 ǀ 849
Chenery et al. (1990) auditory	500	V ǀ N-N	CS, LC, HC	(RTs not published; no deficit)	
Ostrin & Tyler (1993) auditory	250	N-N (associative)	yCS (25)	114*	688
			eCS (13)	117*	763
			BA (DE)	145*	610
			BA (JG)	138*	648
			BA (BN)	108*	927
			BA (GS)	484*	1229
		N-N (semantic)	yCS (25)	92*	763
			eCS (13)	112*	980
			BA (DE)	85*	715
			BA (JG)	56*	757
			BA (BN)	140*	911
			BA (GS)	399*	1565
Prather et al.(1992)/ Stern et al. (1991) auditory	300	X-X-X-X...	yCS (6)	-4	516
	500			-18*	532
	800			9	526
	800			17	450
	1100			9	454
	1500			14	445
	300		ySG (6)	-1	581
	500			35*	573
	800			25	588
	800			21	556
	1100			13	569
	1500			-6	587
	500		BA (LD)	0	695
	800			8	681
	1500			70	675
	800			-8	722
	1500			42*	706
	1800			-12	784

were semantically related to the meaning (*tree*) and secondary meaning of plant (*factory*). In these cases the words *page* and *funeral* respectively served as control items. Note that the targets are presented at a zero-ISI, that is, immediately after the word to be disambiguated. The essential finding is that four Broca's aphasics failed to show semantic priming on both meanings of the ambiguous word when the subdominant target word was presented. Compared to the dominant target word this effect holds good independently of sentential context, that is, whether its content suggested the dominant meaning (-15 ms) or the subdominant meaning (2 ms). In contrast, four Wernicke's aphasics behaved like control subjects and showed significant priming in all four experimental conditions. Again, RTs between experimental groups are comparable with those response patterns found in the studies described above: compared to normal speakers (817.25 ms) the average RTs on all four conditions is for Broca's aphasics considerably longer (1,393.75 ms) and for Wernicke's aphasics about twice as long (1,707.75 ms). Swinney's results seem to support a modified hypothesis of a modular deficit: Broca's aphasics suffer from an automatic access deficit towards the subdominant meaning or meanings of a word.

Finally, the "list priming paradigm" was applied by Prather, Zurif, Stern & Rosen (1992; cf. Prather & Swinney 1988) to minimize the influence of controlled processing. A single case of Broca's aphasia (LD) performed on two types of lists using different ISI. The first list used 500-, 800- and 1500-ISI, and the second list 800-, 1500- and 1800-ISI. Semantically related word sequences were normatively selected. LD showed semantic priming at a 1500-ISI on both lists and failed to show significant priming at the shorter ISI of 500 and 800 ms, and at the longer 1800-ISI. Stern, Prather, Swinney & Zurif's (1991) research was cited as control study because they conducted a similar experiment by examing how elderly normal speakers and young normal speakers perform on a list with 300-, 500- and 800-ISI and on another list with 800-, 1100- and 1500-ISI. In contrast to LD both young and elderly normal speakers showed priming at shorter delays at a 500-ISI. RTs show that young normal speakers performed slightly faster (487.17 ms) than elderly normal speakers (575.67 ms).[3] However, LD reacted more slowly (710.5 ms) but the RTs' differences are not as high as was reported with the pair-priming technique.[4] Thus, Prather et al. found for a single Broca's aphasics a reduction in automatic semantic activation, indicated by the fact that a relatively late priming level was reached (1800-ISI).

5 Some Possible Explanations

In reviewing on-line studies that examine the temporal course of semantic access in normal speakers and aphasic patients it has been shown that the distinction between controlled and automatic semantic processing is a central issue for the interpretation of impaired meaning processes. The findings of several studies indicate that automatic semantic access seems to be preserved in Broca's aphasics; however, with the exception of Swinney et al.'s (1989) experiment, all other priming studies used an ISI of more than 200 ms. Taking into account a psycholinguistic model which differentiates between *pre-lexical, lexical*, and *post-lexical* processing and results with normal

speakers where automatic lexical access occurs in a smaller span than 200 ms, it still might be possible that Broca's aphasics performance results from post-lexical effects. By this we mean that it is not automatic access that has been investigated but rather controlled or "semi-automatic" processing. Experiments are therefore required which examine automatic processes with a zero-ISI. Swinney et al. used a zero-ISI and indeed they were able to demonstrate that automatic access to the subdominant meaning of an ambiguous word seems to be impaired. Let us now summarize the crucial findings of aphasic studies within the semantic priming paradigm.
The hypotheses that Wernicke's aphasics are impaired in controlled semantic processing and Broca's aphasics in automatic semantic processing cannot be excluded. Wernicke's aphasics' RTs are about twice as long as Broca's aphasics' RTs and in off-line tasks they show severe deficits. That they are able to perform successfully in semantic priming tasks is due to an intact automatic access to word meanings. Wernicke's aphasics' long RTs may therefore result from impaired semantic control which takes place when, for example, a 500-ISI is used, as most studies did. They show impairments when sub-dominant meanings of a word are automatically accessed but in off-line tasks they perform much like normal speakers. Because only one priming study used an zero-ISI, the status of automatic processing in Broca's aphasics is quite unclear.
However, that their RTs are about twice as long as those of normal speakers indirectly indicates a deficit in automatic semantic processing. That the RTs of Broca's aphasics are significantly shorter than the RTs of Wernicke's aphasics may result from their preservation of controlled semantic processing. Again, this explains the fact that Broca's aphasics show at an ISI more than 100 ms relatively preserved response patterns when the factor "memory load" is considered.

Notes

1 In contrast to some studies which do not separately analyze Broca's aphasics' and transcortical aphasics' performance or Wernicke's aphasics' and conduction aphasics' performance we avoid in this context to use the terms *fluent* and *non-fluent aphasia*.
2 The data are derived from Milberg & Blumstein's (1981) figures.
3 RTs are averaged across the two types of lists and across the different ISI used.
4 RTs are not completely comparable because the 300-, 1100- and 1800-ISI varied between the experiments with LD and normal speakers.

References

Baker, E., S.E. Blumstein & H. Goodglass (1981): "Interaction between phonological and semantic factors in auditory comprehension". Neuropsychologia 19, 1 – 16.
Balota, D.A. & J.I. Chumbley (1985): "The locus of word-frequency effects in the pronunciation task: Lexical access and/or production?" Journal of Memory and Language 24, 89 – 106.
Balota, D.A. & J.I. Chumbley (1990): "Where are the effects of frequency in visual lexical perception tasks? Right where we said they were!" Comment on Monssell, Doyle, and Haggard (1989). Journal of Experimental Psychology: General 119, 231 – 237.

Balota, D.A. & J.I. Chumbley (1984): "Are lexical decisions a good measure of lexical access? The role of word frequency in the neglected decision stage". Journal of Experimental Psychology: Human Perception and Performance 10, 340 – 357.

Blumstein, S., W. Milberg & R. Shrier (1982): "Semantic processing in aphasia: evidence from an auditory lexical decision task". Brain and Language 17, 301 – 315.

Blutner, R. & R. Sommer (1988): "Sentence processing and lexical access: The influence of the focus-identifying task". Journal of Memory and Language 27, 359 – 367.

Burgess, C., M.K. Tanenhaus & M.S. Seidenberg (1989): "Context and lexical access: Implications of nonword interference for lexical ambiguity resolution". Journal of Experimental Psychology: Learning, Memory, and Cognition 15, 620 – 632.

Butterworth, B. (1989): "Lexical access in speech production". In: W. Marslen-Wilson, ed., Lexical representation and process. Cambridge, MA: MIT Press.

Butterworth, B., D. Howard & P. McLoughlin (1984): "The semantic deficit in aphasia: The relationship between semantic errors in auditory comprehension and picture naming". Neuropsychologia 22, 409 – 426.

Cairns, H.S. (1983): "Current issues in research in language comprehension". In: R. Naremore, ed., Recent advances in language sciences. San Diego: College Hill Press.

Caplan, D. (1987): Neurolinguistics and linguistics aphasiology. Cambridge: Cambridge University Press.

Caramazza, A., R.S. Berndt & H.H. Brownell (1982): "The semantic deficit hypothesis: Perceptual parsing and object classification by aphasic patients". Brain and Language 15, 161 – 189.

Caramazza, A. & M. McCloskey (1988): "The case of single patient studies". Cognitive Neuropsychology 5, 517 – 528.

Chenery, H.J., J.C.L. Ingram & B.E. Murdoch (1990): "Automatic and volitional semantic processing in aphasia". Brain and Language 38, 215 – 232.

Conrad, C. (1974): "Context effects in sentence comprehension: A study of the subjective lexicon". Memory & Cognition 2, 130 – 138.

Dell, G.S. (1986): "A spreading activation theory of retrieval in sentence production". Psychological Review 93, 283 – 321.

DeRenzi, E. & L.A. Vignolo (1962): "The Token Test: A sensitive test to detect receptive disturbances in aphasics". Brain 85, 556 – 678.

Fischler, I. (1977): "Associative facilitation without expectancy in a lexical decision task". Journal of Experimental Psychology: Human Perception and Performance 3, 18 – 26.

Flores d'Arcais, G.B. (1988): "Automatic processes on language comprehension". In: G. Denes, C. Semenza & P. Bisiacchi, eds., Perspectives on cognitive neuropsychology. Hillsdale NJ: LEA.

Fodor, J.A. (1983): The modularity of mind. Cambridge, MA: MIT Press.

Forster, K.I. (1976): "Accessing the mental lexicon". In: R.J. Wales & E.C.T. Walker, eds., New approaches to language mechanisms. Amsterdam: North-Holland.

Forster, K.I. (1979): "Levels of processing and the structure of the language processor". In: W.E. Cooper & E.C.T. Walker, eds., Sentence processing: Psycholinguistic studies presented to Merrill Garrett. Hillsdale, NJ: LEA.

Forster, K.I. (1989): "Basic issues in lexical processing". In: W.D. Marslen-Wilson, ed., Lexical representation and process. Cambridge, MA: MIT Press.

Foss, D.J. & J.R. Ross (1983): "Great expectations: Context effects during sentence processing". In: G.B. Flores d'Arcais & R.J. Jarvella, eds., The process of language understanding. Chichester: Wiley.

Friederici, A.D. (1988): "Autonomy and automaticity: Accessing function words during sentence comprehension". In: G. Denes, C. Semenza & P. Bisiacchi, eds., Perspectives on cognitive neuropsychology. Hillsdale, NJ: LEA.

Friederici, A.D. (1983): "Children's sensitivity to function words during sentence comprehension". Linguistics 21, 717 – 739.

Gainotti, G. (1976): "The relationship between semantic impairment in comprehension and naming in aphasic patients". British Journal of Disorders of Communication 11, 57 – 61.
Gainotti, G., C. Caltagirone & A. Ibba (1975): "Semantic and phonemic aspects of auditory comprehension in aphasia". Linguistics 154/155, 15 – 29.
Gainotti, G., G. Micheli, M.C. Silveri & C. Masullo (1981): "The relationship, between type of naming error and semantic-lexical discrimination in aphasic patients". Cortex 17, 401 – 410.
Garrett, M. (1992): "Disorders of lexical selection". Cognition 42, 143 – 180.
Gerrig, R. (1986): "Process and products of lexical access". Language and Cognitive Processes 1, 187 – 196.
Gerwirth, L.R., A.G. Shindler & D.B. Hier (1984): "Altered patterns of word associations in dementia and aphasia". Brain and Language 21, 307 – 317.
Glucksberg, S., R.J. Kreuz & S.H. Rho (1986): "Context can constrain lexical access: Implications for models of language comprehension". Journal of Experimental Psychology: Learning, Memory, and Cognition 12, 323 – 335.
Goodglass, H. & L. Menn (1985): "Is agrammatism an unitary phenomenon?" In: M.L. Kean, ed., Agrammatism. New York: Academic Press.
Goodglass, H. & E. Baker (1976): "Semantic field, naming, and auditory comprehension in aphasia". Brain and Language 3, 359 – 374.
Grosjean, F. (1980): "Spoken lexical perception processes and the gating paradigm". Perception & Psychophysics 28, 267 – 283.
Hagoort, P. (1993): "Impairments of lexical-semantic processing in aphasia: Evidence from the processing of lexical ambiguities". Brain and Language 45, 189 – 232.
Hakes, D.T. (1972): "Effects of reducing complement constructions on sentence comprehension". Journal of Verbal Learning and Verbal Behavior 11, 278 – 286.
Hillert, D. (1990): Sprachprozesse und Wissensstrukturen. Neuropsychologische Grundlagen der Kognition. Opladen: Westdeutscher Verlag.
Hillert, D.(1992): "Lexical semantics and aphasia: A state-of-the-art review". Neurolinguistics 7 (1/2), 23 – 65.
Hillert, D. (1993): "Semantische Einträge und Konzeptuelle Wissensstrukturen: Psycho- und neurolinguistische Evidenz". Linguistische Berichte 145, 204 – 234.
Hillert, D. (1994): The temporal course of semantic access in aphasia: Some explanations. TENNET V, Montréal.
Hillert, D. (1995): "Linguistics & Cognitive Neuroscience". (forthcoming).
Hogaboam, T.W. & C.A. Perfetti (1975): "Lexical ambiguity and sentence comprehension: The common sense effect". Journal of Verbal Learning and Verbal Behavior 14, 265 – 275.
Howes, D. (1964): "Application of the word-frequency concept to aphasia". In: K. Salzinger & S. Salzinger, ed., Research in verbal behavior and some neuropsychological implications. NY: Academic Press.
Howes, D. (1967): "Some experimental investigation of language in aphasia". In: K. Salzinger & S. Salzinger, ed., Research in verbal behavior and some neurophysiological implications. NY: Academic Press.
Jakimik, J.A. (1980): The interaction of sound and knowledge in lexical perception from fluent speech. Carnegie-Mellon University: dissertation.
Johnson-Laird, P.N. (1983): Mental models: Towards a cognitive science of language, inference, and consciousness. Cambridge: Cambridge University Press.
Jones, J.L.(1989): "Multiple access of homonym meanings: an artifact of backward priming?" Journal of Psycholinguistic Research 18 (4), 417 – 432.
Katz, W.F. (1988): "Note, An investigation of lexical ambiguity in Broca's aphasics using an auditory lexical proming technique". Neuropsychologia 26 (5), 747 – 752.
Kempen, G. & P. Huijbers (1983): "The lexicalization process in sentence production and naming: Indirect selection of words". Cognition 14, 185 – 209.

Kiger, J.I. & A.L. Glass (1983): "The facilitation of lexical decisions by a prime occurring after the target". Memory & Cognition 11, 356 – 365.
Koriat, A. (1981): "Semantic facilitation in lexical decision as a function of prime-target association". Memory & Cognition 9, 587 – 598.
Lesser, R. (1978): Linguistic investigations of aphasia. New York: Elsevier.
Levelt, W.J.M. (1989): Speaking: From Intention to Articulation. Cambridge, MA: MIT Press.
Levelt, W.J.M. (1992): "Accessing words in speech production: Stages, processes and representations". Cognition 42, 1 – 22.
MacKay, D.G. (1973): "Aspects of the theory of comprehension, memory and attention". Quarterly Journal of Experimental Psychology 25, 22 – 40.
Marslen-Wilson, W.D. & L.K. Tyler (1980): "The temporal structure of spoken language understanding". Cognition 8, 1 – 71.
Marslen-Wilson, W.D. & L.K. Tyler (1987): "Against modularity". In: J.L. Garfield, ed., Modularity in knowledge representation and natural-language understanding. Cambridge, MA: MIT Press.
Marslen-Wilson, W.D. & A. Welsh (1978): "Processing interactions and lexical access during word-recognition in continuous speech". Cognitive Psychology 10, 29 – 63.
Marslen-Wilson, W.D. (1984): "Function and process in spoken word-recognition". In: H. Bouma & D.G. Bouwhuis, eds., Attention and Performance X: Control of language processes. Hillsdale, NJ: LEA.
Marslen-Wilson, W.D. (1985): "Speech shadowing and speech comprehension". Speech Communication 4, 55 – 73.
Marslen-Wilson, W.D. (1987): "Functional parallelism in spoken word-recognition". Cognition 25, 71 – 102.
Martin, R.C. (1987): "Articulatory and phonological deficit in short-term memory and their relation to syntactic processing". Brain and Language 32, 159 – 192.
McClelland, J.L. & J. Elman (1986): "The TRACE model of speech perception". Cognitive Psychology 18, 1 – 86.
McClelland, J.L. & D.E. Rummelhart (1981): "An interactive activation model of context effects in letter perception: Part 1. An account of basic findings". Psychological Review 88, 375 – 407.
Mehler, J., J. Segui & P.W. Carey (1978): "Tails of words: Monitoring ambiguity". Journal of Verbal Learning and Verbal Behavior 17, 29 – 35.
Meyer, D.E. & R.W. Schvaneveldt (1971): "Facilitation in recognizing pairs of words: Evidence of a dependence between retrieval operations". Journal of Experimental Psychology 90, 227 – 234.
Milberg, W. & S. Blumstein (1981): "Lexical decision and aphasia: Evidence for semantic processing". Brain and Language 14, 371 – 385.
Milberg, W., S. Blumstein & B. Dworetzky (1987): "Processing of lexical ambiguities in aphasia". Brain and Language 31, 138 – 150.
Morton, J. & J. Long (1976): "Effect of word transitional probability on phoneme identification". Journal of Verbal Learning and Verbal Behavior 12, 431 – 461.
Morton, J. (1969): "Interaction of information in lexical perception". Psychological Review 76, 165 – 178.
Morton, J. (1979): "Lexical perception". In: J. Morton & J.C. Marshall, eds., Psycholinguistic series 2: Structures and processes. London: Elek.
Moss, H.E. & W.D. Marslen-Wilson (1993): "Access to word meanings during spoken language comprehension: Effects of sentential semantic context". Journal of Experimental Psychology: Learning, Memory, and Cognition 19(6), 1254 – 1276.
Neely, J.H. (1977): "Semantic priming and retrieval from lexical memory: Roles of inhibitionless spreading activation and limited-capacity attention!" Journal of Experimental Psychology: General 106, 226 – 254.

Neely, J.H. (1990): "Semantic priming effects in visual lexical perception. A selective review of current findings and theories". In: D. Besner & G. Humphreys, eds., Basic processes in reading: Visual lexical perception. Hillsdale, NJ: LEA.
Norris, D. (1986): "Lexical perception: Context effects without priming". Cognition 22, 93 – 136.
Oden, G.C. & J.L. Spira (1983): "Influence of context on the activation and selection of ambiguous word senses". Quarterly Journal of Experimental Psychology 35A, 51 – 64.
Onifer, W. & D.A. Swinney (1981): "Accessing lexical ambiguities during sentence comprehension: Effects of frequency of meaning and contextual bias". Cognition 9, 225 – 236.
Ostrin, R.K. & M.F. Schwarz (1986): "Reconstructing from a degraded trace: A study of sentence repetition in agrammatism". Brain and Language 28, 328 – 345.
Ostrin, R.K. & L.K. Tyler (1993): "Automatic access to lexical semantics in aphasia: Evidence from semantic and associative priming". Brain and Language 45, 147 – 159.
Posner, M.I. & C.R.R. Snyder (1975): "Attention and cognitive control". In: R. Solso, ed., Information processing and cognition: The Loyola symposium. Hillsdale, NJ: LEA.
Prather, P.A. & D.A. Swinney (1988): "Lexical processing and ambiguity resolution: An autonomous process in an interactive box". In: S.L. Small, G.W. Cottrell & M.K. Tanenhaus, eds., Lexical ambiguity resolution: Perspectives from psycholinguistics, neuropsychology and artificial intelligence. San Mateo, CA: Morgan Kaufmann Publishers.
Prather, P.A., E. Zurif, C. Stern & T.J. Rosen (1992): "Slowed lexical access in nonfluent aphasia: A case study". Brain and Language 43, 336 – 348.
Rinnert, C. & H.A. Whitaker (1973): "Semantic confusions by aphasic patients". Cortex 9, 56 – 81.
Saffran, E.M. & O.S.M. Marin (1975): "Immediate memory for word lists and sentences in a patient with a deficient auditory short-term memory". Brain and Language 2, 420 – 433.
Schneider, W. & R.M. Shiffrin (1977): "Controlled and automatic human information processing: I. Detection, search and attention". Psychology Review 8, 1 – 66.
Schvaneveldt, R.W., D.E. Meyer & C.A. Becker (1976): "Lexical ambiguity, semantic context, and visual lexical perception". Journal of Experimental Psychology: Human Perception and Performance 2, 243 – 256.
Schwanenflugel, P. & K. LaCount (1988): "Semantic relatedness and the scope of facilitation for upcoming words in sentences". Journal of Experimental Psychology: Learning, Memory and Cognition 14, 344 – 354.
Schwanenflugel, P. & E. Shoben (1985): "The influence of sentence constraint on the scope of facilitation for upcoming words". Journal of Memory and Language 24, 232 – 252.
Seidenberg, M.S. & M.K. Tanenhaus (1986): "Modularity and lexical access". In: I. Gopnik, ed., From models to modules: Proceedings of the McGill Cognitive Science Workshop. NJ: Ablex Press.
Seidenberg, M.S. (1985): "The time course of information activation and utilization in visual lexical perception". In: D. Besner, T.G. Wasller & G.E. MacKinon, eds., Reading research: Advances in theory and practice, Vol. 5. New York: Academic Press.
Seidenberg, M.S., M.K. Tanenhaus, J.M. Leimann & M. Bienkowski (1982): "Automatic access of the meanings of ambiguous words in context: Some limitations of knowledge-based processing". Cognitive Psychology 14, 489 – 537.
Seidenberg, M.S., G.S. Waters, M. Sanders & P. Langer (1984): "Pre- and postlexical loci of contextual effects on lexical perception". Memory & Cognition 12, 315 – 328.
Shiffrin, R.M. & W. Schneider (1977): "Controlled and automatic human information processing: II. Perceptual learning, automatic attending and ageneral theory". Psychology Review 84, 127 – 190.
Simpson, G.B. (1981): "Lexical ambiguity and its role in models of lexical perception". Psychological Bulletin 96, 316 – 340.
Stemberger, J.P. (1983): "Inflectional malapropisms: Form-based errors in English morphology". Linguistics 21, 573 – 602.

Stern, C., P. Prather, D.A. Swinney & E. Zurif (1991): "The time course of automatic lexical access and aging". Brain and Language 40, 359 – 372.
Swinney, D.A. & D.T. Hakes (1976): "Effects of prior context upon lexical access during sentence comprehension". Journal of Verbal Learning and Verbal Behavior 15, 681 – 689.
Swinney, D.A. (1979): "Lexical access during sentence comprehension: (Re)consideration of context effects". Journal of Verbal Learning and Verbal Behavior 18, 645 – 660.
Swinney, D.A., W. Onifer, P. Prather & M. Hirshkowitz (1979): "Semantic facilitation across sensory modalities in the processing of individual words and sentences". Memory & Cognition 7, 165 – 195.
Swinney, D.A., E. Zurif & J. Nicol (1989): "The effects of focal brain damage on sentence processing: An examination of the neurological organization of a mental modul". Journal of Cognitive Neuroscience 1 (1), 25 – 37.
Tabossi, P. (1988a): "Accessing lexical ambiguity in different types of contexts". Journal of Memory and Language 27, 324 – 340.
Tabossi, P. (1988b): "Effects of context on the immediate interpretation of unambiguous words". Journal of Experimental Psychology: Learning, Memory and Cognition 14, 153 – 162.
Tabossi, P., L. Colombo & R. Job (1987): "Accessing lexical ambiguity: Effects of context and dominance". Psychological Research 49, 161 – 167.
Tanenhaus, M.K. & M.M. Lucas (1987): "Context effects in lexical processing". Cognition 25, 213 – 234.
Tanenhaus, M.K., C. Burgess & M. Seidenberg (1988): "Is multiple access an artifact of backward priming?" In: S.L. Small, G.W. Cotrell & M.K. Tanenhaus, eds., Lexical ambiguity resolution. San Maeto, CA: Morgan Kaufmann.
Tanenhaus, M.K., G.N. Carlson & M. Seidenberg (1985): "Do listeners compute linguistic representations?" In: D.R. Dowty, L. Kartunnen & A.M. Zwicky, ed., Natural language parsing: Psycholinguistic, theoretical and computational perspectives. Cambridge: Cambridge University Press.
Tanenhaus, M.K., G.S. Dell & G. Carlson (1987): "Context effects in lexical processing: A connectionist approach to modularity". In: J.L. Garfield, ed., Modularity in knowledge representation and natural-language understanding. Cambridge, MA: MIT Press.
Tanenhaus, M.K., J.M. Leiman & M. Seidenberg (1979): "Evidence for multiple stages in the processing of ambiguous words in syntactic contexts". Journal of Verbal Learning and Verbal Behavior 18, 427 – 440.
Treisman, A.M. (1960): "Contextual cues in selective listening". Quarterly Journal of Experimental Psychology 12, 242 – 248.
Tyler, L.K. (1988): Spoken Language Comprehension. An experimental approach to disordered and normal processing. Cambridge, MA: MIT Press.
Tyler, L.K. & U.H. Frauenfelder (1987): "The process of spoken lexical perception: An introduction". In: U.H. Frauenfelder & L.K. Tyler, eds., Spoken lexical perception. A Cognition special issue. Cambridge, MA: MIT Press.
Williams, J.N. (1988): "Constraints upon semantic activation during sentence comprehension". Language and Cognitive Processes 3 (3), 165 – 206.
Wundt, W. (1907): Outlines of psychology. London: Williams & Norgate.
Zwitserlood, P. (1989): "The locus of the effects of sentential-semantic context in spoken-word processing". Cognition 32, 25 – 64.

The Authors

Elizabeth Bates, Ph.D.
Center for Research in Language
Department of Cognitive Science
University of California, San Diego
La Jolla, CA 92093-0526
U.S.A.

Pr. François Boller, M.D., Ph.D.
Unité 324 – INSERM
Neuropsychologie et Neurobiologie
du Vieillissement Cérébral
Centre Paul Broca
2ter, rue d'Alésia
75014 Paris
France

Douglas F.G. Burrington
University of Manchester
Institute of Science and Technology
Centre for Computational Linguistics
P.O. Box 88
Manchester M60 1QD
U.K.

Prof. Dr. Angela D. Friederici
Cognitive Science Lab Berlin
Institut für Psychologie
Freie Universität Berlin
Habelschwerdter Allee 45
14195 Berlin
F.R.G.

Jean Gagnon, Ph.D.
Laboratoire Théophile-Alajouanine
Centre de Recherche du
Centre Hospitalier Côte-des-Neiges
4565 Reine-Marie
Montréal, Québec
Canada, H3W 1W5

Harold Goodglass, Ph.D.
Psychology Service
Boston VA Medical Center
150 South Huntington Ave.
Boston, MA 02130
U.S.A.

Pierre Goulet, Ph.D.
École d'orthophonie et d'audiologie
Faculté de médicine
Université de Montréal
c.p. 6208, succ. A
Montréal, Québec
Canada, H3C 3T4

Gautam A. Gupta
University of Manchester
Institute of Science and Technology
Centre for Computational Linguistics
P.O. Box 88
Manchester M60 1QD
U.K.

Arturo Hernandez, Ph.D.
Center for Research in Language
Department of Cognitive Science
University of California, San Diego
La Jolla, CA 92093-0526
U.S.A.

PD Dr. Dieter Hillert
University of Manchester
Institute of Science and Technology
Centre for Computational Linguistics
P.O. Box 88
Manchester M60 1QD
U.K.

Yves Joanette, Ph.D.
Laboratoire Théophile-Alajouanine
Centre de Recherche du
Centre Hospitalier Côte-des-Neiges
4565 Reine-Marie
Montréal, Québec
Canada, H3W 1W5

Jörg Keller, M.A.
Institut für Deutsche Sprache und
Literatur II
Johann Wolfgang Goethe-Universität
Gräfstraße 79
Postfach 11 19 32
60054 Frankfurt/Main
F.R.G.

Kerry Kilborn, Ph.D.
Department of Psychology
University of Glasgow
56 Hillhead Street
Glasgow G12 9YR
U.K.

Helgard Kremin
Pavillon Clérambault (U. 302)
Hôpital de la Salpétrière
47 Blvd de l'Hôpital
75013 Paris
France

Prof. Dr. Helen Leuninger
Institut für Deutsche Sprache und
Literatur II
Johann Wolfgang Goethe-Universität
Gräfstraße 79
Postfach 11 19 32
60054 Frankfurt/Main
F.R.G.

Pierre Marcie Ph.D.
Unité 324 – INSERM
Neuropsychologie et Neurobiologie
du Vieillissement Cérébral
Centre Paul Broca
2ter, rue d'Alésia
75014 Paris
France

Penny A. Prather, Ph.D.
Psychology, m/c 116B
Boston VA Medical Center
150 South Huntington Ave.
Boston, MA 02130
U.S.A.

Michel Roudier, M.D., Ph.D.
Unité 324 – INSERM
Neuropsychologie et Neurobiologie
du Vieillissement Cérébral
Centre Paul Broca
2ter, rue d'Alésia
75014 Paris
France

PD Dr. Herbert Schriefers
Cognitive Science Lab Berlin
Institut für Psychologie
Freie Universität Berlin
Habelschwerdter Allee 45
14195 Berlin
F.R.G.

Lewis P. Shapiro, Ph.D.
Department of Psychology
Florida Atlantic University
P.O. Box 3091
Boca Raton, FL 33431-0991
U.S.A.

David Swinney, Ph.D.
Department of Psychology
University of California, San Diego
La Jolla, CA 92093-0109
U.S.A.

Cynthia K. Thompson, Ph.D.
Speech and Language Pathology
Northwestern University
2299 Campus Dr. North
Evanston, IL 60208
U.S.A

Professor Lorraine K. Tyler
Centre for Speech and Language
Department of Psychology
Birkbeck College
University of London
Malet Street
London WC1E 7HX
U.K.

Edgar Zurif, Ph.D.
Brandeis University
Program in Linguistics and Cognitive Science
Brown 125
Waltham, MA 02254-9110
U.S.A.

Aus dem Programm Sprachwissenschaft

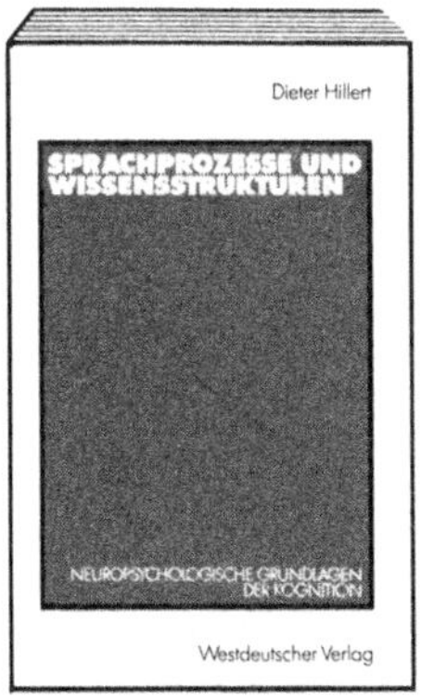

Dieter Hillert

Sprachprozesse und Wissensstrukturen

Neuropsychologische Grundlagen der Kognition

1990. 314 S. Kart.
ISBN 3-531-12217-7

Dieses Buch stellt aktuelle Fragen der Aphasieforschung vor und analysiert gestörte Sprachprozesse auf der Grundlage psycholinguistischer Modellvorstellungen. Mit dieser Konzeption lassen sich divergierende Befunde, die sowohl bei Broca- als auch bei Wernicke-Aphasikern hinsichtlich der On- und Off-line-Verarbeitung gefunden werden, vereinbaren: Während Off-line-Untersuchungen einen Vergleich zwischen interaktiven Prozessen des Experimentators und des Probanden überprüfen und daher aus methodischer Sicht einen solipsistischen Ansatz implizieren, ermöglichen zeitgebundene On-line-Untersuchungen eine Einblick in die Funktionsweise modular organisierter und dem Bewußtsein nicht direkt zugänglicher Systeme.

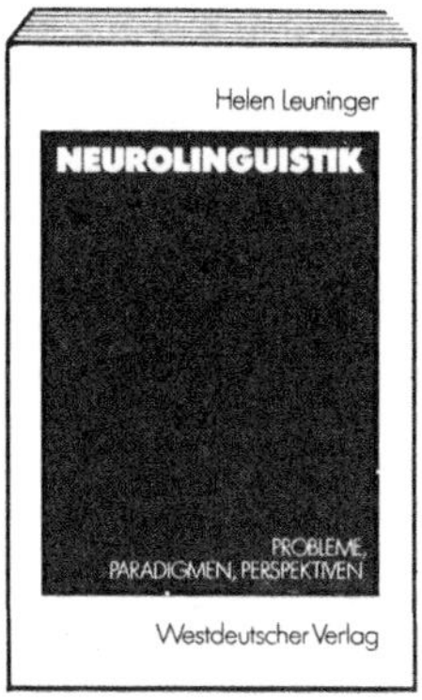

Helen Leuninger

Neurolinguistik

Probleme, Paradigmen, Perspektiven

1989. X, 207 S. Kart.
ISBN 3-531-11866-8

Der erste Teil des Buches handelt von eher traditionellen Beschreibungen von Sprachstörungen und den mit ihnen verbundenen erkenntnistheoretischen und empirischen Problemen. Der zweite Teil zeigt, daß einige dieser Probleme präzisiert und z. T. gelöst werden konnten aufgrund der paradigmatischen Ansätze, die heute in der Neurolinguistik erkenntnisleitend sind. Schließlich wird im dritten Teil unter Zugrundelegung heute gültiger sprachtheoretischer Auffassungen über das Sprachsystem und sprachliche Verarbeitungsprozesse und Entwicklungen eine perspektivische Synthese vorgestellt.

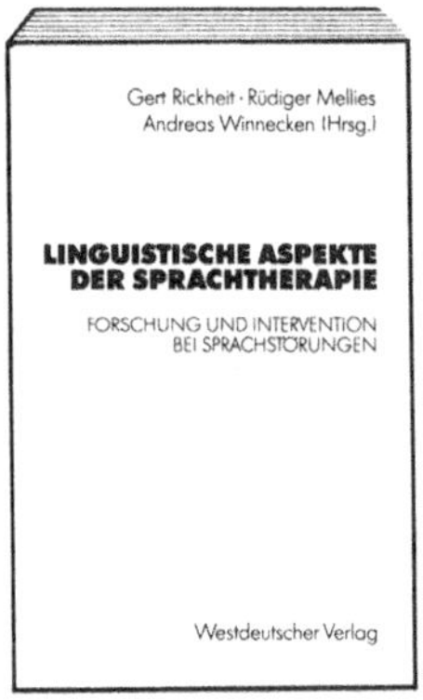

Gert Rickheit / Rüdiger Mellies / Andreas Winnecken (Hrsg.)

Linguistische Aspekte der Sprachtherapie

Forschung und Intervention bei Sprachstörungen

1992. VI, 309 S.
(Psycholinguistische Studien; hrsg. von Gert Rickheit und Dieter Metzing) Kart.
ISBN 3-531-12345-9

Die therapeutische Behandlung von Aphasikern stand im Mittelpunkt einer Fachtagung, die vom Bundesverband „Klinische Linguistik" initiiert und von der Universität Bielefeld durchgeführt worden ist. Die auf dieser Tagung gehaltenen Vorträge sind in überarbeiteter und erweiterter Form in diesen Band aufgenommen worden. Sie geben einen guten Überblick über den derzeitigen Stand der Aphasieforschung, wobei Fragen der Therapie im Vordergrund stehen, aber auch Probleme der Aphasiediagnose behandelt werden.

WESTDEUTSCHER VERLAG
OPLADEN · WIESBADEN

GPSR Compliance

The European Union's (EU) General Product Safety Regulation (GPSR) is a set of rules that requires consumer products to be safe and our obligations to ensure this.

If you have any concerns about our products, you can contact us on ProductSafety@springernature.com

In case Publisher is established outside the EU, the EU authorized representative is:

Springer Nature Customer Service Center GmbH
Europaplatz 3
69115 Heidelberg, Germany

Batch number: 10809636

Printed by Printforce, the Netherlands